Microsatellite Markers
http://dx.doi.org/10.5772/62560
Edited by Ibrokhim Y. Abdurakhmonov

Contributors

Narasimha Reddy Parine, Mohammad Alanazi, Hongyu Ma, Eugenia Barrandeguy, Maria Victoria Garcia, Yoshiaki Kikkawa, Yuta Seki, Kenta Wada, Jamila Bernardi, Matteo Busconi, Licia Colli, Virginia Ughini, Emil Hernández, Evonnildo Costa Gonçalves, Artur Silva, Rodolfo Aureliano Salm, Isadora França, Maria Paula Cruz Schneider, Pascale Besse, Rodolphe Gigant, Michel Grisoni, Narindra Rakotomanga, Chloé Goulié, Nicolas Barre, Gervais Citadelle, Daniel Silvestre, Denis Da Silva, Richard Halberg, Jeff Bacher, Linda Clipson, Leta Steffen, Justyna Nowakowska, Amelework Beyene Assefa, Hussein Shimelis, Mark Laing, Demissew Abakemal, Ibrokhim Y. Abdurakhmonov

Published by InTech

Janeza Trdine 9, 51000 Rijeka, Croatia

Publishing Process Manager Iva Lipovic

Technical Editor SPi Global

Cover InTech Design team

First published December, 2016

Printed in Croatia

Additional hard copies can be obtained from orders@intechopen.com

Microsatellite Markers, Edited by Ibrokhim Y. Abdurakhmonov

p. cm.

Print ISBN 978-953-51-2797-0
Online ISBN 978-953-51-2798-7

Meet the editor

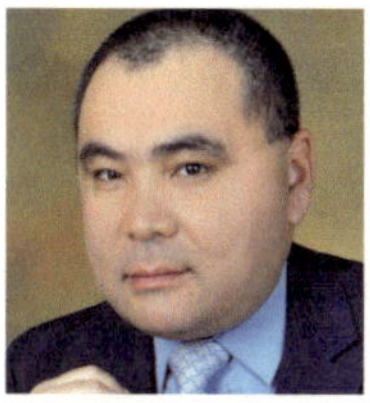

Ibrokhim Y. Abdurakhmonov received his BS degree (1997) in *biotechnology* from the National University of Uzbekistan, MS degree in *plant breeding* (2001) from Texas A&M University, USA, PhD degree (2002) in *molecular genetics*, Doctor of Science degree (2009) in *genetics*, and full professorship (2011) in *molecular genetics and molecular biotechnology* from the Institute of Genetics and Plant Experimental Biology, Academy of Sciences of Uzbekistan. He founded (2012) and is currently leading the Center of Genomics and Bioinformatics of Uzbekistan. He serves as an associate editor/editorial board member of several international and national journals on plant sciences. He received the following government awards: chest badge "Sign of Uzbekistan" (2010), The World Academy of Sciences (TWAS) prize (2010), and "ICAC Cotton Researcher of the Year 2013" for his outstanding contribution to cotton genomics and biotechnology. He was elected The World Academy of Sciences (TWAS) Fellow (2014) in *Agricultural Science* and a co-chair/chair of "Comparative Genomics and Bioinformatics" workgroup (2015) of International Cotton Genome Initiative (ICGI).

Contents

Foreword

Molecular marker technologies are efficient, accurate, and extensively exploited tools to solve puzzles of genetics and life forms, helping us understand the basis of genetic process in living organisms. The development of molecular markers has shed light into many features of genomes and biological complexities in early studies without recently available "omics" platforms. Among most favored and widely used molecular markers are microsatellites. This Microsatellite Markers book, edited by a distinguished plant genomics scientist Prof. Ibrokhim Y. Abdurakhmonov, provides an excellent addendum on the utilization of microsatellite markers in the era of current abundance of many molecular marker technologies and in the period of emerging high-throughput platforms.

Microsatellites are short tandem DNA repeats that detect polymorphisms in both prokaryotes and eukaryotes. Over the past decades, microsatellites were at the frontier of DNA-based investigations into genetics and molecular biology worldwide. They have facilitated numerous applications, including genetic mapping, molecular breeding, and studies of evolutionary relationships among species and populations.

This Microsatellite Markers book, composed of research studies and review chapters from an international group of researchers, covers the basics of microsatellite markers, their development and utilization. It highlights continuous benefits of microsatellite markers to genetic studies and applications despite recent misperception on decreased use as a genetic marker of choice. The book provides useful information to all life science researchers, educators, students, and others who are interested in applications of molecular markers. There is no doubt that all, as this volume emphasizes, will enjoy the benefits of microsatellite markers far into the future.

John Z. Yu, Ph.D.
Research Geneticist
USDA-ARS
Adjunct Professor of Genetics
Texas A&M University
College station, Texas, USA

Preface

The pattern and "spelling" of DNA variations among individuals, contributing beneficial and diseased phenotypes, are very useful to differentiate organisms in molecular level. One of such abundantly dispersed DNA variations in a genome is variable number of tandem repeats (VNTRs) that include both minisatellite and microsatellite repeat arrays. The VNTRs with more than nine nucleotide core repeats are categorized into minisatellites, while those repeats less than nine nucleotides (usually 2–6 bp) arrays belong to microsatellites.

According to the field of usage (i.e. plant science or biomedical fields), microsatellites are also called simple sequence length polymorphisms (SSLP), simple sequence repeats (SSRs), or short tandem repeats (STRs), which are used interchangeably among researchers. As a genetic marker, microsatellites have been widely applied for almost three decades to complete a numerous type of genetic tasks. These include the construction of genetic linkage groups and integrated maps; correlation of phenotypic and genotypic variations; analyses of parentage and/or ancestry; DNA barcoding for plant varieties and germplasm; evaluation of gene flow and variety/seed purity; breeding using marker-assisted selection tools; analyses of genetic diversity; conservation and restoration of biodiversity; assessment of molecular evolution, taxonomy, and phylogenetic features of biological species; population genetics including analyses of genetic strata, kinship, and differentiation of native plant populations and crop germplasm resources, origin, and domestication of crop species, migration, and demographic process, that is, changes in population size and structure through time; and forensic and disease diagnostics.

The emergence of cost-effective and large-scale next-generation sequencing, SNP detection, and genotyping methodologies has circumvented a rapid shift of SSR-based molecular marker studies toward SNP-based marker studies. However, microsatellite markers will continue to be useful and favorable markers because of their multiallelic nature, simplicity of genotyping procedures, cost-effectivity, and their suitability, especially for small-scale laboratories with limited budget. Therefore, the objective of this *Microsatellite Markers* book is to rehighlight and provide some updates on previous and recent utilization of microsatellite markers for various applications in environmental, agricultural, and biomedical sciences, which invalidate emerging opinion on "full death" of microsatellites as useful genetic markers.

Addressing these, in this edited volume, we gathered 11 chapters including an introductory chapter that described and discussed the basic characterization and exploitation of microsatellites in various genetic studies, which covered previous efforts and recent updates, advantages, and disadvantages as well as future perspectives of microsatellites in plants and genetic diversity research, animal genetics and breeding, and cancer research. I trust that, being a useful addendum to published literature worldwide, the chapter materials presented in this book should be useful for university students, life science researchers, and interested readers.

I thank the InTech book department and its publication managers Ms. Iva Lipovic and Ms. Iva Simcic for the book editing opportunity and help during the entire editorial process of this book. I am thankful to all authors of the book chapters for their chapter contributions and cooperation.

Ibrokhim Y. Abdurakhmonov
Center of Genomics and Bioinformatics
Academy of Sciences of Uzbekistan
Tashkent, Uzbekistan

Section 1

Introduction

Chapter 1

Introduction to Microsatellites: Basics, Trends and Highlights

Ibrokhim Y. Abdurakhmonov

Additional information is available at the end of the chapter

http://dx.doi.org/10.5772/66446

1. Introduction

A genome is written in four chemical letters (nucleotides designated as A, T, G, and C). Various combinations of these letters as a stretch of DNA molecule provide specificity and uniqueness of each gene sequence, cell types, and each individual genotype. Magic is that the order of each triplet (known as genetic code) of these four-letter DNA sequence stretches corresponds to one of 20 amino acids. A "spelling" order of nucleotides encodes the specific protein sequences determining a life function. Therefore, variations in these four-letter DNA sequences in a genome make the meaning and differentiation of the living organisms on Earth that generated biological diversity. Because of degeneracy of genetic code, some spelling changes in coding parts of a sequence (exons) may have no meaning and still code the same amino acid although changes may have evolutionary role and contribute to the biodiversity levels of populations. However, other changes may lead to generate novel proteins with new function and characteristics, stop the gene function and protein synthesis, or generate a partial protein sequences that is not sufficient for its functional activity—all these alter the function of the cell and generate a difference.

The pattern of DNA variations among individuals, generating beneficial and diseased phenotypes, is very useful to differentiate organisms in molecular level and to understand the evolutionary path of important genes as well as their functional and adaptive roles in the different eco-geographic environments. One of such abundant spelling variations in a genome is the 5- to 50-fold repetitions of the two to six nucleotide base pair (bp) motifs of DNA, such as $(GA)_n$ or $(GTACGT)_n$, which are called as microsatellites [1–4]. These tandem repeats are referred to as microsatellites, simple sequence length polymorphisms (SSLP), simple sequence repeats (SSR), or short tandem repeats (STR), which are used interchangeably among researchers. Microsatellites are abundantly found in all prokaryote and eukaryote genomes.

Litt and Luty [4] first coined the term "microsatellite" in 1989, where the word "satellite" was used due to fact that density gradient centrifugation separates DNA fragments with repetitive sequences into the upper "satellite" fraction with less density. As a genetic marker, microsatellites have been widely used in DNA-based genetic analyses for the past 25 years. Since the first paper by Litt and Luty [4] in 1989, as of October 2016, *Pubmed* [5] database search with the quoted keyword "microsatellite" found almost 44,000 research publications that have used or discussed microsatellites (**Figure 1**). Hodel et al. [1] reported that as of April 2016, they have found almost 225,000 published articles by searching Web of Science (WOS) database. Searching the WOS core collection for plant science-related articles, Vieira et al. [2] reported that for the past 5-year period from 2010 to 2015, there were 993 unique crop-related publications using microsatellites that demonstrate a wide utilization of SSRs in plant sciences. In this introductory chapter, I aimed to give an overview of definition, distribution, utility, and future of microsatellites, briefly highlighting chapter contents of this book.

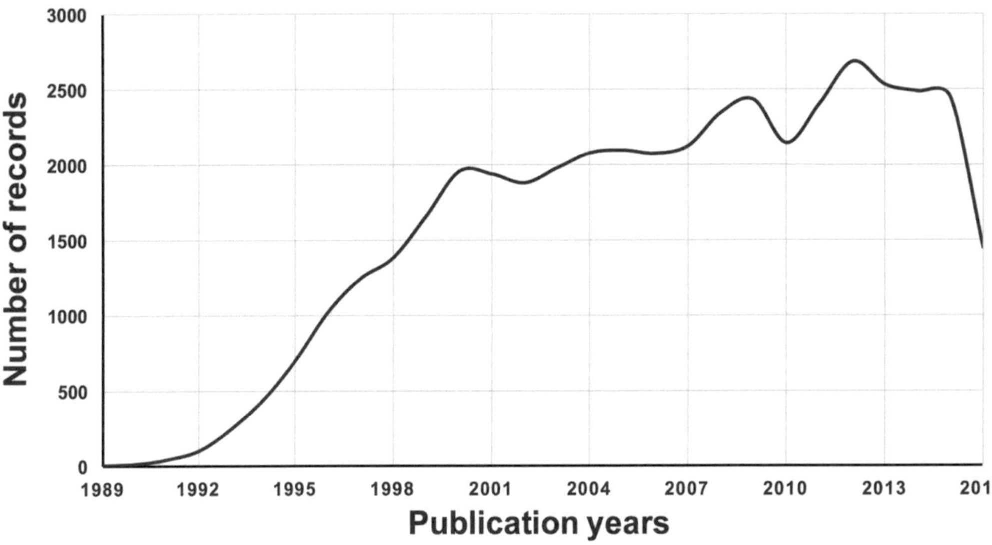

Figure 1. Number of publications retrieved with "microsatellite" keyword from PubMed [5].

2. Definition, occurrence, types, distribution, and density

A variable number tandem repeats (VNTRs) include both mini- and microsatellite DNAs. Minisatellites are the heterogeneous array of 10–60/100 core bp repeat motif sequences such as $(GGGCAGGTNG)_n$ that have repeat size of 1–15 kilobases (kb). In contrast, microsatellites, commonly, consist of a homogeneous array of core mono, di, tri, tetra, penta, and hexanucleotide motifs with repeat size of less than or around 1 kb. Controversially, some reports include all repeat arrays less than 9 bp into microsatellite category and those above nine core repeats into minisatellite group [1–3, 6]. However, the suggested core array of repeat motifs for microsatellites are 2–6 bp, which non-randomly distributed throughout the genome [7] and vary largely in different regions of a genome or on different taxa [2]. Microsatellites can be found abundantly in non-coding parts of the genome such as introns, untranslated regions (UTR), and intergenic spaces, but they also occur in coding exonic sequences. Microsatellites also located within transposons and other dispersed repetitive elements [1–3, 6, 7].

Density of microsatellites considered to be highest in UTRs and in decreasing order in promoters, introns, intergenic regions, and coding sequences. Microsatellite repeat lengths in coding, non-coding and intergenic regions are reported to be species specific. For instance, generally, vertebrates (e.g., turtles) tend to have more and longer array microsatellites compared to plants and then invertebrates [6]. Although vary organism to organism and may not be true for all genomes under consideration, commonly trinucleotide motifs are more frequent than other types, being highest in plants to 61–73%, except Arabidopsis and potato (>30%) [6]. The distribution of di-nucleotide repeat microsatellites is higher in mammals (31%) and rodents (33%) than plants (in average ~24%) although Arabidopsis and potato have >30 and 50% dinucleotide repeats [6]. Plants have less frequency of GA dinucleotide repeat SSRs, while animal genomes abundantly contain these types of repeats. GC dinucleotide arrays are less frequent in coding sequences, but GC-rich trinucleotide arrays frequently occurred in exons, while AT-rich trinucleotides evenly distributed throughout all genomic regions. For example, ATT repeats are abundant in introns of genes of most organisms although some genomes like rodents tend to have AAG abundance in introns. Generally, ACG, ACC, ACT repeat SSRs are rare in all organisms [6].

Interestingly, there is a predominance of tri- and hexanucleotides in coding regions that is explained as a result of selection forces to keep reading frame not altered. However, microsatellites of such triplet expansions can cause harmful phenotypes such as Fragile X syndrome (FXS) and Huntington's disease [7]. Tetranucleotide motif SSRs located predominantly in noncoding regions with abundance of AT-rich motifs. Mammals have more tetranucleotide microsatellites compared to other organisms [6]. Similarly, pentanucleotide motif microsatellites abundantly represented in intronic regions of animal genomes compared to bacteria and plants.

According to a repeat motif pattern, microsatellites can be classified as (1) perfect with continuous repeat of single motif, (2) imperfect with a base pair disruption between repeats, (3) interrupted with insertion of a stretch of sequence of few nucleotides within repeats, or (4) composite with multiple SRR motif repeat types that vary among different taxa [2]. The density of SSRs also vary among different taxa and occurred one SSR in about 6.04 kb for Arabidopsis, 6–7 kb in mammals and could be less than 1 kb in puffer fish [2] or up to 212–292 kb in hexaploid wheat [8]. Microsatellites can be genomic, i.e., developed from genomic DNAs (gSSRs) or can be expressed, referred to as EST-SSRs, derived from expressed sequence tags (ESTs) [2, 9]. EST-SSRs have high power because of their associations with expressed genes, directly contributing to a phenotype [10]. In plants, SSRs can also be classified as nuclear SSRs if they occurred in nuclear DNA (nuSSRs) and chloroplast SSRs (cpSSRs), if they occurred in chloroplast DNA. cpSSR loci were first introduced by Powel et al. [11, 12] in 1995 as useful genetic markers with broad applications in plants, in particular for measuring the cytoplasmic diversity and introgression in plant species, although there are some limitations highlighted below [12].

3. Origin, evolution, and mutation mechanisms and rates

Due to sequence mutation, the genesis of microsatellite locus can be started from a mutated site with minimum of eight nucleotide repeats or from de novo points without repeat motifs leading to formation of "proto-microsatellites/SSRs" sites. Some reports discuss the potential of minisatellites as a progenitor of SSRs, while others suggest the contribution of transposons to the birth of SSRs although it is not evident in birds and plants [6]. Following the next generation of DNA replication process, "proto-SSR" sites can get expanded due to errors caused by DNA polymerase strand slippage [2, 3, 6, 7]. Moreover, based on "transposon-mediated" microsatellite birth, SSRs can be born due to transposon movement, exemplified by the origin of *Alu* element-derived AT-rich SSRs [3, 6, 7].

Replication slippage is considered the main mechanism [2, 3, 6, 7] of microsatellite genesis, repeat expansion or reduction, and generating a variability that all are contributing to the molecular evolution of microsatellites. Besides replication-associated slippage, the birth of microsatellites can occur during transcription-coupled DNA repair and/or repair of double-stranded breaks where repetitive sequences are preferably used for filling the gaps [6]. Further, insertion and deletions (indels) or single nucleotide substitutions, which occur in increased rates [13, 14], can generate new repeat arrays in microsatellites. For instance, a comparative human and primate genome analysis revealed that the repeat number change in short microsatellites mostly occurs because of single nucleotide polymorphism (SNP) mutations rather than slippage [15].

Microsatellite mutations can simultaneously change one, two, or more repeat unit(s), providing a higher mutation rates of 10^{-2} to 10^{-6} per microsatellite locus per generation [6] than other mutation types, such as point mutation rates, which is approximately 10^{-9} nucleotides per generation for entire genome in eukaryotes [1]. The base position relative to the microsatellite, genomic location, repeat type and number, base identity, flanking sequence, speed of recombination and transcription, and heterozygosity of microsatellite alleles greatly affect the microsatellite mutation rates [6, 16]. In particular, microsatellites in noncoding regions tend to mutate frequently than those in coding regions, and/or changes in perfect repeats can generate new SSRs [6]. In addition, recombination with unequal-length SSR alleles can increasingly cause SSR instability during meiosis [15, 16]; dinucleotide repeats mutate frequently than tri- and tetra-nucleotide arrays, and/or longer and purer repeats can mutate in high rate than shorter repeats with low purity [2]. SSR mutation rate is species and gender specific where human males have higher SSR mutation rate ($0–7 \times 10^{-3}$ per locus per gamete per generation) compared to females [17].

The rate of both repeat motif expansion and contraction is also species specific. For example, repeat expansion mutations are faster in humans than chimpanzees, or there is a loss of two repeat units per mutation in yeast compared to a loss of 1.4 repeats in Drosophila [6]. Repeat expansion mutations predominantly found in primates, while bacteria have repeat contractions. Longer repeat arrays in SSRs are considered to be recent origin and long repeat SSRs are biased toward repeat expansion mutation. Statistically, the patterns of variation in SSR loci can be studied and predicted using "Stepwise Mutation Model" (SMM) or its two-step modification and "Infinite Allele Model" (IAM) [6].

4. Biological function

Due to common understanding that repetitive DNAs are "junk" and nonfunctional, tandem repeat microsatellites have been considered as neutral elements in a genome without distinct biological function although there were numerous observations that microsatellite mutations can lead to many diseased phenotypes and change the function of proteins. The occurrence of microsatellites in coding and regulatory gene regions (as well as introns or in intergene regions) supported the biological function of microsatellites in such processes as (1) gene expression including transcription and translation, (2) gene silencing, (3) alternative splicing and mRNA transport, (4) chromatin organization, and (5) regulation of cell cycle [2, 6]. Involvement of microsatellite repeat motives in these key biological processes of cell life not only leads to the cell phenotype change and cause disease and unwanted traits but also determines the evolutionary fate, survival, plasticity, and adaptation of organisms in changing and potentially harmful environments [2, 3, 6]. Discovery of the co-localization of SSR with pre-microRNAs and influence of CUU repeat numbers to the loop size of pri-microRNAs in orange plants [6, 18] or involvement of certain r(CGG)-derived microRNAs such as miR-fmr1s in FXS-pathogenesis demonstrated a possible role of microsatellites in many developmental processes regulated by microRNAs [19].

There are many examples for distinctive phenotypic changes that directly associated with the increases or decreases of microsatellite repeat arrays. For instance, more than 40 neurological diseases in humans, such as FXS and spinocerebellar ataxia (SCA1) with a polyglutamine tracts, are caused by microsatellite motif length changes in trinucleotide arrays [20]. Microsatellite repeat changes determine morphological features, for example, repeat expansion of microsatellite stretches in the *aristaless-like 4 (ALX-4)* and *runt-related transcription factor 2 (RUNX2)* genes of domesticated dogs (*Canis familiaris*) is associated with limb and skull morphology [21] with interesting correlation between longer sequence lengths of *RUNX2* microsatellites and longer faces of dogs, which is observed in 30 naturally evolving Carnivora species [22]. Microsatellite repeat polymorphism in control regions of the *Vasopressin 1a receptor* gene affects social behavior, level of monogamy [23], and autism and socialization skills [24] in humans, and the courtship behaviors in other mammals [25]. Repeat number changes in microsatellites control the duration of its circadian clock cycles in a fungus *Neurospora crassa* [26]. SSR expansions in noncoding regions also generate diseased phenotypes. For instance, Friedreich Ataxia is caused by a GAA triplet expansion in the first intron of the *X25* gene that is explained by its influence with transcription [27]. Repeat number expansions/reductions in introns of several genes such as *Asparagine synthetase, NOS3*, and *EGRF* genes cause acute lymphoblastic leukemia [28], hypertension [29], and osteosarcomas [30], respectively.

5. Utility of microsatellites as genetic markers

As a genetic marker, microsatellites can be widely applied for solving a numerous type of different tasks. These include the construction of genetic linkage groups and integrated maps; correlation of phenotypic and genotypic variations using quantitative trait locus (QTL) and/or linkage disequilibrium (LD)-based association mapping approaches; analyses of parentage and/or ancestry; DNA barcoding for plant varieties and germplasm; evaluation of gene flow and variety/seed purity; breeding using marker-assisted selection tools; estimation of genetic diversity, phylogeography, conservation and restoration of biodiversity, molecular evolution, taxonomy, and phylogenetic features of biological species; detection of genetic structure of native plant populations and crop germplasm, origin and domestication of crop species, migration, demographic process, population differentiation and kinship; assessment of impacts of mutagenic contaminants; and application in forensics and disease diagnostics [1, 2, 31].

5.1. Marker development

Microsatellites are polymerase chain reaction (PCR)-based markers and require a prior knowledge on sequence structure before using them as a genetic marker. There are two ways to develop SSR markers: (1) necessary genome or its part should be sequenced following screening for microsatellite repeat arrays; or (2) preliminary sequenced genomes databases can be mined using variety of *in silico* bioinformatics software packages. As further steps, both approaches, however, require designing and synthesis of marker primers, genotyping, scoring, and assessing the polymorphism levels in diverse genotypes under study using PCR to apply for a specific genetic study. There are various methods and approaches [1, 2] available for construction/enrichment (e.g., selective hybridization or biotin-captured) and sequencing [e.g., Sanger or next generation sequencing (NGS)-based] of genomic libraries for SSRs as well as genotyping (e.g., agarose, polyacrylamide (PAG), and capillary electrophoresis with fluorescent detection), which we skip the details here. These approaches have been historically well optimized and used depending on the purpose of study, expertise, availability of necessary equipment and reagents, and targeted types of SSR arrays.

When sequences are generated de novo or available as genome databases in the National Center of Biotechnology Information NCBI [32], most important step is to efficiently screen microsatellite containing sequences and design markers. For this purpose, there are many SSR array searching algorithms available such as tandem repeat finder (TRF), MIcroSAtellite identification tool (MISA), SSRFinder, and PALFinder [1, 2]. Besides there are several web servers based online tools such as CID [33] and WebSat [34]. Each of these bioinformatics tools has its advantages and disadvantages, can address various aspects of microsatellite mining and marker development and be used according to study/task objectives, expertise and availability. There is some recommended software for efficient screening microsatellite repeats from DNA sequences such as MISA or Phobos [1]. Further, there is a list of many other useful bioinformatics resources for the genetic analyses of microsatellite data [35].

5.2. Advantages

Among all other type of molecular markers, for past three decades, microsatellite markers were the marker of choice because they are PCR based; abundant and dispersed throughout a genome; highly mutagenic, polymorphic, and informative; co-dominant, suitable for detecting heterozygotes, and multi-allelic; experimentally reproducible; transferable among related taxa; cost-effective and easy to detect; amplified from low quality and low quantity of DNAs; and presumably neutral markers. In addition, microsatellites are of particularly useful to construct a genetic map of large genomes when a reference genome is absent [1]. They are favored markers for small-scale genetic studies with limited budget, potentially detecting large genetic information and physiological parameters of a genome [3], do not require high marker density, especially if LD block sizes of a genome are long [31] and benefit from inclusion of additional samples for the project without significant costs [1]. Microsatellites can be also used for testing non-neutrality and subjected to automated florescent dye-based band scoring through multiplexed genotyping for large-scale studies, which help to cut the time and cost of the study [2]. Unipartental cytoplasmic inheritance with presumably no recombination history of cpSSR [12] further provide a great advantage to develop universal primers to genotype and genetically analyze distantly related plant taxa although there are some limitations, too (see below). Importantly, EST-SSR markers developed from coding genes can be a great tool to directly tag and map-based cloning of functionally meaningful "candidate genes" through genotype to phenotype correlations in genetic mapping studies [10].

5.3. Disadvantages

There are various concerns and caveats to use microsatellites, too. Some of these include but not limited to (1) need for a priori genomic sequence information that is not available for most prokaryotes where specific effort can be costly and time consuming; (2) PCR failure due to point mutations in primer sequences resulting in 'null' alleles and falsely hiding the reality when applying PCR primers across different species with mutated primer binding sites, or because of environmental degradation of long repeat arrays; (3) PCR stutters of short SSR arrays giving multiple bands from single locus; (4) abundance for rare, private or minor alleles; (5) issues with assigning of multiple band SSRs alleles in the absence of correct parentage and pedigree information; and (6) size homoplasy, heteroplasmy and cytoplasmic introgression (in particular with cpSSR) due to back mutations during replication slippage [1, 2, 3, 9, 12]. All these complicate and bias downstream genetic analyses, inflate F-statistics or p-values, falsify the diversity levels, relatedness, divergence, and true evolution or phylogenetic grouping. Due to homoplasy and high rate of polymorphism in SSRs, phylogenetic studies should be carried with cautiousness for distantly related species [1].

However, these all do not void the usefulness of SSR markers, rather call attention of researchers using this marker system. There are several approaches to take into consideration of these caveats when SSRs are used that include verification of size homoplasy, heteroplasmy and primer site point mutations using additional cloning and re-sequencing including NGS [12]; exclusion of problematic, rare, and private alleles from the analyses based on specific objective

[29] (e.g., haplotype networks due to high potential of repeated evolution [12]); use of more samples and markers for genotyping rather concluding based on few samples and small number of markers; and reanalysis of the results with or in combination of different type DNA markers such as RFLPs, SNPs, etc. [12].

5.4. Future utilization

Because of past 5 years' successful and wide application of SNP markers for genome-wide applications and the emergence of cost-effective and large-scale sequencing, as well as SNP detection and genotyping methodology such as NGS, NGS-based genotyping by sequencing (GBS), and restriction site–associated DNA sequencing (RAD-Seq) techniques circumvented a rapid shift of SSR-based molecular marker studies to SNP-based research. This was evidenced by sharp decrease of a number of publications using microsatellites in crop species during 2010–2015 [2]. However, as discussed and highlighted by Hodel et al. [1], microsatellite markers will continue to be useful and favorable markers. This is due to the fact that (1) not all studies require in-depth genotyping as provided by NGS-based approaches where SSRs remain a suitable choice, and (2) sample size can be largely expanded without significant cost when SSRs are used, which is costly with NGS-based approaches. Further, (3) additional large sample inclusion can increase the power of microsatellite-based studies, which perform similarly with SNPs; (4) existed SSR-marker data can be readily incorporated and used with new studies; (5) multi-allelic nature of SSRs makes them highly suitable for studying small subpopulations; and (6) microsatellites are the best markers of choice for small-scale laboratories with limited budget.

Additionally, SSRs are still efficient markers for (1) marker-assisted selection (MAS) programs to mobilize QTL blocks using small number of SSR markers based on LD information, (2) germplasm characterization using evenly spaced core set of few SSRs, (3) seed or variety purity testing, and (4) SSR indexing of cultivars (barcoding) and plant germplasm resource. All these invalidate any emerging opinion on prospective total "death" of microsatellites as useful genetic markers and demonstrate the future benefit of microsatellites in many genetic studies. Highlights and some updates on advantages, disadvantages, and usefulness of SSRs for various applications in agricultural and biomedical fields have been presented in following book chapters of this book, which I provide a brief information below to introduce them to readers.

6. Highlights from chapters

In this context, with the objective to provide current updates on microsatellite applications in genetic studies as well as re-highlight the usefulness of microsatellites in current and future genetic analyses, in this edited volume, we compiled 10 chapters describing the wide utilization of microsatellite markers in different biological taxa. Generally, chapters presented research studies and review discussions on following three directions: (1) microsatellite markers in plants and genetic diversity research, (2) microsatellite markers in animal genetics and breeding, and (3) microsatellites in cancer research.

In the first section, the chapter by Jamila Bernardia and her team, Universita Cattolica del Sacro Cuore, Piacenza, Italy, presents the use of microsatellites in livestock and illustrated exploitation and versatility of microsatellites for the characterization of agricultural diversity and food traceability. Authors studied the assessment of genetic diversity in apple, pear, and sweet and sour cherry trees and explored the molecular authentication of wheat food chain of plant cultivars and farm animals. The chapter discusses that a small number of SSR markers can be efficiently used to differentiate and link each tree cultivar to its corresponding genotypic profile and be useful for molecular traceability of the whole production chain from durum wheat raw material to processed pasta despite food processing degrades DNAs.

Further, the chapter by Maria Eugenia Barrandeguy and Maria Victoria Garcia, Universidad Nacional de Misiones, Instituto de Biologia Subtropical Nodo Posadas, Argentina, has covered the development of microsatellite markers, genotyping, data analysis, and interpretation of obtained results in the examples of nuSSRs and cpSSRs. The chapter discusses the usefulness of microsatellite markers for the analysis of past and present microevolutionary forces in native forest pant populations and making inferences about future of these natural populations.

In their chapter, Rodolphe Laurent Gigant and his team from France have assessed the mating system of the natural populations of *Vanilla mexicana* (Orchidaceae) in the island of Guadeloupe. Using only six transferable SSRs out of 33 developed in other *Vanilla* species, authors successfully genotyped a set of 51 *V. mexicana* samples, which helped to differentiate *V. mexicana* samples, assess the genetic diversity and other genetic characteristics, determine a heterozygote deficiency, and estimate self-pollination rates. Results showed that "*V. mexicana* is mainly reproducing by autogamy via spontaneous self-pollination in Guadeloupe," which is reported as a useful trait for interspecific breeding of *Vanilla* species. Justyna Anna Nowakowska, from Forest Research Institute, Poland, has studied genetic structure of fourteen Scots pine populations from North-eastern Poland using SSR markers that revealed high genetic indices for the mean polymorphic information content, genetic diversity and heterozygosity. There was low population differentiation identified among stands, which were clustered into one genetically similar group. The chapter concludes that the present distribution of genetically related populations of Scots pine in North-eastern Poland seems to reflect the historical events such as post-glacial colonization of Poland from different European refugia and/or human management carried out in the past.

The last chapter in this section by Beyene Amelework, University of KwaZulu-Natal, South Africa, and Ethiopian Institute of Agricultural Research, Ethiopia, reviewed the use of microsatellite markers in genetic diversity analysis and heterotic grouping of sorghum and maize through the estimation of molecular-based genetic distance. The chapter also discusses the existing challenges with the use of SSR markers in heterotic grouping in studied crops.

The second section of the book covers microsatellite marker application in animal sciences. The chapter by Yuta Seki and his colleagues, Tokyo Metropolitan Institute of Medical Science and Tokyo University of Agriculture, Japan, has provided a review on the currently available studies on domestic goat (*Capra hircus*) breeding using microsatellite markers to demonstrate exploitation of these markers for the assessment of intra- and inter-population genetic diversity, QTL mapping, and marker-assisted selection of favorable phenotypes. Authors also stated that despite SNPs may be favorable marker for animal studies because of their large-scale genomic converge, microsatellites remain as a marker of choice for small scale genetic studies, owing to economic concerns such as cost, time and labor as well as because of their genotyping simplicity.

Further, Emil J. Hernandez-Ruz and his colleagues, Federal University of Para (UFPA), Brazil, presented a research study on microsatellite marker development and evaluation of the genetic structure of the Amazonian fish *Hypophthalmus marginatus* from the Tocantins and Araguaia River in the Eastern Amazonia. Although genetic analyses were performed using only two polymorphic microsatellite loci out of 17 developed for this fish species, results not only provided evidence on the existence of (1) low levels of genetic diversity in H. marginatus of the Tocantis basin possibility related to the Dam construction and 2) a gene flow mainly in the upstream or downstream directions but also were consistent with data from mitochondrial markers. Authors recommend the use of more markers to validate the influence of dam for reduction of genetic diversity of the Amazonian fish species.

In the chapter by Hongyu Ma and his colleagues, Shantou University and Chinese Academy of Fishery Sciences, China, authors presented a research study on the development and characterization of microsatellite markers for genetic study of the mud crab (*Scylla paramamosain*). Efforts have helped to isolate and characterize 302 polymorphic microsatellite markers. Authors have evaluated polymorphism and genetic differentiation of the mud crab wild populations, established microsatellite-based parentage assignment of the mud crab offspring, identified a marker associated with growth performance, and constructed a first preliminary genetic linkage map for *S. paramamosain* using microsatellite and amplified fragment length polymorphism (AFLP) markers. The chapter concludes that these findings should provide novel insights into genome biology, wild resource background, and molecular marker-assisted selection in S. paramamosain

The third section of the book includes two similar topic chapters that describe the impact of microsatellite instability (MSI) in causing the cancer diseases. In particular, Jeffery W. Bacher and his team from Promega Corporation and University of Wisconsin, Madison, USA, provided a detailed review on the role and significance of MSI in hereditary and sporadic type of cancers. They have discussed the discovery of MSI and its association with colorectal cancer or Lynch syndrome, and the use of SSR marker in disease screening. In addition, emerging and alternative NGS-based methods in detecting both tumor MSI status and germline mutations in a single test for LS are reviewed. The chapter concludes that MSI detection is poised to take on an even greater role in prediction of responses to the new immunotherapies targeted at MSI-positive tumors Similarly, the following chapter by Narasimha Reddy Parine and Mohammad

http://dx.doi.org/10.5772/66446

Saud Alanazi, King Saud University, Saudi Arabia, described the role of genetic instability, including MSI in colorectal cancer. Differing from previous chapter, this chapter reviews the major molecular mechanisms causing genomic and microsatellite instability, including a mismatch repair (MMR) system and cancer formation.

7. Conclusions

Microsatellite markers have been one of the most reliable molecular markers derived from the DNA molecule, which were widely and successfully used for life science research directions including agriculture and biomedical fields. As a molecular marker, microsatellites have many advantages suitable for the wide types of genetic analyses, but do present concerns and caveats that require attention and corrections for the results and their interpretation in specific analyses, which were highlighted by chapters of this book. Although the trends of molecular marker application and use for past 5 years show a decreased utilization of microsatellite markers and present a shifted growth toward the use of SNP markers, that is due to the emergence of novel generation NGS-based genotyping technologies, microsatellite markers remain to be useful and choice of marker system for the specific genetic studies. This is because of multi-allelic nature, simplicity of genotyping procedures, cost-effectivity, and suitability of microsatellite markers for small-scale laboratories with limited budget. In this book, all chapters re-highlighted the usefulness of microsatellites in genetic analyses of various life science fields, providing updated discussions and reviews on current use and future prospects of these markers, which invalidate emerging opinion on "full-death" of microsatellites as useful genetic markers.

Acknowledgements

I am thankful to the Academy of Sciences of Uzbekistan, Committee for Coordination of Science and Technology Development, the Office of International Research Programs (OIRP) of the United States Department of Agriculture (USDA)—Agricultural Research Service (ARS), Texas A&M University, and U.S. Civilian Research & Development Foundation (CRDF) for financial support of SSR marker–based research of cotton in Uzbekistan.

Author details

Ibrokhim Y. Abdurakhmonov

Address all correspondence to: genomics@uzsci.net

Center of Genomics and Bioinformatics, Academy of Science of the Republic of Uzbekistan, Tashkent, Uzbekistan

References

[1] Hodel RG, Segovia-Salcedo MC, Landis JB, Crowl AA, Sun M, Liu X, Gitzendanner MA, Douglas NA, Germain-Aubrey CC, Chen S, Soltis DE, Soltis PS. The report of my death was an exaggeration: A review for researchers using microsatellites in the 21st century. Appl Plant Sci. 2016;4:1600025. DOI:10.3732/apps.1600025

[2] Vieira ML, Santini L, Diniz AL, Munhoz CF. Microsatellite markers: what they mean and why they are so useful. Genet Mol Biol. 2016;39:12–328. DOI: 10.1590/1678-4685-GMB-2016-0027

[3] Saeed AF, Wang R, Wang S. Microsatellites in pursuit of microbial genome evolution. Front Microbiol. 2016;6:1462. DOI: 10.3389/fmicb.2015.01462

[4] Litt M, Luty JA. A hypervariable microsatellite revealed by in vitro amplification of a dinucleotide repeat within the cardiac muscle actin gene. Am J Hum Genet. 1989;44:397–401

[5] PubMed database [Internet]. 2015. Available from: http://www.ncbi.nlm.nih.gov/pubmed [Accessed from 2016-10-14]

[6] Trivedi S. Microsatellites (SSRs): Puzzles within puzzle. Indian J Biotechnol. 2004;3:331–347

[7] Richard GF, Kerrest A, Dujon B. Comparative genomics and molecular dynamics of DNA repeats in eukaryotes. Microbiol Mol Biol Rev. 2008;72:686–727. DOI:10.1128/MMBR.00011-08

[8] Ma ZQ, Röder M, Sorrells ME. Frequencies and sequence characteristics of di-, tri-, and tetra-nucleotide microsatellites in wheat. Genome. 1996;39:123–30

[9] Ellis JR, Burke JM. EST-SSRs as a resource for population genetic analyses. Heredity (Edinb). 2007;99:125–132

[10] Varshney RK, Graner A, Sorrells ME. Genic microsatellite markers in plants: features and applications. Trends Biotechnol. 2005;23:48–55.

[11] Powell W, Morgante M, Andre C, McNicol JW, Machray GC, Doyle JJ, Tingey SV,Rafalski JA. Hypervariable microsatellites provide a general source of polymorphic DNA markers for the chloroplast genome. Curr Biol. 1995;5:1023–1029

[12] Wheeler GL, Dorman HE, Buchanan A, Challagundla L, Wallace LE. A review of the prevalence, utility, and caveats of using chloroplast simple sequence repeats for studies of plant biology. Appl Plant Sci. 2014;2:1400059. DOI: 10.3732/apps.1400059.

[13] Pumpernik D, Oblak B, Borstnik B. Replication slippage versus point mutation rates in short tandem repeats of the human genome. Mol Genet Genomics. 2008;279:53–61. DOI: 10. 1007/s00438-007-0294-1

[14] Siddle KJ, Goodship JA, Keavney B, Santibanez-Koref MF. Bases adjacent to mononucleotide repeats show an increased single nucleotide polymorphism frequency in the human genome. Bioinformatics. 2011;27:895–898. DOI: 10.1093/bioinformatics/btr067

[15] Amos W. Mutation biases and mutation rate variation around very short human microsatellites revealed by human-chimpanzee-orangutan genomic sequence alignments. J Mol Evol. 2010;71:192–201. DOI: 10.1007/s00239-010-9377-4

[16] Amos W. Heterozygosity increases microsatellite mutation rate. Biol Lett. 2006;12: 20150929. DOI:10.1098/rsbl.2015.0929

[17] Brinkmann B, Klintschar M, Neuhuber F, Hühne J, Rolf B. Mutation rate in human microsatellites: influence of the structure and length of the tandem repeat. Am J Hum Genet. 1998;62:1408–1415

[18] Liu Y, Wang L, Chen D, Wu X, Huang D, Chen L, Li L, Deng X, Xu Q. Genome-wide comparison of microRNAs and their targeted transcripts among leaf, flower and fruit of sweet orange. BMC Genomics. 2014;15:695. DOI: 10.1186/1471-2164-15-695

[19] Lin SL. microRNAs and Fragile X Syndrome. Adv Exp Med Biol. 2015;888:107–121. DOI: 10.1007/978-3-319-22671-2_7

[20] Pearson CE, Nichol Edamura K, Cleary JD. Repeat instability: mechanisms of dynamic mutations. Nat Rev Genet. 2005;6:729–742

[21] Fondon JW 3rd, Garner HR. Molecular origins of rapid and continuous morphological evolution. Proc Natl Acad Sci U S A. 2004;101:18058–18063. DOI: 10.1073/pnas.0408118101

[22] Sears KE, Goswami A, Flynn JJ, Niswander LA. The correlated evolution of Runx2 tandem repeats, transcriptional activity, and facial length in carnivora. Evol Dev. 2007;9:555–565.DOI:10.1111/j.1525-142X.2007.00196.x

[23] Hammock EA, Young LJ. Microsatellite instability generates diversity in brain and sociobehavioral traits. Science. 2005;308:1630–1634

[24] Yirmiya N, Rosenberg C, Levi S, Salomon S, Shulman C, Nemanov L, Dina C, Ebstein RP. Association between the arginine vasopressin 1a receptor (AVPR1a) gene and autism in a family-based study: mediation by socialization skills. Mol Psychiatry. 2006;11:488–94

[25] Graham BM, Solomon NG, Noe DA, Keane B. Male prairie voles with different avpr1a microsatellite lengths do not differ in courtship behaviour. Behav Processes. 2016;128:53–57. DOI: 10.1016/j.beproc.2016.04.006

[26] Michael TP, Park S, Kim TS, Booth J, Byer A, Sun Q, Chory J, Lee K. Simple sequence repeats provide a substrate for phenotypic variation in the *Neurospora crassa* circadian clock. PLoS One. 2007;2:e795

[27] Bidichandani SI, Ashizawa T, Patel PI. The GAA triplet-repeat expansion in Friedreich ataxia interferes with transcription and may be associated with an unusual DNA structure. Am J Hum Genet. 1998;62:111–21

[28] Akagi T, Yin D, Kawamata N, Bartram CR, Hofmann WK, Song JH, Miller CW, den Boer ML, Koeffler HP. Functional analysis of a novel DNA polymorphism of a tandem repeated sequence in the asparagine synthetase gene in acute lymphoblastic leukemia cells. Leuk Res. 2009;33:991–996. DOI: 10.1016/j.leukres.2008.10.022

[29] Jemaa R, Ben Ali S, Kallel A, Feki M, Elasmi M, Taieb SH, Sanhaji H, Omar S, Kaabachi N. Association of a 27-bp repeat polymorphism in intron 4 of endothelial constitutive nitric oxide synthase gene with hypertension in a Tunisian population. Clin Biochem. 2009;42:852–856. DOI:10.1016/j.clinbiochem.2008.12.002

[30] Kersting C, Agelopoulos K, Schmidt H, Korsching E, August C, Gosheger G, Dirksen U, Juergens H, Winkelmann W, Brandt B, Bielack S, Buerger H, Gebert C. Biological importance of a polymorphic CA sequence within intron 1 of the epidermal growth factor receptor gene (EGFR) in high grade central osteosarcomas. Genes Chromosomes Cancer. 2008;47:657–64. DOI: 10.1002/gcc.20571

[31] Abdurakhmonov IY, Abdukarimov A. Application of association mapping to understanding the genetic diversity of plant germplasm resources. Int J Plant Genomics. 2008;2008:574927. DOI: 10.1155/2008/574927

[32] The National Center of Biotechnology Information (NCBI) [Internet]. 2016. Available from: http://www.ncbi.nlm.nih.gov [Accessed: 2016-10-14]

[33] Freitas PD, Martins DS, Galetti PM Jr. cid: a rapid and efficient bioinformatic tool for the detection of SSRs from genomic libraries. Mol Ecol Resour. 2008;8:107–108. DOI: 10.1111/j.1471-8286.2007.01950.x

[34] Martins WS, Lucas DC, Neves KF, Bertioli DJ. WebSat—a web software for microsatellite marker development. Bioinformation. 2009;3:282–283

[35] SoftLinks [Internet]. 2016. Available from: http://softlinks.amnh.org/microsatellites.html [Accessed: 2016-10-14]

Section 2

Microsatellite Markers in Plants and Genetic Diversity Research

Chapter 2

Use of Microsatellites to Study Agricultural Biodiversity and Food Traceability

Jamila Bernardi, Licia Colli, Virginia Ughini and Matteo Busconi

Additional information is available at the end of the chapter

http://dx.doi.org/10.5772/64863

Abstract

Molecular markers are useful tools for measuring the genetic diversity among agricultural species. In plants, microsatellites are still the most used markers for germplasm characterization, conservation, and traceability purposes, while in the livestock sector, although having represented the standard for at least two decades, they are still used only for minor farm animal species. In this work, together with a review on the use of microsatellites in livestock, we also illustrate the use of these markers for the characterization of agricultural diversity and food traceability through two case studies: (i) the analysis of genetic diversity in ancient fruit tree cultivars of apple (*Malus × domestica* Borkh.), pear (*Pyrus communis* L.), sweet cherry (*Prunus avium* L.), and sour cherry (*Prunus cerasus* L.) from Northern Italy and (ii) the molecular authentication of wheat food chain. In the former case, a high genetic variability as well as the presence of different ploidy levels were detected, while in the latter microsatellite markers were shown to be useful for traceability and product authentication along the whole food chain. Overall, the presented evidence confirms the versatility of microsatellites as markers for both agrobiodiversity characterization and food traceability in cultivated plants and farm animals.

Keywords: agrobiodiversity, fruit tree, livestock, microsatellites, traceability

1. Introduction

Molecular characterization has various purposes in plant and animal genetic resource management, such as elucidating relationships between breeds/varieties, characterizing new genotypes, monitoring shifts in population genetic structure, and exploiting associations among traits and markers [1–3]. A well-recognizable molecular profile is a key factor for the protection and conservation of any genetic resource. Researchers can properly exploit plant and animal genetic resources if the materials are well characterized. Low assay cost, affordable hardware, throughput, convenience and ease of assay development, and automation are important factors when choosing DNA-based technology.

Microsatellites, or simple sequence repeats (SSRs), are polymorphic loci that derive from the repetition of short sequence motives of one to six base pairs in length. Microsatellites are among the most useful markers mainly because they are single locus co-dominant markers [4]. In the plant field, the availability of co-dominant markers is important in the analysis of hybrids. Furthermore, with respect to some categories of multi-locus markers (e.g. RAPD), microsatellites are characterized by higher reproducibility. Microsatellites have been largely used for DNA fingerprinting in several species, both wild and domesticated, although in recent years they have been increasingly replaced by single nucleotide polymorphisms (SNPs), particularly in the livestock genetic field [5].

Microsatellites have a series of characteristics that make them ideal to analyze plant genomes: (1) co-dominance that makes possible the analysis of hybrids of plant commercial varieties; (2) the amplified fragments are usually small in size (100 and 300 base pairs) resulting in positive PCR amplifications even in highly degraded DNA; (3) because of the polyploid nature of the genome of several important crop species, a small number of selected SSRs are able to provide a high discrimination capacity, as reported in the section on plant biodiversity; (4) SSRs are automatable, reproducible between different laboratories (provided that some precautions are taken to uniform allele size scoring, such as sharing of standard samples between labs), easily multiplexed, and easy to score; (5) SSRs usually show a high level of polymorphism and several alleles can be detected for a single SSR locus. This latter aspect makes SSRs extremely useful also for organisms with limited or no information on the genomic sequence because a small number of markers can be enough to clearly discriminate between a large number of samples. Compared to SNP markers, SSRs are less numerous in the genome but present a higher number of alleles per locus (SNPs are usually bi-allelic); therefore, a small number of SSRs can result in a discrimination capacity similar to that obtained with a large number of SNPs [6].

Biological diversity—or biodiversity—is a term used to describe the variety of life on Earth. It refers to the wide variety of ecosystems and living organisms: animals, plants, their habitats, and their genes [7]. While biodiversity can be considered as the foundation of life on Earth, it is crucial for the functioning of ecosystems providing us with products and services without which we could not live. Biodiversity is also the foundation of agriculture. In presence of biodiversity, men can select the genetic material available and gradually improve varieties and breeds. Preservation of biodiversity is, therefore, recognized worldwide as a topic of great concern both in wild and agricultural species, and with respect to the latter, recently, there has been an increasing interest in preserving local plant germplasms. Local varieties as breeds, landraces, ecotypes, and ancient varieties, which have been rarely subjected to breeding, are usually characterized by high genetic variability and genotypes. These germplasm resources are well adapted to both local needs and environmental conditions with good fitness for the anthropic and natural environments in which they have evolved [2, 3].

Local germplasms, as ancient fruit tree cultivars or traditional livestock breeds, frequently face strong genetic erosion starting from the twentieth century. Genetic erosion refers to "the loss of individual genes and the loss of particular combinations of genes (i.e., gene complexes) such as those maintained in locally adapted landraces" [8]. Therefore, the term "genetic erosion" refers to both the loss of genes or alleles and the loss of varieties. Conservation of genetic materials, both using *in-situ* or *ex-situ* strategies, is expensive and needs infrastructure not always available. Because of these constraints, correct management of the different agricultural resources strongly relies on molecular information that can be generated using molecular markers.

Microsatellites have been used to evaluate crop germplasm and genetic diversity in several species, including rye [9], grape [10], sugarcane [11], rice [12], and olive [13]. Agrobiodiversity of fruit tree is of increasing concern mainly because repositories still remain a valuable source of allelic variation for many traits and can be exploited for breeding in the near future. Studying the genetic diversity of germplasm resources is not only significant for the protection of species, but also necessary for the development and utilization of germplasm resources for crop improvement and to face existing and future biotic and abiotic constraints with respect to sustainable production in the context of global environmental change [14]. Examples include apple landraces (*Malus* × *domestica* Borkh.) that represent the main fruit crop in temperate regions. It is not surprising that many studies concerning apple biodiversity were performed, both in Europe [3, 15] and in Asia [16].

In the livestock sector, microsatellite markers have been widely used for more than a decade for the characterization and conservation of livestock biodiversity and for the traceability of food products. In livestock, current genotyping standards are represented by standardized SNP panels that allow the characterization of tens or hundreds of thousand markers per sample [5]; but due to the low costs and to the possibility of in-house implementation of genotyping protocols, microsatellite markers still represent a useful resource to characterize livestock breeds in several developing countries, in which the access to SNP typing or other high throughput technologies can be difficult or too expensive [17–19]. Some years ago, FAO published recommendations for standardized sets of microsatellite loci to be used for studying diversity in the major livestock species [20] in order to make possible the comparison of results across different research projects [17–19].

The good resolution power and frequent occurrence of SSR within plant and farm animal genomes make this type of marker very useful in the food sector also. Food traceability is a milestone of EU food safety policy. The European Commission has agreed to establish a 'Reference Centre' to combat food fraud and ensure the "authenticity and integrity" of the EU food supply chain [21]. EU enhances and supports projects related to food safety as the recently approved project Food Integrity, comprising 38 participants from 18 European countries and one from China [22]. Furthermore, the addition of products without prior declaration on the label, besides representing fraud and adulteration, can also bring health risks, in particular to allergic consumers. In recent years, food traceability has become a topical field mainly to prevent fraud, adulteration, and sophistication. A database of food ingredient fraud issues was developed by [23]. The food products more subject to fraud are, in order, olive oil, milk, honey, saffron, orange juice, coffee, apple juice and wine [23]. Most of the processed foods contain very low quality and quantity of DNA, because thermal or chemical treatments determine its degradation. Being microsatellites short repeats of 1–6 nucleotides, they are the most useful markers for DNA recovered from a treated food matrix and combined with *in vitro* DNA amplification (PCR); they allow the analysis of low amount of starting material. Indeed, as the amplified fragments are short, they can also be obtained from highly fragmented DNA.

Apart from adulteration and fraudulent procedures, traceability is of great importance to authenticate the quality and integrity of European high value food. A biochemical and genetic approach using microsatellites was useful to discriminate the geographical origin of Italian red wines obtained from Campania region native red grape varieties [10]. Several DNA-based analytical methods have been developed and applied to identify and quantify cereal species and to fingerprint and identify varieties to verify their authenticity [24, 25] developed a microsatellite-based method to verify the presence of the four required durum wheat cultivars in "Altamura" bread, and which are cultivated in a restricted geographical area close to the town of Altamura. Altamura bread, according to its European mark of protected designation of origin (PDO), at least 80% of the total flour used for Altamura bread preparation must derive from the aforementioned traditional durum wheat cultivars used alone or in combination.

In livestock, breed discrimination is useful to detect fraud and to protect and valorize typical productions. Girgentana goat (*Capra hircus* L.), an ancient breed reared in a restricted area of Sicily (southern Italy) and its dairy products were traced by the use of a specific panel of microsatellites [26]. The potential of microsatellites for determining the origin of meat products was also important for traceability of nine Portuguese breeds with PDO products [27], while four Italian cattle breeds were identified by microsatellite markers using different statistical approaches to certify the origin of their typical products [28].

The aim of this paper is to highlight the utility of microsatellite markers to study both genetic diversity of domesticated plants and animals and food traceability. Some examples have been provided in the following sections.

2. Agrobiodiversity: the case study of fruit tree species in Northern Italy

Researchers [29] reported that 940 crop plants species are threatened globally and genetic erosion was described in different crop groups, such as cereals and grasses or fruits and nuts [8]. When a species, or the diversity within a species, is lost, the genes important for improving crops are also lost. Preserving local germplasms, landraces, ecotypes, and ancient varieties, means preserving not only our history and culture (such populations represented for centuries an important source of food for local people) but also an extremely useful reserve of genes usable to introduce new characteristics in modern varieties. In order to preserve the local germplasm of ancient fruit tree cultivars, a systematic recovering and characterization of the traditional material of the western part of the Emilia Romagna region was carried out. In this area the tradition of pear (*Pyrus communis* L.), apple (*M.* × *domestica* Borkh.), sweet and sour

http://dx.doi.org/10.5772/64863

cherry (*Prunus avium* L. and *Prunus cerasus* L.) cultivation is well established. Seventeen accessions belonging to ancient varieties of sweet cherry, 7 of sour cherry, 20 of apple, and 32 of pear have been sampled (**Tables 1–3**), and an example of some accessions is shown in **Figures 1–3**.

Species	Cultivar name—accessions	Origin	Microsatellite markers and size of the amplicons (bp)[a]				
			EMPA 015	EMPA 018	UDP 97/402	UCDCH 17	UCDCH 31
P. avium	Selvaticona di Magnano	PC	253/219	101/92	140/118	187/185	141
	Mora piacentina	PC	253/219	101/92	140/118	187/185	141
	Picaion acc.1	PC	238	92	118	185	141/130
	Picaion acc.2	PC	238	92	118	185	141/130
	Smirne	PC	253/219	92	118	185/187	130/123
	Pavesi acc. A	PC	253/249	101/96	118	197/183	128/125
	Pavesi acc. C1	PC	253/249	101/96	118	197/183	128/125
	Pavesi acc. C2	PC	253/249	101/96	118	197/183	128/125
	Mori	PC	221/219	92	118	187/185	141/132
	Raffaella	PC	238	101	118	185	141
	Flamengo acc.A	PC	238	92	118	185	141/130
	Flamengo acc.B	PC	238	92	118	185	141/130
	Flamengo acc.C	PC	238	92	118	185	141/130
	Duroncina della goccia	PC	221/219	92	118	197/185	141
	Prima	PC	253/249	96/92	118/114	185	145/130
	Mora di Vignola	PC	221/219	101	126/114	197/185	128/123
	Giambella	PR	251/219	96/92	126/118	187/185	128/123
P. cerasus	Marasca dal peduncolo lungo	PC	249/247/221/195	96	126/112	185/179/155	130/113
	Marasca Villanova	PC	249/238/225/195	92	126/112	195/185/175/169	141/130/123
	Marinone I acc. A	PC	251/225/195	105/92	140/126/114/112	195/185/175/167	141/130/123
	Marinone II acc. A	PC	225/221/195	92	126/118/112	193/185/175/167	141/130/123
	Marinone II acc. C	PC	251/225/195	105/92	140/126/114/112	195/185/175/167	141/130/123
	Amarena Piacentina	PC	249/247/225/195	92	126/112	193/185/175/167	141/130/123
P. × gondouini	Visciola	PC	225/211/195	105/99	126/122/118/110	197/191/187/171	130/123

Microsatellite profiles are reported for each cherry cultivar. Columns from left to right indicate: (i) the species, (ii) the local name, (iii) the accession, (iv) the origin of the accession, Piacenza (PC) or Parma (PR), and (v) the size of the PCR amplified product.

Table 1. Molecular characterization of cherry varieties.

In addition, DNA analysis was carried out using SSR markers in order to obtain a preliminary fingerprint of each sampled accession and to eventually solve controversies of synonyms (different names for a single genotype) and homonyms (a single name for different genotypes). Genetic variability of the samples was evaluated using five SSR markers for each species: EMPA015, EMPA018 [30], UDP97-402 [31], UCDCH17, and UCDCH31 [32] for sweet and sour cherry; GD96, GD100 and GD162 [33] for apple; KA14, KA16 and BGT23b [34] for pear; GD142, GD147 [33] for both apple and pear (**Tables 1–3**). DNA extraction from young leaves and PCR amplification have been carried out as previously reported [35]. Analysis of PCR products was performed using an ABI Prism 3100 Genetic Analyzer (Applied Biosystem—Thermofisher). Expected heterozygosity and discrimination power were calculated as described in [35], while observed heterozygosity was calculated as the ratio between heterozygous genotypes over the total number of the samples (*Nh*/*Ntot*). Results are shown in **Table 4**.

Species	Cultivar name—accessions	Origin	Microsatellite markers and size of the amplicons (bp)[a]				
			GD96	GD100	GD147	GD162	GD142
	Ruggine acc. I	PC	178/172	230/222	150/129	219/210	138/132
	Ruggine acc. II	PC	178/172	230/222	150/129	219/210	138/132
	Fior d'acacia	PC	180/172	224	146/129	230	140/138
M. × *domestica*	Verdone	PC	176/172	234/224	148/135/129	228/210	144/126
	Rustaio	PC	178/174	224	135/129	228/210	131
	Rustajò	PC	176/174/168	226/224/222	135	230/228/210	154/144/126
	Restajo	PC	174/150	226/219	142/135	210	144/138
	Carraia acc. I	PC	170/168/150	234/230/224	148/146/135	234/230/222/210	140/138
	Carraia acc. II	PC	174/150	232/230	148/135	228/222/210	140/138
	Salame	PC	172	224	148/146	222/210	144
	Rosa	PR	178/174/168	230/226/224	148/137/135	230/219/210	148/144/138
	Mela Rosa	PR	187/185/164	NA	139	226/210	144/132/126
	Bella di Maggio	PR	174	226	127	219/210	144/140
	Cavic	PR	178/172	224	148/135	230/228	144
	Seriana	PR	176/170/168	226	148/137/129	230/226/210	148/144/126
	Melo Olio	PR	194/176	222	142/137	234/228	152/140
	Cucumero	PR	172	224	148	222/210	144
	Ghiacciata	PR	176/172	224	135/129	210	132/126
	Musona	PR	178/172	234/224	135/129	230/228	144/142
	Codaro	PR	172/166	224/222	135	228/210	152/126

Microsatellite profiles are reported for each apple cultivar. Columns from left to right indicate: (i) species, (ii) the local name, (iii) the accession, (iv) the origin of the accession, Piacenza (PC) or Parma (PR), and (v) the size of the PCR amplified product.
a: NA means null allele and it refers to the absence of the amplification product in a specific sample.

Table 2. Molecular characterization of apple varieties.

Species	Cultivar name—Accessions	Origin	Microsatellite markers and size of the amplicons (bp)[a]				
			BGT23b	KA16	GD147	KA14	GD 142
P. communis							
	Lauro acc. I	PC	213/195	129	132/120	194/176	166/158
	Lauro acc. II	PC	213/195	129	132/120	194/176	166/158
	Limone acc. I	PC	209	129/115	118	184/178	156/152
	Limone acc. II	PC	209	129/115	118	184/178	156/152
	Limone acc. III	PC	209	129/115	118	184/178	156/152
	Rossetto	PC	193/191	147	118	184	158/148
	Macagn	PC	213/195	145/129	128/118	188	174/160
	Sburdacen	PC	191	129/123	128/118	184	182/180/176/174
	Sburdacion acc. I	PC	NA	129/123	122/118	222/190/184	178/160/156
	Sburdacion acc. II	PC	NA	129/123	120/118	190/184	178/160/156
	Coda torta acc. I	PC	505/488	147/129	124/118	194/176	174/172/146
	Coda torta acc. II	PC	505/488	147/129	124/118	194/176	174/172/146
	Nigrò	PC	NA	129/125	134/128	194/184/166	174/164/146
	Colar	PC	213	147/129	126/120/118	194/186/184	174/160/146
	Bianchetto	PC	543/509	129	124/120	184/180	180/158
	Nobile acc. I	PR	213/195	129	132/120	194/176	166/158
	Nobile acc. II	PR	213/195	129	132/120	194/176	166/158
	Butirra Polesine	PR	235/231	145/129	138/118	190/176	166
	San Giovanni	PR	191	129/125	125/118	194/184	168/160
	San Germano	PR	209/203	147/131	118	186	160/158
	San Pietro	PR	209	139/129	122/118	184/186	164/136
	Cipolla	PR	209/193	145/129/123	132/118	186/184/176	166/150/136
	Bergamotto	PR	203	131/129	122/118	184	160/156
	Nigrer	PR	179	131/129	126/118	184	164/148
	Carlet	PR	179	139/129	128/118	194/186	148/146
	Moscato	PR	209	129	124/118	184	170/160
	Spadone	PR	179	151/115	136/126/120	184/176	178/174/164
	Ingurien	PR	169	129/125	118	NA	164/148
	Svirgolato	PR	223/213	129/119	126/120	184/176	166/158
	Colar	PR	213	147/129	120/118	194/186/184	174/160/146
	Pavia	PR	209/195	145/131/123	128/118	186	158/148
	Ducale	PR	209/195	129/125	118	184/176	164/136
	Butirra Ruggina	PR	195	129/115	128/120/118	NA	174/166

Microsatellite profiles are reported for each pear cultivar. Columns from left to right indicate: (i) the species, (ii) the local name, (iii) the accession, (iv) the origin of the accession, Piacenza (PC) or Parma (PR) and (v) the size of the PCR amplified product.

a: NA means null allele and it refers to the absence of the amplification product in a specific sample.

Table 3. Molecular characterization of pear varieties.

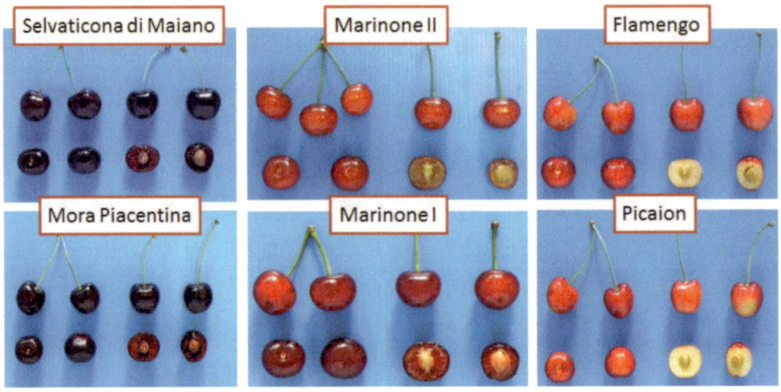

Figure 1. Fruit morphology of some ancient varieties of sweet cherry.

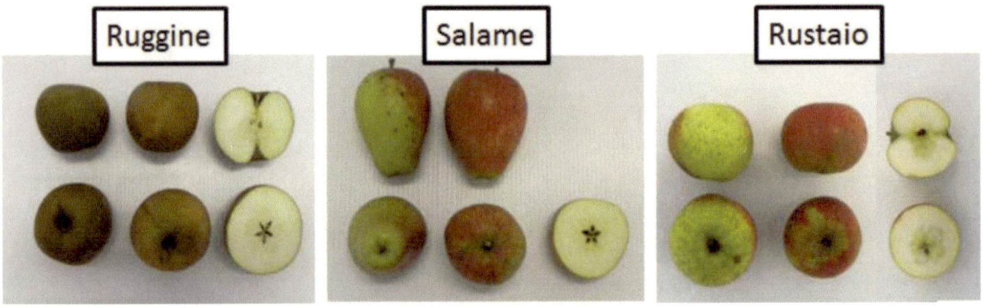

Figure 2. Fruit morphology of some ancient varieties of apple.

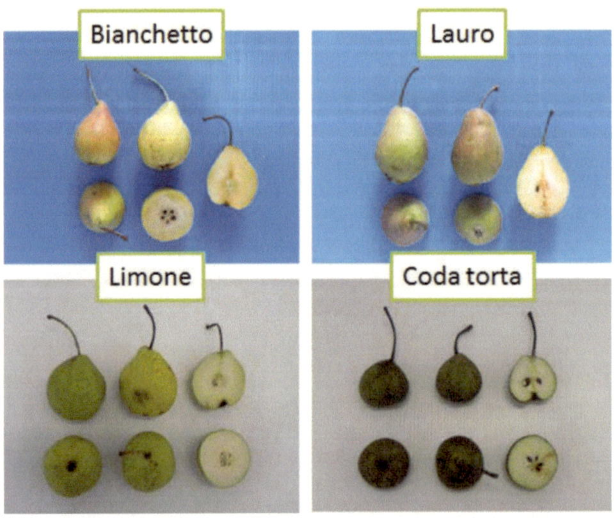

Figure 3. Fruit morphology of some ancient varieties of pear.

Species	Markers	No. of alleles	Expected heterozygosity	Discrimination power
Prunus avium Prunus cerasus	EMPA015	10	0.881	0.861
	EMPA018	5	0.668	0.743
	UDP97/402	7	0.753	0.712
	UCDCH 17	13	0.815	0.712
	UCDCH 31	8	0.775	0.854
	Average	8.6	0.778	0.776
Malus domestica	GD96	13	0.868	0.905
	GD100	8	0.788	0.867
	GD147	9	0.818	0.920
	GD162	7	0.779	0.905
	GD142	10	0.839	0.915
	Average	9.4	0.818	0.902
Pyrus communis	BGT23b	16	0.888	0.915
	KA16	10	0.723	0.898
	GD147	11	0.778	0.894
	KA14	11	0.807	0.907
	GD 142	18	0.921	0.935
	Average	13.2	0.823	0.909

Table 4. Statistical analysis of the microsatellite markers.

Sweet cherry (*P. avium* L., Rosaceae, 2n = 16) is widely cultivated in temperate regions because of the edible fruit. Likely originated in the area of the Caspian and Black Seas, sweet cherry cultivation spread through Europe during the Roman Empire. The spread of sweet cherry cultivation across Western Europe, initially, was probably the consequence of the domestication of wild individuals that were well adapted to each area of cultivation [36]. Sour cherry (*P. cerasus* L.), originated in the same area as sweet cherry, is an allotetraploid (2n = 4x = 32), that might have arisen from a cross between *P. avium* and *P. fruticosa* Pall. Finally, duke cherry is an allotetraploid species originated subsequently from natural hybridization of sweet and sour cherry. More precisely, it originated from the fertilization of sour cherry by unreduced gametes of sweet cherry [37]. In the Northern Italy, the province of Piacenza has a long history of cherry cultivation and several local varieties have been selected after centuries of use.

The microsatellite analysis revealed a different scenario regarding sour, sweet, and duke cherry accessions (**Table 1**). The number of different alleles detected is reported in **Table 4**, the average number of alleles is 8.6, the lowest number of alleles is 5 for EMPA018, and the highest is 13 for UCDCH17. The expected heterozygosity ranged between 0.668 (EMPA018) and 0.881 (EMPA015) (**Table 4**). Based on the frequencies of the different alleles, the probability to obtain a particular genotype by chance was evaluated. Despite the use of a small set of markers, we had very low probability values ranging from 10^{-6} to 10^{-9} for diploid varieties and 10^{-12} to 10^{-19} for polyploid varieties. The smallest value was obtained for the variety Visciola, this is likely a consequence of its hybrid nature (data not shown). These results confirm what had already been shown in the case of *Vitis vinifera* L., in which a small set (six) of SSR markers was able to successfully discriminate between varieties and to identify the starting material used to produce the must [38].

The three accessions belonging to the sweet cherry cultivar Pavesi have the same molecular profile, indicating that they derived from a unique mother plant. The same could be noted for the accessions of the cultivars Flamengo and Picaion. Two cultivars, namely Mora piacentina and Selvaticona di Magnano, have the same SSR profile. This situation, with all the caution due to the small number of markers used, could be a typical case of synonymy and the two names could be two different local designations for plants anciently derived from the same genetic material and then vegetatively propagated. Concerning sour cherry, the cultivars Marasca and Marasca di Villanova, despite a similar name, had a different genetic profile suggesting that they belong to two different cultivars and they are a case of homonymy. A similar situation was found within the three accessions belonging to Marinone: Marinone I acc. A and Marinone II acc. C had the same profile while Marinone II acc. A was clearly different. Very likely, the first two accessions derived from the same mother plant while the last one had a different origin resulting in a case of homonymy. Comparing the profiles of the different markers in sweet and sour cherries, sweet cherries had a simple profile with the different loci having just one (homozygous) or two (heterozygous) alleles. On the contrary, sour cherries had a more complicated allelic combination and it was common to find, for each marker, the presence of single loci having three or four different alleles. This high number of alleles at the level of the single locus could be a consequence of local duplications of genomic regions or, more likely, of different ploidy levels. In this respect it is reported that sweet cherries are diploids while sour cherries are polyploids (such as tetraploids).

To have a better representation of the relationships among the different accessions analysis, principal component analysis (PCA) was carried out (**Figure 4**). Two clearly separated groups could be defined: the first including sweet cherry accessions and the second including sour cherry accessions. Among the sour cherry accessions, the one being closest to the sweet cherry group was the variety Visciola. The term Visciola is used to refer to a variety of duke cherry that originated by natural hybridization between a sweet and a sour cherry variety. This hybrid nature can determine the intermediate position of this sample between the sweet and sour cherry groups.

Apple and pear are among the most economically important fruit tree crops of the temperate zones. According to the FAO report on the state of world's plant genetic resources for food and agriculture, at least 97,500 apple accessions and 1140 pear accessions are present in worldwide *ex-situ* collections [35]. Moreover, apple is the most common fruit crop of temperate areas. The wild Central Asian species *Malus sieversii* (Ledeb) M. Roem was identified as the main contributor to the genome of the cultivated apple [39] but, recently, it has been demonstrated that multiple species have contributed to the genetic makeup of domesticated apples [40]. Concerning pear, there are two centers of domestication and primary origin, one located in

China and the second in the area stretching from Asia Minor to the Middle East, in the Caucasus Mountains. Also, a third secondary center is located in Central Asia [41].

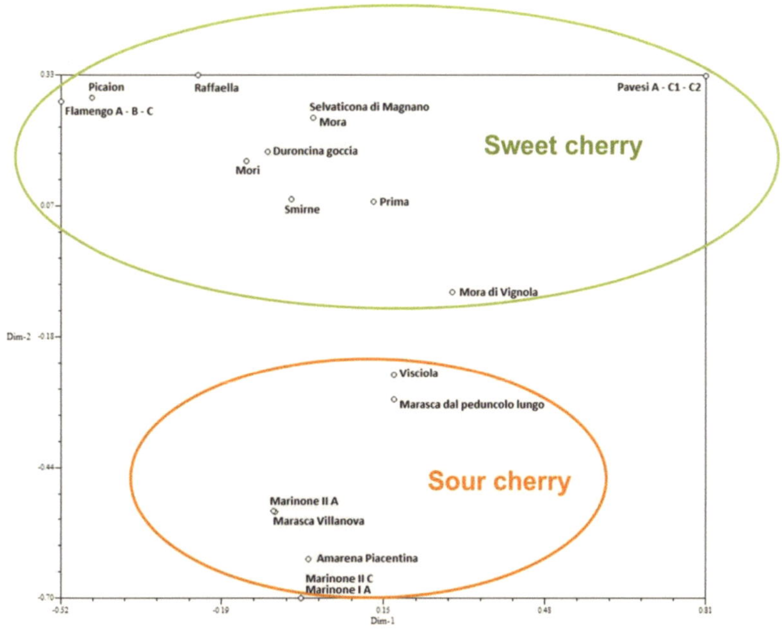

Figure 4. Principal component analysis of the cherry varieties based on the SSR profiles. The PCA based on SSR results, clearly evidence the differences between the groups of sweet and sour cherries. It is interesting to note that, in the sour cherry group, the accession of Visciola (*P.* × *gondouini*) is the closest to the sweet cherry group. This can be a consequence of the hybrid nature of the species, likely a cross between *P. avium* and *P. cerasus*.

The provinces of Parma and Piacenza have a long tradition of apple and pear cultivation, and a wide diversity of cultivars, well adapted to the local environmental conditions, was grown in this area since ancient times. In apple, as in cherry, the number of alleles highlighted at a single locus in the different samples, ranged from one to four supporting the presence of different ploidy levels (**Table 2**).

Along with cultivars having just one or two alleles at each locus, such as Ruggine, Fior d'Acacia, and Salame, there were some cultivars with three alleles per locus, such as Seriana, Rosa, and Rustajò. These results supported diploidy and triploidy as the main ploidy levels in local apple germplasm and they agree with what is generally reported in literature concerning apple varieties: most of the apples grown commercially are diploid (2n), although there are many triploid varieties (3n) [42]. The presence of four different alleles, in a single locus, was a rare event and it was found just in a single case (marker GD162, first accession of variety Carraia). While the high number of currently cultivated varieties is diploid or triploid, the presence of tetraploid forms not cultivated but useful for breeding was reported too [43]. It cannot be excluded that after centuries of vegetative propagation, some tetraploid forms could be originated and unintentionally cultivated. The number of different alleles detected by the five

SSRs is reported in **Table 4**; the average value was 9.4, the lowest value was 7 for GD162, while the highest was 13 for GD96. The expected heterozygosity ranged between 0.779 (GD162) and 0.868 (GD96). The probabilities to obtain a particular genotype by chance were very low ranging from 10^{-7} to 10^{-10} for diploid varieties and 10^{-9} to 10^{-16} for polyploid varieties (data not shown). Also in apple there were cases of homonymy: i) the two accessions of the variety Carraia were clearly different at the genetic level and, very likely, they originated from different mother plants, ii) despite very similar denominations, the varieties Rustaio, Rustajò, and Restajo had different genetic profiles, so they can be effectively considered as different cultivated varieties.

In pear, as in the previous species, it was possible to detect the presence of loci with more than two alleles (**Table 3**). As for apple and cherry, this evidence suggested the presence of different ploidy levels in the local pear germplasm. Based on the results, diploid varieties were the most diffused followed by triploids. Tetraploidy was rarer, being evidenced just a single time in cultivar Sburdacen with marker GD142. The presence of varieties of pear characterized by different ploidy level, diploids, triploids, and tetraploids was already reported in the literature [44]. The number of different alleles detected by the five SSRs is reported (**Table 4**): the average value was 13.2, the highest among the three species, while the average expected heterozygosity and discrimination power were similar to the values of apple. The lowest allele number was 10 for KA16 while the highest was 19 for GD142. The expected heterozygosity ranged between 0.723 (KA16) and 0.921 (GD142) (**Table 4**). Based on the frequencies of the different alleles, we evaluated the probability to obtain any particular genotype. Once again, the probability values were very low ranging from 10^{-8} to 10^{-11} for diploid varieties and 10^{-10} to 10^{-14} for polyploid varieties (data not shown).

A clear case of synonymy was present concerning the two names Lauro and Nobile. By comparing the genetic profiles, it was possible to see that the different accessions had the same alleles showing that they derived from a common mother ancestor. In this case, the two names are linked to the different provinces, with the name Lauro diffused in the province of Piacenza and the name Nobile in the province of Parma. The three accessions belonging to the variety Limone had the same genetic profile, confirming that they derived from the same mother plant. The same was found for the two accessions of the variety Coda torta. On the contrary, the two accessions of the variety Sburdacion were slightly different, being a case of homonymy. Probably these accessions derived from a common ancestor that encountered some genetic changes (as somatic mutations). Despite the similar names, varieties Nigrò and Nigrer and varieties Butirra Polesine and Butirra ruggina had different genetic profiles and they can be considered as different cultivars. With respect to cherry and apple, in pear a higher frequency of null alleles, i.e. five cases in pear against one case in apple and none in cherry, was observed. To verify this, the amplifications were replicated at least five independent times and the amplicons were always absent. The two accessions of the variety Sburdacion with the marker BGT23b were both characterized by the absence of amplification, supporting close genetic relationships.

This study confirmed the utility of microsatellite markers for biodiversity evaluation and for all conservation actions that can follow the preliminary analysis of genetic variability. Despite the use of a small number of markers, several cases were highlighted: (1) synonymy in sweet cherry (Mora piacentina and Selvaticona di Magnano) and pear (Lauro and Nobile); (2) homonymy inside the Marinone and Marasca (sour cherry), Carraia (apple), and Sburdacion (pear); (3) accessions belonging to the same cultivated variety characterized by high genetic uniformity as a consequence of the derivation from a common ancestor; (4) high biodiversity in the old local germplasm; (5) different levels of ploidy: diploidy in sweet cherry, apple, and pear; triploidy in apple and pear; tetraploidy, rare in apple and pear, and mainly present in sour cherry.

3. Microsatellite markers in the livestock sector

For more than a decade, microsatellites have been one of the most popular types of markers used in the livestock sector for various purposes [45], e.g., the characterization and conservation of diversity [46, 47], the reconstruction of the post-domestication evolutionary history of farm animals [48, 49], parentage testing [50], mapping of quantitative trait loci (QTL) [51, 52] or other causative mutations [53], and traceability of food products [26, 54, 55]. The average number of microsatellite loci used in livestock research varied between 15 and 30 [45], even if a lower number of highly informative loci have been adopted for specific purposes. For example, the International Society for Animal Genetics has established that panels of as few as 12 microsatellite loci have enough resolution for the routine identification of individuals and parentage testing in cattle and horse [56].

A large number of national and international projects aiming at the description of farm animal species diversity have relied on the use of microsatellites. These markers have been used to estimate diversity (both within and between breeds) and genetic admixture even among closely related breeds, usually by means of clustering approaches, principal coordinate analysis, or phylogenetic inference [46]. Comprehensive microsatellite-based studies of livestock diversity have been carried out in European chicken [57], goats from Europe and the middle East [58], Eurasian sheep [59], and African cattle [48], just to mention a few.

One of the major drawbacks of microsatellite genotyping is that the use of different PCR-amplification protocols and genotyping techniques may result in different allele size scoring at the same locus in different labs or experiments, thus hampering the possibility to combine microsatellite genotypes obtained from different projects. To circumvent this, the use of the same set of markers (or at least of a common subset of markers) and genotyping of standard samples across projects has been recommended [60]. In particular, to promote the use of common marker panels, the ISAG-FAO Advisory Group on Animal Genetic Diversity has published guidelines and ranked lists of microsatellite loci to be used for studying diversity in major livestock species [20]. Using these markers in order of ranking should maximize the overlap and increase the possibility of merging data from different investigations.

Concerning allele size standardization through the inclusion of standard samples, for some species (e.g. sheep and goats) the standards adopted in the course of large-scale projects have also been shared with research initiatives in different continents to permit merging of the results. This is the case of the European project Econogene [61] whose sheep and goat standard samples have been made available to other large-scale investigations in Africa and Asia. Acknowledging the usefulness of a joint analysis of different datasets to obtain a global view of livestock diversity, as in the case of the meta-analysis performed by the EU project Global-Div [62, 63], a number of statistical methods have been devised that allow merging and analyzing datasets even when they have only a few breeds and/or markers in common. The method developed by [64], for example, estimates population genetics parameters (e.g., heterozygosity, allelic richness, and admixture) by means of a double regression approach and has been successfully applied to the meta-analysis of microsatellite data of cattle populations from Europe, Africa, and Asia [45]. [65], instead, have devised a method based on iterative regression to infer the contribution given by each missing allele/breed combination, which allows calculating genetic distances also on merged datasets with missing information (see [45] and figures therein).

Gaining a global view on the worldwide patterns of diversity of livestock genetic resources may allow to highlight (i) the presence of gaps, i.e., areas in which livestock characterization is incomplete or lacking, (ii) local diversity hotspots which may deserve particular attention or conservation efforts, (iii) geographical trends of clonal variation or discontinuities that can shed further light on the evolutionary history and post-domestication migration routes of farm animal species.

In livestock, current genotyping standards are represented by standardized SNP panels that allow the characterization of tens or hundreds of thousand markers per sample at the same time and at a reasonable cost. Commercial SNP chips at varying levels of marker density are already available for the major livestock species, e.g. for cattle at medium density [66] and high density [67], for sheep and goats at medium density [68, 69]. Being highly standardized, SNP panels do not suffer from allele scoring differences and thus permit an immediate comparison and merging of data produced in different labs [70]. A comparative evaluation of the effectiveness of microsatellites vs. SNP markers for individual identification and parentage assessment has recently shown that 2–3 SNPs per microsatellite were necessary to obtain a comparable exclusion power value in a highly consanguineous Angus cattle herd [71]. Therefore, in a similar context the use of, e.g. 50K SNP chip panel might be equivalent to typing of 16–25K microsatellite loci. Nevertheless, due to the low costs and to the possibility of in-house implementation of genotyping protocols, microsatellite markers still represent a useful resource, e.g. to characterize livestock breeds in several developing countries [72, 73], in which the access to SNP typing or other high throughput technologies can be difficult or just too expensive, or to set priorities for conservation at the local or regional scale [74, 75].

4. Traceability of food

Food traceability is of primary importance to avoid fraudulent procedures and to authenticate the origin of particular products. Dishonest producers may substitute, partially or totally, some food products with others less expensive to increase the profit. For this reason, certifying the origin and composition of a certain food is becoming more and more important [76–78]. Molecular analysis is one of the most recently developed methods to trace food products. Molecular traceability is useful to distinguish traditional varieties with specific high quality traits and to protect the PDO and "Protected Geographical Indication" (PGI) marks. Italian products represent 20% of protected food in Europe and the certified "made in Italy" is important for Italian product exportation. DNA is present in every food product and its analysis makes possible to recover a lot of information about the identity of the ingredients in foods and feed. It is often reported that DNA is relatively more resistant than other classes of biological molecules (e.g. proteins) to the degradation caused by food processing. Despite this, as a consequence of processes such as cooking, fermentation etc., degradation of DNA occurs anyway and, generally, the stronger the treatment the shorter the DNA fragments become. Thus, the possibility to analyze small DNA fragments is very important for traceability purposes.

An additional problem, when working with plant-derived products is that along with the DNA, a high number of different inhibitors of polymerase reactions can be recovered from a food matrix. Plants are very rich in carbohydrates and polyphenols, which tend to be co-extracted with the DNA. Their presence can prevent the activity of polymerases hindering the analysis of DNA by PCR reaction. Different commercial kits or customized protocols can be considered to tackle this problem and usually DNA extracted from most food matrixes can be analyzed using molecular tools. Molecular markers make it possible to discriminate, not only the species from which the food is originated, but also the variety (cultivar) or population of origin [79–81]. Among the different classes of markers, some are more suitable than others for traceability purposes. Recently, the two main classes of markers that have been adopted are SNPs and microsatellites. While SNPs are becoming the most used markers for animal-based product analysis and identification, microsatellites are still the election markers for genetic traceability of plant-based products.

The final goal of DNA analysis in the agro-food sector is the comparison of the molecular profile of a sample with a reference profile to evidence the presence of congruencies or discrepancies. When the SSR profile of the sample is congruent with what is expected (similar to the reference profile), the two profiles are matching and it is possible to speculate that the sample under investigation has the same origin as the reference. However, in any final conclusion that is reached in certain cases, it is also important to evaluate the probabilities that the two profiles are identical because they derive from the same genetic material and not just by chance. This requires deep knowledge of the genetic base of the species under investigation and the probability level to obtain the same marker profile, using a set of SSRs, in two independent samples just by chance. This is very important for plant species in which it is often not enough to detect the presence of a particular species in a processed product. For several plant-derived products, as for extra virgin olive oil and wine, the final price on the market is highly dependent on the cultivated variety of the species that has been used as raw material. In this situation, a possible fraud could be represented by the substitution of a declared cultivar with another one with a smaller commercial value but with similar organoleptic properties (different cultivars of olive or of grapevine).

Sample	Xgwm 46	Xgwm 408	WMS 376	Xgwm 459	Xgwm 577	WMS5	WMS 120
Type A seed	180	97	142/96	129/113	127/150	167/165	160/129
Type B seed	180	97	142/96	113	127	154/152	160
Type C seed	180	97	142/96	117	127	154/152	129
Type A treated seed	180	97	142/96	117	127	154/152	129
Type B treated seed	180	97	142/96	129/113	127/250	167/165	160/129
Type C treated seed	180	97	142/96	113	127	154/152	160
Type A flour	180	97	142/96	117	127	154/152	129
Type B flour	180	97	142/96	117	127/150	154/152	129
Type C flour	180	97	142/96	113	127	154/152	160
Type A Pasta	180	97	142/96	113	127	154/152	160/129
Type B Pasta	180	97	142/96	129/113	127/150	167/165	160/129
Type C Pasta	180	97	142/96	113	127	154/152	160

Table 5. Molecular profile of the wheat samples and derived products for traceability purposes.

Correct identification and authentication of processed food is more challenging than that of fresh food mainly because of the presence of inhibitors and of DNA degradation. To face these problems, PCRs for food traceability are usually low template-DNA PCRs (LT-DNA PCRs), because increasing the amount of DNA may consequently increase the quantity of inhibitors and determine the failure of the amplification. These PCRs are usually carried out using very small amount of DNA (in the order of few dozens of picograms) and high numbers of amplification cycles (>35) to have a visible signal. While it is reported that PCR can theoretically work even with amounts of template DNA lower than the aforementioned ones, usually LT-DNA PCRs suffer from several limitations. Concerning SSRs, LT-DNA PCRs can be characterized by marker profiles showing a higher heterozygote peak imbalance between the signals of the observed alleles in a specific sample with respect to standard PCR or by the stochastic disappearance of some allele signals (allelic drop-out, mainly a problem for the bigger size alleles). This outcome is mainly a consequence of the small amount and of the degradation of the template DNA. In these conditions, the final result of the PCR can be strongly influenced by the effect of a random selection of the template molecules during the first cycles of the amplification. Other factors that can make the interpretation of the molecular profiles difficult are the presence of: (1) stutter bands; (2) split peaks, deriving from the incomplete adenylation of the PCR products; (3) allelic drop-in, deriving often from contamination and mainly present in the multiplexing amplifications; (4) triploid profile, deriving from the unexpected amplification of three peaks (three loci) from a diploid genome.

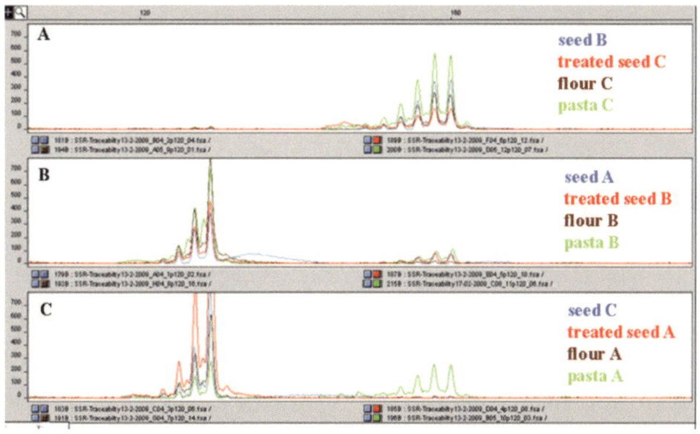

Figure 5. The electropherograms obtained with the microsatellite marker WMS120 are shown. The superimposition of the profiles has been done based on the highest level of correspondence among the different samples. In the upper panel are reported, with different color, the profile of samples seeds B (blue), treated seeds C (red), flour C (brown), and pasta C (green). In the intermediate and lower panels are reported, using the same colors as for the upper panel, respectively: samples seeds A (blue), treated seeds B (red), flour B (brown), and pasta B (green); seeds C (blue), treated seeds A (red), flour A (brown), and pasta A (green). Similarities and differences are clearly evident.

In recent years, our laboratory dealt with the extraction and analysis of DNA from different kinds of food matrices with different purposes and different markers technologies [82–86]. In this section, as an example, the results on traceability of wheat-derived products will be provided. These SSR analyses were carried out as a work under contract for which a third party commissioned us. The samples were collected from the whole supply chain of durum wheat (*Triticum durum* Desf.), starting from grain and ending with pasta and finally provided to us. In detail, DNA was isolated from seeds, vacuum-sealed (treated) seeds, flour, and pasta. Three different sample sets labeled as A, B, and C were received and analyzed in blind. Each labeled set was made of a sample of seed (seeds A, B, and C), treated seed (treated seed A, B, and C), flour (flour A, B, and C) and pasta (pasta A, B, and C). The aim of the analysis was to show the capacity and utility of SSRs to follow, along all the food chain from the raw material to the final product, the presence of a specific DNA, in this case the DNA of the cultivar used to produce the pasta. At the same time, for each labeled set, the presence or absence of correspondence among the genetic profiles of the seeds, treated seeds, flours and pasta was investigated. The DNA was extracted using different commercial kits. Some preliminary trials were carried out to determine the best kit available for our purpose, attempting to find the one providing the highest amount of PCR-grade DNA. The best results were obtained using the GenElute Plant Genomic DNA kit from SIGMA-Aldrich. As expected, high quality DNA was recovered from seeds and treated seeds; in flours some traces of degradation were present and evident as a faint smear in an agarose gel electrophoresis and, finally, from pasta, DNA was always highly degraded as evident by the more intense smear and the absence of any band indicating the presence of high molecular weight DNA. DNA with an estimated average concentration of 60 ng/μl was recovered from the first three kinds of samples (seeds, treated seeds, and flours). Because of the low amount and high degradation, it was not possible to correctly quantify the DNA in pasta. Seven SSRs were used for the analysis: Xgwm46, Xgwm186, Xgwm408, Xgwm459, Xgwm577, WMS5, and WMS120. Three microsatellites

Xgwm46, Xgwm186, and Xgwm408 were monomorphic but polymorphic signals were obtained with the remaining four markers making possible the distinction between different samples (**Table 5**).

From the results obtained, it was not possible to find correspondence between the different samples within each label. As an example, seeds A did not correspond to treated seeds A, flour A, and pasta A. On the contrary, seeds A had the same profile as treated seed B and pasta B. Similarly, seeds B had the same profile as treated seeds C, flour C, and pasta C (**Figure 5**). Concerning the last samples, the presence of correspondence between seeds C, treated seeds A, and flour A was evidenced. Absence of correspondence was found for type A pasta whose genetic profile was more similar to the genetic profile of pasta B and for flour B whose genetic profile was unique and different from the other profiles. As previously stated, samples were received in blind without any knowledge about the origin of the different labeled samples.

Based on this, it was possible to conclude that the seeds of cultivar B (the exact name of the variety was unknown) were used to produce treated seeds C, flour C, and pasta C; seeds of cultivar A were used to produce treated seeds B and pasta B; seeds of cultivar C were used to produce treated seeds A and flour A (**Figure 5**). Pasta A was likely produced by mixing flour A with flour C in almost identical percentages and this was explained by the appearance of the signal corresponding to flour C allele (**Figure 5**). The only incongruence was about flour B. This sample had a genetic profile different from the other samples: it had the same profile of flour A with just an extra allele with SSR Xgwm577. This means that flour B was obtained from a fourth and different cultivated variety, but the possibility of contamination cannot be excluded. Concerning the sample pasta B, the amplification with marker Xgm459 was replicated four times and two times just the 113 bp allele was obtained, while the other two times both the 129 and 113 bp alleles were amplified. As reported previously, working with food-derived DNA is challenging also because of the allelic drop-out: the stochastic disappearance of one of the alleles, usually the biggest one, can be observed as a consequence of DNA degradation, which can explain the results obtained for pasta B.

The results obtained were a clear indication of the utility of SSR markers in following the whole wheat chain, despite the DNA degradation determined by processing.

5. Conclusions

The recent development of high throughput genotyping methods has prompted SNPs as desired markers for several applications in agricultural research, in particular in the livestock sector. Despite this, microsatellites, because of their characteristics, can still be considered as markers of choice for numerous studies, in particular concerning plant genomes, both for biodiversity studies and for molecular traceability of plant-derived food products. In a biodiversity study of local ancient germplasm of fruit tree species, using a small number of markers, we obtained important indications as the presence of synonymy and homonymy, high biodiversity, and different levels of ploidy. Furthermore, the high polymorphism of microsatellite loci together with the different ploidy levels detected increased the probability to link each cultivar to its corresponding genotypic profile. This is particularly interesting because it means that few properly selected SSRs can be enough to obtain robust results. In the same time, microsatellites can be very useful for molecular traceability as it was evidenced from our results of the whole production chain from durum wheat raw material to processed pasta. Indeed, despite the degradation of DNA caused by food processing, SSRs were able to find the correspondence between blind samples and genotypes highlighting some incongruences.

Acknowledgements

The study of fruit tree biodiversity was funded by Misura 214, and Azione 7 of the Emilia Romagna regional development plan.

Author details

Jamila Bernardi[1*], Licia Colli[2,3], Virginia Ughini[1] and Matteo Busconi[1,2]

*Address all correspondence to: jamila.bernardi@unicatt.it

1 Department of Sustainable Crop Production, Catholic University of the Sacred Heart, Piacenza, Italy

2 Research Center on Biodiversity and Ancient DNA – BioDNA, Catholic University of the Sacred Heart, Piacenza, Italy

3 Institute of Zootechnics, Catholic University of the Sacred Heart, Piacenza, Italy

References

[1] Ahrens CW, James EA. Conserving the small milkwort, *Comesperma polygaloides*, a vulnerable subshrub in a fragmented landscape. Conserv Genet. 2016;17:891–901. DOI 10.1007/s10592-016-0830-9

[2] Martins S, Simões F, MendonÇa D, Matos J, Silva AP, Carnide V. Western European wild and landraces hazelnuts evaluated by SSR markers. Plant Mol Biol Report. 2015;33:1712–1720. DOI 10.1007/s11105-015-0867-9

[3] Liang W, Dondini L, De Franceschi P, Paris R, Sansavini S, Tartarini S. Genetic diversity, population structure and construction of a core collection of apple cultivars from Italian Germplasm. Plant Mol Biol Report. 2015;33:458–473. DOI 10.1007/s11105-014-0754-9

[4] Powell W, Morgante M, Andre C, Hanafey M, Vogel J, Tingey S, Rafalski A. The comparison of RFLP, RAPD, AFLP and SSR (microsatellite) markers for germplasm analysis. Mol Breed. 1996;2:225–238.

[5] Nicoloso L, Bomba L, Colli L, Negrini R, Milanesi M, Mazza R, and the Italian Goat Consortium. Genetic diversity of Italian goat breeds assessed with a medium-density SNP chip. Genet Sel Evol. 2015;47:62. DOI 10.1186/s12711-015-0140-6

[6] Scarano D, Rao R. DNA markers for food products authentication. Diversity. 2014; 6:579–596. DOI:10.3390/d6030579

[7] IUCN, International Union for Conservation of Nature [Internet]. 2016. Available from: http://www.iucn.org [Accessed: 2016-07-05]

[8] The Second Report on the state of the World's Plant Genetic Resources for Food and Agriculture [Internet]. 2010. Available from: http://www.fao.org/agriculture/crops/thematic-sitemap/theme/seeds-pgr/sow/sow2/en/[Accessed: 2016-07-05]

[9] Targońska M, Bolibok-Brągoszewska H, Rakoczy-Trojanowska M. Assessment of genetic diversity in *Secale cereale* based on SSR markers. Plant Mol Biol Rep. 2016;34:37–51. DOI: 10.1007/s11105-015-0896-4

[10] Muccillo L, Gambuti A, Frusciante L, Iorizzo M, Moio L, Raieta K, Rinaldi A, Colantuoni V, Aversano R. Biochemical features of native red wines and genetic diversity of the corresponding grape varieties from Campania region. Food Chem. 2014;143:506–513. DOI: 10.1016/j.foodchem.2013.07.133

[11] Lu X, Zhou H, Pan Y, Chen C, Zhu J, Chen P, Li Y, Cai Q, Chen R. Segregation analysis of microsatellite (SSR) markers in sugarcane polyploids. Genet Mol Res. 2015;14:18384–18395. DOI: 10.4238/2015.December.23.26

[12] Ahmad F, Hanafi MM, Hakim MA, Rafii MY, Arolu IW, Abdullah SNA. Genetic divergence and heritability of 42 coloured upland rice genotypes (*Oryza sativa*) as revealed by microsatellites marker and agro-morphological traits. PLoS One. 2015;10. DOI: 10.1371/journal.pone.0138246

[13] Doveri S, Gil F, Díaz A, Reale S, Busconi M, Machado A, Martín A, Fogher C, Donini P, Lee D. Standardization of a set of microsatellite markers for use in cultivar identification studies in olive (*Olea europaea* L.). Sci Hortic. 2008;116:367–373. DOI:10.1016/j.scienta.2008.02.005

[14] Dwivedi SL, Ceccarelli S, Blair MW, Upadhyaya HD, Are AK, Ortiz R. Landrace germplasm for improving yield and abiotic stress adaptation. Trends Plant Sci. 2016;21:31–42. DOI: 10.1016/j.tplants.2015.10.012

[15] Lassois L, Denancé C, Ravon E, Guyader A, Guisnel R, Hibrand-Saint-Oyant L, Poncet C, Lasserre-Zuber P, Feugey L, Durel C-E. Genetic diversity, population structure, parentage analysis, and construction of core collections in the French apple germplasm based on SSR markers. Plant Mol Biol Rep. 2016:1-18. DOI: 10.1007/s11105-015-0966-7

[16] Gao Y, Liu F, Wang K, Wang D, Gong X, Liu L, et al. Genetic diversity of Malus cultivars and wild relatives in the Chinese National Repository of Apple Germplasm Resources. Tree Genet Genom. 2015;11. DOI: 10.1007/s11295-015-0913-7

[17] Zaman G, Shekar MC, Aziz A. Molecular characterization of Meghalaya Local pigs (Niang Megha) using microsatellite markers. Indian J Sci Technol. 2013;6:5302-5306. DOI: 10.17485/ijst/2013/v6i10/38777

[18] Colombo E, Strillacci MG, Cozzi MC, Madeddu M, Mangiagalli MG, Mosca F, Zaniboni L, Bagnato A, Cerolini S. Feasibility study on the FAO chicken microsatellite panel to assess genetic variability in the Turkey (*Meleagris gallopavo*). Ital J Anim Sci. 2014;13:887–890. DOI: 10.4081/ijas.2014.3334

[19] Radhika G, Raghavan KC, Aravindakshan TV, Thirupathy V. Genetic diversity and population structure analysis of native and crossbred goat genetic groups of Kerala, India. Small Ruminant Res. 2015;131:50–57. DOI: 10.1016/j.smallrumres.2015.08.008

[20] DADÂIS Domestic Animal Diversity Information System (DADÂIS), Food and Agriculture Organization of the United Nations [Internet]. 2016. Available from: http://www.fao.org/dad-is/[Accessed: 2016-07-05]

[21] Traceability - EU Food Law [internet]. 2016. Available from: http://www.eurofood-law.com/food-safety-and-standards/traceability [Accessed: 2016-07-05]

[22] Food Integrity [Internet] Available from: https://secure.fera.defra.gov.uk/foodintegrity [Accessed: 2016-07-05]

[23] Moore J, Spink J, Lipp M. Development and application of a database of food ingredient fraud and economically motivated adulteration from 1980 to 2010. J Food Sci. 2012;77:R118–R126. DOI: 10.1111/j.1750-3841.2012.02657.x

[24] Terzi V, Morcia C, Gorrini A, Stanca AM, Shewry PR, Faccioli P. DNA-based methods for identification and quantification of small grain cereal mixtures and fingerprinting of varieties. J Cereal Sci. 2005;41:213–220. DOI: 10.1016/j.jcs.2004.08.003

[25] Pasqualone A, Alba V, Mangini G, Blanco A, Montemurro C. Durum wheat cultivar traceability in PDO Altamura bread by analysis of DNA microsatellites. Eur Food Res Technol. 2010;230:723–729. DOI: 10.1007/s00217-009-1210-1

[26] Sardina M, Tortorici L, Mastrangelo S, Gerlando R, Tolone M, Portolano B. Application of microsatellite markers as potential tools for traceability of Girgentana goat breed dairy products. Food Res Int. 2015;74:115–122. DOI: 10.1016/j.foodres.2015.04.038

[27] Mateus JC, Russo-Almeida PA. Traceability of 9 Portuguese cattle breeds with PDO products in the market using microsatellites. Food Control. 2015;47:487–492. DOI: 10.1016/j.foodcont.2014.07.038

[28] Dalvit C, De Marchi M, Dal Zotto R, Gervaso M, Meuwissen T, Cassandro M. Breed assignment test in four Italian beef cattle breeds. Meat Sci. 2008;80:389–395. DOI: 10.1016/j.meatsci.2008.01.001

[29] Khoshbakht K, Hammer K. Threatened and rare ornamental plants. J Agr Rural Dev Trop Subtrop. 2007;108:19–39.

[30] Clarke JB, Tobutt KR. Development and characterization of polymorphic microsatellites from *Prunus avium* 'Napoleon'. Mol Ecol Notes. 2003;3:578–580. DOI: 10.1046/j.1471-8286.2003.00517.x

[31] Cipriani G, Lot G, Huang W-G, Marrazzo MT, Peterlunger E, Testolin R. AC/GT and AG/CT microsatellite repeats in peach [*Prunus persica* (L) Batsch]: isolation, characterisation and cross-species amplification in Prunus. Theor Appl Genet. 1999;99:65–72. DOI: 10.1007/s001220051209

[32] Turkoglu Z, Bilgener S, Ercisli S, Bakır M, Koc A, Akbulut M, Gercekcioglu R, Gunes M, Esitken A. Simple sequence repeat-based assessment of genetic relationships among *Prunus* rootstocks. Genet Mol Res. 2010;9:2156–2165. DOI: 10.4238/vol9-4gmr957

[33] Hokanson SC, Szewc-McFadden AK, Lamboy WF, McFerson JR. Microsatellite (SSR) markers reveal genetic identities, genetic diversity and relationships in a *Malus* × *domestica* Borkh: core subset collection. Theor Appl Genet. 1998;97:671–683. DOI: 10.1007/s001220050943

[34] Yamamoto T, Kimura T, Sawamura Y, Manabe T, Kotobuki K, Hayashi T, Ban Y, Matsuta N. Simple sequence repeats for genetic analysis in pear. Euphytica. 2002;124:129–137. DOI: 10.1023/A:1015677505602

[35] Martinelli F, Busconi M, Camangi F, Fogher C, Stefani A, Sebastiani L. Ancient *Pomoideae* (*Malus domestica* Borkh. and *Pyrus communis* L.) cultivars in "Appennino Toscano" (Tuscany, Italy): molecular (SSR) and morphological characterization. Caryologia. 2008;61:320–331. DOI: 10.1080/00087114.2008.10589643

[36] Wünsch A, Hormaza JI. Molecular characterisation of sweet cherry (*Prunus avium* L.) genotypes using peach [*Prunus persica* (L.) Batsch] SSR sequences. Heredity. 2002;89:56–63. DOI: 10.1038/sj.hdy.6800101

[37] Höfer M, Peil A. Phenotypic and genotypic characterization in the collection of sour and duke cherries (*Prunus cerasus* and × *P.* × *gondouini*) of the Fruit Genebank in Dresden-Pillnitz, Germany. Genet Resour Crop Evol. 2015;62:551–566. DOI: 10.1007/s10722-014-0180-8

[38] Pereira L, Martins-Lopes P, Batista C, Zanol GC, Clímaco P, Brazão J, Eiras-Dias JE, Guedes-Pinto H. Molecular markers for assessing must varietal origin. Food Anal Method. 2012;5:1252–1259. DOI: 10.1007/s12161-012-9369-7

[39] Velasco R, Zharkikh A, Affourtit J, Dhingra A, Cestaro A, Kalyanaraman A, Fontana P, Bhatnagar SK, Troggio M, Pruss D et al. The genome of the domesticated apple (*Malus* × *domestica* Borkh.). Nat Genet. 2010;42:833–839. DOI: 10.1038/ng.654

[40] Cornille A, Gladieux P, Smulders M, Roldán-Ruiz I, Laurens F, Le Cam B, Nersesyan A, Clavel J, Olonova M, Feugey L, Gabrielyan I, Zhang X, Tenaillon M, Giraud T. New insight into the history of domesticated apple: secondary contribution of the European wild apple to the genome of cultivated varieties. PLoS Genet. 2012;8:e1002703. DOI: 10.1371/journal.pgen.1002703

[41] Silva GJ, Souza TM, Barbieri RL, Costa de Oliveira A. Origin, domestication, and dispersing of Pear (*Pyrus* spp.). Adv Agr. 2014; 2014:541097. DOI: 10.1155/2014/541097

[42] Höfer M, Meister A. Genome size variation in *Malus* species. J Bot. 2010; 2010:480873. DOI:10.1155/2010/480873.

[43] Sedysheva GA, Gorbacheva NG. Estimation of new tetraploid apple forms as donors of diploid gametes for selection on a polyploidy level. Univ J Plant Sci. 2013;1:49–54. DOI: 10.13189/ujps.2013.010204

[44] Cao Y, Huang L, Li S, Yang Y. Genetics of ploidy and hybridized combination types for polyploid breeding in pear. Acta Hortic. 2002;587:207–210. DOI: 10.17660/ActaHortic.2002.587.24

[45] Lenstra JA, Groeneveld LF, Eding H, Kantanen J, Williams JL, Taberlet P, Nicolazzi EL, Sölkner J, Simianer H, Ciani E, Garcia JF, Bruford MW, Ajmone-Marsan P, Weigend S. Molecular tools and analytical approaches for the characterization of farm animal genetic diversity. Anim Genet. 2012;43:483–502. DOI: 10.1111/j.1365-2052.2011.02309.x

[46] Groeneveld LF, Lenstra JA, Eding H, Toro MA, Scherf B, Pilling D, Negrini R, Finlay EK, Jianlin H, Groeneveld E, Weigend S; GLOBALDIV Consortium. Genetic diversity in farm animals: a review. Anim Genet. 2010;41 S1:6–31. DOI: 10.1111/j.1365-2052.2010.02038.x

[47] Colli L, Perrotta G, Negrini R, Bomba L, Bigi D, Zambonelli P, Verini Supplizi A, Liotta L, Ajmone-Marsan P. Detecting population structure and recent demographic history in endangered livestock breeds: the case of the Italian autochthonous donkeys. Anim Genet. 2013;44:69–78. DOI: 10.1111/j.1365-2052.2012.02356.x

[48] Hanotte O, Bradley DG, Ochieng JW, Verjee Y, Hill EW, Rege JE. African pastoralism: genetic imprints of origins and migrations. Science. 2002;296:336–339. DOI: 10.1126/science.1069878

[49] Cymbron T, Freeman AR, Isabel Malheiro M, Vigne JD, Bradley DG. Microsatellite diversity suggests different histories for Mediterranean and Northern European cattle populations. Proc Biol Sci. 2005;272:1837–1843. DOI: 10.1098/rspb.2005.3138

[50] da Silva EC, McManus CM, de Paiva Guimarães MP, Gouveia AM, Facó O, Pimentel DM, Caetano AR, Paiva SR. Validation of a microsatellite panel for parentage testing of locally adapted and commercial goats in Brazil. Genet Mol Biol. 2014;37:54–60. DOI: 10.1590/S1415-47572014000100010

[51] Uemoto Y, Sato S, Ohnishi C, Hirose K, Kameyama K, Fukawa K, Kudo O, Kobayashi E. Quantitative trait loci for leg weakness traits in a Landrace purebred population. Anim Sci J. 2010;81:28–33. DOI: 10.1111/j.1740-0929.2009.00713.x

[52] Dayo GK, Gautier M, Berthier D, Poivey JP, Sidibe I, Bengaly Z, Eggen A, Boichard D, Thevenon S. Association studies in QTL regions linked to bovine trypanotolerance in a West African crossbred population. Anim Genet. 2012;43:123–132. DOI: 10.1111/j.1365-2052.2011.02227.x

[53] Georges M, A B Dietz, A Mishra, D Nielsen, L S Sargeant, A Sorensen, M R Steele, X Zhao, H Leipold, J E Womack. Microsatellite mapping of the gene causing weaver disease in cattle will allow the study of an associated quantitative trait locus. Proc Natl Acad Sci U S A. 1993;90:1058–1062. DOI: 10.1073/pnas.90.3.1058

[54] Lenstra JA. Primary identification: DNA markers for animal and plant traceability. In: Smith I, Furness T (Eds.) Improving Traceability in Food Processing and Distribution. Woodhead Publ., Cambridge; 2005. p. 147–164.

[55] Orrú L, Napolitano F, Catillo G, Moioli B. Meat molecular traceability: how to choose the best set of microsatellites? Meat Sci. 2006;72:312–317. DOI: 10.1016/j.meatsci.2005.07.018

[56] International Society of Animal Genetics. [Internet]. 2006. Available from http://www.isag.us/index.asp?autotry=true&ULnotkn=true [Accessed: 2016-07-05]

[57] Berthouly C, Bed'Hom B, Tixier-Boichard M, Chen CF, Lee YP, Laloë D, Legros H, Verrier E, Rognon X. Using molecular markers and multivariate methods to study the genetic diversity of local European and Asian chicken breeds. Anim Genet. 2008;39:121–129. DOI: 10.1111/j.1365-2052.2008.01703.x

[58] Cañón J, García D, García-Atance MA, Obexer-Ruff G, Lenstra JA, Ajmone-Marsan P, Dunner S; ECONOGENE Consortium. Geographical partitioning of goat diversity in Europe and the Middle East. Anim Genet. 2006;37:327–334. DOI: 10.1111/j.1365-2052.2006.01461.x

[59] Tapio M, Ozerov M, Tapio I, Toro MA, Marzanov N, Cinkulov M, Goncharenko G, Kiselyova T, Murawski M, Kantanen J. Microsatellite-based genetic diversity and population structure of domestic sheep in northern Eurasia. BMC Genet. 2010;11:76. DOI: 10.1186/1471-2156-11-76

[60] The State of the World's Animal Genetic Resources for Food and Agriculture. In: Rischkowsky B, Pilling D (Eds.). FAO 2007 Rome. [Internet]. 2007. http://www.fao.org/docrep/010/a1250e/a1250e00.htm [Accessed: 2016-07-05]

[61] Sustainable conservation of animal genetic resources in margin rural areas: integrating molecular genetics socio-economic and geostatistical approaches. [Internet]. 2002. Available from http://www.econogene.eu [Accessed: 2016-07-05]

[62] The Second Report on the State of the World's Animal Genetic Resources for Food and Agriculture. In Scherf BD, Pilling D (Eds.). FAO Commission on Genetic Resources for

Food and Agriculture Assessments. [Internet]. 2015. Available from http://www.fao.org/3/a-i4787e/index.html [Accessed: 2016-07-05]

[63] Ajmone-Marsan P and The GLOBALDIV Consortium: a global view of livestock biodiversity and conservation – GLOBALDIV. Anim Genet. 2010;41:1–5. DOI: 10.1111/j.1365-2052.2010.02036.x

[64] Freeman AR, Bradley DG, Nagda S, Gibson JP, Hanotte O. Combination of multiple microsatellite data sets to investigate genetic diversity and admixture of domestic cattle. Anim Genet. 2006;37:1–9. DOI: 10.1111/j.1365-2052.2005.01363.x

[65] Taeubert H, Bradley D, Simianer H. Estimation of genetic distances from two partly overlapping microsatellite marker data sets. Proceedings of 30th International Conference on Animal Genetics, 20–25 August, 2006; Porto Seguro, Brazil. p.28

[66] Matukumalli LK, Lawley CT, Schnabel RD, Taylor JF, Allan MF, Heaton MP, O'Connell J, Moore SS, Smith TP, Sonstegard TS, Van Tassell CP. Development and characterization of a high density SNP genotyping assay for cattle. PLoS One. 2009;4:e5350. DOI: 10.1371/journal.pone.0005350

[67] Cañas-Álvarez JJ, González-Rodríguez A, Munilla S, Varona L, Díaz C, Baro JA, Altarriba J, Molina A, Piedrafita J. Genetic diversity and divergence among Spanish beef cattle breeds assessed by a bovine high-density SNP chip. J Anim Sci. 2015;93:5164–5174. DOI: 10.2527/jas.2015-9271

[68] Kijas JW, Lenstra JA, Hayes B, Boitard S, Porto Neto LR, San Cristobal M, Servin B, McCulloch R, Whan V, Gietzen K, Paiva S, Barendse W, Ciani E, Raadsma H, McEwan J, Dalrymple B; International Sheep Genomics Consortium Members. Genome-wide analysis of the world's sheep breeds reveals high levels of historic mixture and strong recent selection. PLoS Biol. 2013;10:e1001258. DOI: 10.1371/journal.pbio.1001258

[69] Tosser-Klopp G, Bardou P, Bouchez O, Cabau C, Crooijmans R, Dong Y, Donnadieu-Tonon C, Eggen A, Heuven HC, Jamli S, Jiken AJ, Klopp C, Lawley CT, McEwan J, Martin P, Moreno CR, Mulsant P, Nabihoudine I, Pailhoux E, Palhière I, Rupp R, Sarry J, Sayre BL, Tircazes A, Jun Wang, Wang W, Zhang W; International Goat Genome Consortium. Design and characterization of a 52K SNP chip for goats. PLoS One. 2014;9:e86227. DOI: 10.1371/journal.pone.0086227

[70] Bruford MW, Ginja C, Hoffmann I, Joost S, Orozco-terWengel P, Alberto FJ, Amaral AJ, Barbato M, Biscarini F, Colli L, Costa M, Curik I, Duruz S, Ferenčaković M, Fischer D, Fitak R, Groeneveld LF, Hall SJG, Hanotte O, Hassan F, Helsen P, Iacolina L, Kantanen J, Leempoel K, Lenstra JA, Ajmone-Marsan P, Masembe C, Megens H-J, Miele M, Neuditschko M, Nicolazzi EL, Pompanon F, Roosen J, Sevane N, Smetko A, Štambuk A, Streeter I, Stucki S, Supakorn C, Telo Da Gama L, Tixier-Boichard M, Wegmann D, Zhan X. Prospects and challenges for the conservation of farm animal genomic resources, 2015-2025. Front Genet. 2015;6:314. DOI: 10.3389/fgene.2015.00314

[71] Fernández ME, Goszczynski DE, Lirón JP, Villegas-Castagnasso EE, Carino MH, Ripoli MV, Rogberg-Muñoz A, Posik DM, Peral-García P, Giovambattista G. Comparison of

the effectiveness of microsatellites and SNP panels for genetic identification, traceability and assessment of parentage in an inbred Angus herd. Genet Mol Biol. 2013;36:185–191. DOI: 10.1590/S1415-47572013000200008

[72] Azam A, Babar ME, Firyal S, Anjum AA, Akhtar N, Asif M, Hussain T. DNA typing of Pakistani cattle breeds Tharparkar and Red Sindhi by microsatellite markers. Mol Biol Rep. 2012;39:845–849. DOI: 10.1007/s11033-011-0807-1

[73] Yadav AS, Gahlot K, Gahlot GC, Asraf M, Yadav ML. Microsatellite DNA typing for assessment of genetic variability in Marwari breed of Indian goat. Vet World. 2015;8:848–854. DOI: 10.14202/vetworld.2015.848-854.

[74] Medugorac I, Veit-Kensch CE, Ramljak J, Brka M, Marković B, Stojanovic S, Bytyqi H, Kochoski L, Kume K, Grünenfelder HP, Bennewitz J, Förster M. Conservation priorities of genetic diversity in domesticated metapopulations: a study in taurine cattle breeds. Ecol Evol. 2011;1:408–420. DOI: 10.1002/ece3.39

[75] Ginja C, Gama LT, Cortes O, Delgado JV, Dunner S, García D, Landi V, Martin-Burriel I, Martinez-Martinez A, Penedo MCT, Rodellar C, Zaragoza P, Canon J and Biobovis Consortium. Analysis of conservation priorities of Iberoamerican cattle based on autosomal microsatellite markers. Genet Sel Evol. 2013;45:35. DOI: 10.1186/1297-9686-45-35

[76] Testolin R; Lain O. DNA extraction from olive oil and PCR amplification of microsatellite markers. Food Chem Toxicol. 2005;70:108–112. DOI: 10.1111/j.1365-2621.2005.tb09011.x

[77] Alba V, Sabetta W, Blanco A, Pasqualone A, Montemurro C. Microsatellite marker to identify specific alleles in DNA extracted from monovarietal virgin olive oils. Eur Food Res Technol. 2009;229:375–382. DOI: 10.1007/s00217-009-1062-8

[78] Soffritti G, Busconi M, Sánchez RA, Thiercelin JM, Polissiou M, Roldán M, Fernández JA. Genetic and epigenetic approaches for the possible detection of adulteration and auto-adulteration in Saffron (*Crocus sativus* L.) Spice. Molecules. 2016;21:E343. DOI: 10.3390/molecules21030343

[79] Caramante M, Corrado G, Monti LM, Rao R. Simple sequence repeats are able to trace tomato cultivars in tomato food chains. Food Cont. 2011;22(3–4):549–554. DOI: 10.1016/j.foodcont.2010.10.002

[80] Corrado G, Imperato A, la Mura M, Perri E, Rao R. Genetic diversity among olive varieties of southern Italy and the traceability of olive oil using SSR markers. J Hortic Sci Biotech. 2011;86:461–466. DOI: 10.1080/14620316.2011.11512789

[81] Pasqualone A, Montemurro C, Summo C, Sabetta W, Caponio F, Blanco A. Effectiveness of microsatellite DNA markers in checking the identity of protected designation of origin extra virgin olive oil. J Agric Food Chem. 2007;55:3857–3862. DOI: 10.1021/jf063708r

[82] Busconi M, Foroni C, Corradi M, Bongiorni C, Cattapan F, Fogher C. DNA extraction from olive oil and its use in the identification of the production cultivar. Food Chem. 2003;83:127–134. DOI: 10.1016/S0308-8146(03)00218-8

[83] Pafundo S, Busconi M, Agrimonti C, Fogher C, Marmiroli N. Storage-time effect on olive oil DNA assessed by amplified fragments length polymorphisms. Food Chem. 2010;123:787–793. DOI: 10.1016/j.foodchem.2010.05.027

[84] Bracci T, Busconi M, Fogher C, Sebastiani L. Molecular studies in olive (*Olea europaea* L.): Overview on DNA markers applications and recent advances in genome analysis. Plant Cell Rep. 2011;30:449–462. DOI: 10.1007/s00299-010-0991-9

[85] Busconi M, Reggi S, Dallolio G, Fogher C. Food microbiota diversity. In: Grillo A, Venora G (Eds.). Changing Diversity in Changing Environment. Intech, Croatia 2011; p. 17–32. DOI: 10.5772/24841

[86] Busconi M, Zacconi C, Scolari G. Bacterial ecology of PDO Coppa and Pancetta Piacentina at the end of ripening and after MAP storage of sliced product. Int J Food Microbiol. 2014;172:13–20. DOI: 10.1016/j.ijfoodmicro.2013.11.023

Chapter 3

Microsatellites as a Tool for the Study of Microevolutionary Process in Native Forest Trees

Maria Eugenia Barrandeguy and
Maria Victoria Garcia

Additional information is available at the end of the chapter

http://dx.doi.org/10.5772/65042

Abstract

The main aim of this work is an attempt to help researchers that use microsatellite markers to analyze microevolutionary forces in natural populations of native forest species. This kind of studies drives the researchers to make decisions regarding management or conservation of such species. This chapter pays attention to the entire process—from development of microsatellite markers, going through data analysis and ending with interpretation of these results. This work helps to researchers that are not familiarizing with methods and population genetics theories to analyze nuclear and chloroplast microsatellite data. These methods allow quantification of genetic variation and genetic structure in native forest species, and theoretical content allows knowledge about the past and the present genetic states of populations for making inferences about the future of these populations.

Keywords: cpSSRs, nuSSRs, native forest trees, population genetics

1. Introduction

Patterns of distribution of genetic variation in the landscape reflect the responses of species to evolutionary forces operating within current and past environments, and it can tell us much about how species have evolved and may continue to evolve in the future [1]. Most studies on genetic variation patterns within tree species were primarily motivated by attempts to improve our understanding of biodiversity at the intraspecific level or the evolutionary dynamics within plant species in an early stage of domestication [2]. However, forest tree species have many valuable subjects to be explored, and problems could be solved using microsatellite markers in combination with appropriate statistical analyses to make recommendations for conservation of forest genetic resources [3], infer the origin of forest plants and woods [2], and conduct molecular tree improvements [4].

The main aim of this work is an attempt to help researchers that use microsatellite markers to analyze microevolutionary forces in natural populations of native forest species. This kind of studies drives the researchers to make decisions regarding management or conservation of such species.

2. The challenge to work with microsatellite markers in species without economical interest

Native forest species are interesting models of biodiversity study because they give valuable information about current and past conditions that could have influence on the amount and distribution of genetic variation in natural populations. Hence, long-lived tree species have witnessed climatic, demographic, and/or ecological changes, and all these changes left genetic traces that can be studied using microsatellite markers (Simple Sequence Repeats - SSRs). However, every interesting point about working with native species has its unfavorable counterpart because of low economic value of native forest species. One of the limitations is the lack of DNA sequence information needed to develop and use simple sequence repeats (SSRs). Unfortunately, SSRs are not universal markers, and species specificity of SSR loci in plants is a major constraint to their ubiquitous adoption [5], although limited cross-species transferability of SSR loci of closely related taxa is possible.

The starting point of a genetic study using SSRs in native forest trees is getting species-specific SSRs, e.g., searching in the nucleotide section of GeneBank public database. In the case of unavailability of species-specific SSRs, an alternative is to search SSR primers developed for a phylogenetically closely related species because as mentioned above, empirical studies have demonstrated that cross-species transfer of nuclear microsatellite markers is possible [6]. Using latter methodology, SSRs developed for one species can be used to detect polymorphism at homologous sites in related species. However, the repeat sequence and the flanking regions-containing primer binding sites must be conserved across taxa to detect polymorphism at homologous sites in related species [5].

The success of heterologous PCR amplification will depend upon evolutionary distance between the source and the target species because empirical studies have shown an inverse relationship between primer site conservation and evolutionary relationship between tested taxa [5]. Cross-species transferability of polymorphic markers in plants is mainly successful within genera (success rate close to 60% in eudicots and close to 40% in the reviewed monocots), whereas between genera, cross-species transfer rates are approximately 10% for eudicots [6]. There are studies with native forest tree species in which cross-species transfer were successful, e.g., *Quercus* [7–9], *Prosopis* [10], *Eucalyptus* [11], *Enterolobium* [12], *Pithecellobium* [13], *Araucaria* [14], and *Taxus* [15].

In the worst of cases, cross-species transfer of SSRs may not work. Hence, we propose two nonmutually excluding alternatives: the development of species-specific microsatellites for nuclear genome (nuclear Simple Sequence Repeats – nuSSRs) and the use of chloroplast microsatellite markers (chloroplast Simple Sequence Repeats - cpSSRs). These alternatives are very different regarding to genetic information they provide and its cost in terms of time and money. Many laboratories have enough resources and expertise for conducting SSR-based research but not for characterizing new loci [5].

Microsatellite markers are present in chloroplast genome but particular traits of this genome provide different population genetic information than nuSSRs. Organelle genomes are typically nonrecombinant, uniparentally inherited, and effectively haploid [16]. Unlike the conventional approach for obtaining nuclear microsatellites, when cpSSRs primers designed for one species can regularly cross-amplify in related species, giving an opportunity to develop efficient "universal" SSR primers that show widespread intraspecific polymorphism. Chloroplast SSR primers developed by Weising and Gardner [17] are the most popular in Angiosperms. However, the low mutation rates associated with the chloroplast genome meant that detection of enough variation represents a major technical barrier for the widespread application of a particular marker [16].

3. Development of species-specific nuclear microsatellite markers

Population geneticists, forestry breeders, and ecologists starting a new research that must contend with a dichotomous decision: the isolation of species-specific microsatellite markers or application of multilocus fingerprinting approaches. The advantages of hypervariable, codominant markers as SSRs are well documented [18], but in many cases, the perceived difficulties of SSRs isolation act as a deterrent for the utilization of this class of markers [19].

In recent years, publications of new species-specific nuSSRs in forest tree species and in other plant taxa are frequent in most of journals. However, development of species-specific nuSSRs is time and cost consuming. Also, specific laboratory and technical conditions are needed, costly and laborious cloning and screening procedures limit the number of species that can be studied.

As a consequence of the diverse publications and techniques for nuSSRs development, in this section, we will exclusively focus on the SSR development procedure in plants addressing to describe the typical situation that the researchers must consider when working with nonmodel organisms. Our own experience comes from the development of specific nuSSRs for *Anadenanthera colubrina* var. *cebil* (Mimosoideae, Leguminosoideae), a native forest tree species from South America [20]. Laboratory work was started to cross-species transfer of nuSSRs developed for other legume tree species because SSR primers from species of the same genera were not available. Eighteen primer pairs from six different species were tested including *Koompasia malascensis, Acacia nilotica, Geoffroea spinosa, Prosopis sp., Dinizia excelsa*, and *Parkia panurensis*. Results of cross-species transfer were unsatisfactory, and development of species-specific nuSSRs was necessary.

The successful isolation of SSRs involves several steps: (1) preparation of a microsatellite-enriched genomic library, (2) cloning and sequencing of fragments containing microsatellites,

(3) primer design, and (4) testing the functionality of SSR primers and polymorphisms in tested genotypes. There is a potential loss of loci at each stage. A number of loci that will finally constitute the working primer set are a fraction of the original number of sequenced clones, which is called attrition rate [19]. Microsatellite markers were developed from two microsatellite-enriched genomic libraries screening for an increase in the variability of microsatellite motifs. The results were notoriously different as only one library gave positive results. The libraries were developed using the enrichment procedure proposed by Fischer and Bachmann [21] and modified by Prinz et al. [22]. **Table 1** shows the attrition rates for this work. The development of specific nuSSRs for *A. colubrina* var. *cebil* demanded 3 months of work in a fully equipped laboratory. Human resources involved in the development of SSRs included a technical assistant, a doctoral student, and an experienced researcher.

		Efficiency of enrichment			Efficiency of primer design					Functionality	
Library	Oligo pool	N° of inserts sequenced	N° of inserts with SSRs	High quality sequences with SSRs	Sequences with flanking region suitable to design primers	Sequences with a unique SSRs locus	Sequences without restriction site inside the SSRs region	Primers designed	Tested primers	Clearly amplified loci	Polymorphic loci
A	$(GA)_{10}$	106	77 (73%)	56 (73%)	84%	70%	98.2%	30 (52%)	30 (52%)	16 (51.7%)	8(50%)
B	$(CA)_{10}$ $(GAA)_8$ $(CAA)_8$	98	20 (20.5%)	6 (30%)	100%	100%	100%	6 (100%)	1 (17%)	0(0%)	–
Total		204	97 (47.6%)	62 (64%)	85.5%	72.6%	98.4%	36 (56.5%)	30 (48.4%)	16(50%)	8(50%)

Table 1. Attrition rates for *A. colubrina* var. *cebil* specific nuSSRs development.

From our experience, we suggest to pay attention on the following: starting the process with DNA of good quality and enough quantity; ensuring good conditions of sterility during enrichment procedure and in the whole process; making two simultaneous libraries using different sets of repeated motifs for enrichment; avoiding repetitive bases in primer sequences; analyzing the primer sequences directly in the electropherograms to ensure that primers were designed on sequences of good quality with high peaks; resequencing amplified products after functionality tests; and aligning the original fragment obtained from the enrichment procedure.

New and revolutionary sequencing methods, referred to as next-generation sequencing (NGS), are extremely high-throughput technologies that produce thousands or millions of sequences at once at a fraction of the cost of traditional Sanger methods [23]. A specific application of this new technology in plants is the possibility of rapid and cost-effective discovery of microsatellite loci [23]. Despite this modern technology is more cost effective than traditional enrichment procedures, currently it is not yet widely used for nuSSRs development in plant species. A commonly cited weakness of microsatellites is their high development cost and relatively low-throughput when compared to SNPs but the same technologies that have widened the use of SNPs have also benefited microsatellite development processes [24].

Once a set of nuSSRs primers was developed, the final step was the statistical analyses of data to confirm the utility of these markers to population genetic studies. These analyses consist of: (1) estimation of observed and expected heterozygosity, (2) test of Hardy-Weinberg equilibrium, (3) test of genotypic linkage disequilibrium, (4) test of null alleles and genotyping errors, and (5) perform neutrality test. There are free software available for these analyses, e.g., Genalex [25], Genepop [26], and/or Microchecker [27]. Expected good results for these analyses include high heterozygosity, high number of loci in Hardy-Weinberg equilibrium and linkage disequilibrium, low number of loci with null alleles and absence of genotyping errors, and lack of traces of selection.

4. What do microsatellite markers say us about natural populations of forest tree species?

The development of molecular genetic markers has had a great impact on our understanding of the processes that determine structure and variation within and among natural populations [16]. Microsatellites, as other molecular markers, are particular characteristics of DNA molecule that enable the identification of individuals at DNA level. However, a molecular marker must be considered as genetic marker when its particular genetic features are known. The knowledge on precise molecular basis and a mode of inheritance of a genetic polymorphism are crucial for the appropriate interpretation of molecular marker data in a population context [28].

Plants show a remarkable variety of inheritance modes, and further, some of their reproductive patterns permit genetic study with means not available in other types of organisms [29]. The mitochondrial genome in plants shows a large size, slow nucleotide substitution rates and extensive levels of intramolecular recombination, and has been of limited use in genetic diversity studies. The chloroplast genome shows conserved gene order and a general lack of heteroplasmy and recombination, and it is an attractive tool for demographic and phylogenetic studies [16]. There is considerable potential for hypervariable chloroplast microsatellites to provide markers with uniparental inheritance for indirect measures of seed or pollen gene flow. Studies of angiosperms, where chloroplast DNA (cpDNA) is predominantly maternally inherited, might offer further insights and provide information on the patterns and extent of localized seed dispersal [16]. Furthermore, its uniparental mode of inheritance makes it possible to elucidate the relative contributions of seed and pollen gene flow to the genetic structure of natural populations by comparing nuclear and chloroplast markers [16].

The use of genetic markers with uni- and biparental inheritance (i.e., cpSSRs and nuSSRs) differentiates the historical contributions of the movement of seed and pollen on the levels of gene flow. This information is relevant to distinguish between genetic consequences of colonization by seed and the exchange of genes through pollen between established populations [30, 31]. Given haploid genome of organelles, effective population size in hermaphrodite outcrossing plants is half that of diploid nuclear genome, and as a result, chloroplast-specific markers should be good indicators of historical bottlenecks, founder effects, and genetic drift [16].

Differences in mutation rates, ploidy levels, and recombination presence or absence between nuclear and chloroplast genomes make cpSSRs and nuSSRs valuable tools for the study of the effects of historical and recent fragmentation on the contemporary genetic variation and current population genetic structure. This allows contrasting the relative role of genetic drift and gene flow as microevolutionary process that shapes population genetic structure [32].

In addition, due to their high rate of polymorphism, nuclear microsatellites are often cited as being very useful for studying recent evolutionary events among subpopulations within an individual species [24].

Microevolutionary process	**cpSSRs**	**Both**	**nuSSRs**
Gene flow	Gene flow by seeds	–	Gene flow by pollen and seed
Genetic drift	Historical fragmentation	–	Recent fragmentation
Genetic drift vs. gene flow	–	Relative contributions of seed and pollen flow to the genetic structure of natural populations	–
Factor			
Demographic events	Colonization/ expansion Historical bottlenecks Founder effects	–	–

Table 2. Microevolutionary processes and demographic events that can be studied by microsatellite markers.

The movement of alleles within and between natural populations and their interaction with genetic drift, mutation, and natural selection determine the genetic composition of a population, including its genetic diversity and genetic structure [28]. Microsatellites allow taking a high-resolution snapshot of a given allelic composition at a given time for certain loci, and the studying of mechanisms that generate and maintain genetic variability is possible by means of population genetics theories and methods.

Great potential exists for the application of coalescent-based models to cpSSRs [16]. Coalescent approaches can be extremely useful in assessing a range of demographic histories but their application to intraspecific studies in plants has been hampered by the slow mutation rate of the nonrecombinant genomes, such as chloroplast DNA. Although limitations exist, cpSSRs represent a potentially informative data source with which coalescent-based approaches can be explored [16]. Microevolutionary processes and demographic events that can be studied by microsatellite markers are showed in **Table 2**.

5. Population genetic data analysis

This section attempts to guide the researchers to make decisions regarding the statistical analysis of nuclear and chloroplast microsatellite data. Nevertheless, those attempting to use these analyses for the first time will need to read the cited bibliography here for each particular analysis. Advances in computing technology have inspired the use of intensive statistical approaches such as maximum likelihood, Bayesian probability theory, and Markov chain Monte Carlo simulation contributing to the recent technical advancements of molecular ecology [33].

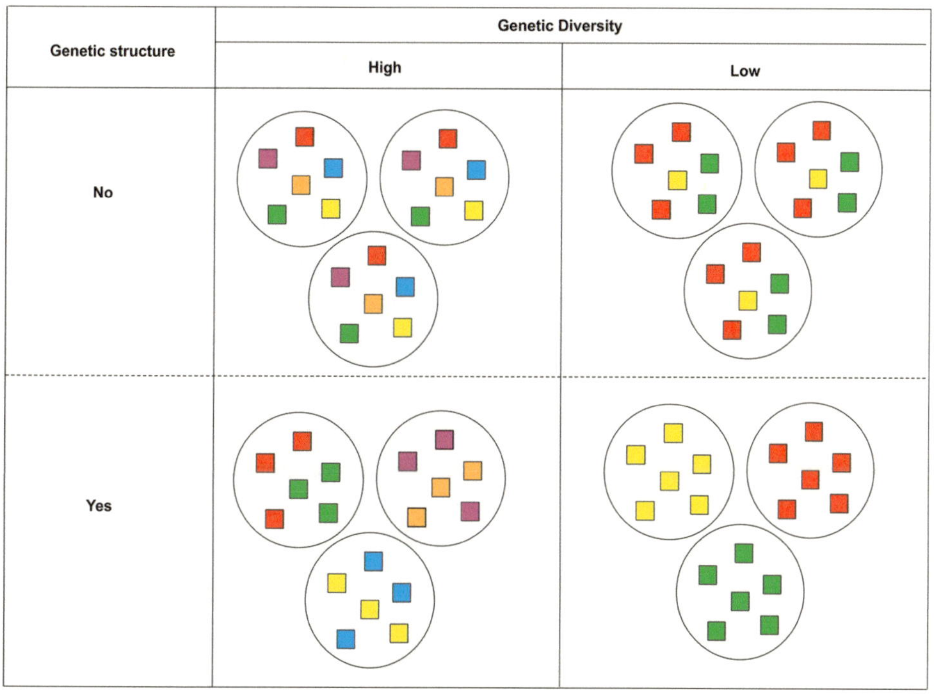

Figure 1. Extreme states of allelic configuration of one theoretical population integrated by three subpopulations. Circles: subpopulations; Squares: nuSSRs genotypes or cpSSRs haplotypes. Colors show differences in the allelic compositions.

Fourth extreme and simple states of allelic configuration of a theoretical population integrated by three subpopulations are showed in **Figure 1**. Each state was defined from the relationship between genetic diversity levels and genetic structure of the theoretical population. In the nature, these extremes are exceptions while complex allelic configurations are the usual situations. Statistical analyses are the most appropriate tools to infer levels and distribution patterns of genetic variation while population genetic theory gives the knowledge for interpreting statistical data analysis results.

5.1. Genetic diversity

A prerequisite for starting population studies is to detect the genetic diversity underlying phenotypic variation, and understand the genetic diversity as the total genetic variation among individuals within a population. Several measures of genetic diversity have been developed over the years. The simplest measure of genetic diversity from molecular data is the number of alleles at a given locus (N_A), which is also known as gene multiplicity [34]. At the same time, these alleles have their own frequencies in each population, which represent their abundance. As multiplicity and abundance vary independently, genetic diversity can be expressed as the effective number of alleles (N_E) [35]. N_E will be equal to N_A if alleles show the same frequency. In case that allele frequency distribution is not uniform, N_E will be lower than N_A. The number of alleles that can be found in only one population is defined as private alleles (N_P) [36]. In this way, N_P is a simple measure of genetic distinctiveness. Private alleles can also have low frequencies being able to call them rare alleles. These kinds of alleles are very informative because their presence and frequency allow quantification of gene flow levels.

Since the number of detected alleles in a population depends on its size, it is not advisable to compare genetic diversity parameters among subpopulations with different sizes. An useful parameter to compare the number of alleles between samples that differ in size is the allelic richness (R). This parameter predicts the expected number of alleles if samples have the same size using the rarefaction method [37]. However, the original and most important measure of genetic diversity is Nei's gene diversity index (h) estimated as $h = \Sigma_1^n\left(1 - x_i^2\right)$, where x_i indicates the allele frequency [38]. This parameter represents the probability that two alleles randomly and independently selected from a gene pool will represent different alleles. This index analyzes allele frequency variation directly in the terms of heterozygosity without consideration of the number of alleles at a given locus or the pattern of evolutionary forces [38]. In this way, the treatment of this index is biologically most appropriate because it has been formulated entirely in terms of allele and genotype frequencies [39].

Since particular genetics features of chloroplast genome, combination of cpSSRs alleles from different loci allows determining the chloroplast haplotypes. Hence, haplotype genetic multiplicity could also be characterized from haplotype number, genetic abundance from haplotype frequencies, genetic distinctiveness from the number of private haplotypes, and genetic diversity from Nei´s haplotypic diversity index (H) estimated as $H = \left\{\left[\frac{n}{n-1}\right]\left[1 - \Sigma_1^n p_i^2\right]\right\}$, where n is the number of analyzed individuals and p_i is the frequency of haplotypes in the population [40, 41] (**Table 3**).

http://dx.doi.org/10.5772/65042

Population genetic measure	Objective of analysis	Analysis		Statistical estimation	Suggested software[a]
Genetic diversity	Characterization	Genetic multiplicity		Number of alleles (N_A) Number of chloroplast haplotypes (N_H)	Genalex [25]
		Genetic abundance		Allele frequencies Haplotype frequencies	Genalex [25] Arlequin [59]
		Multiplicity vs. abundancy		Effective number of alleles (N_E)	Genalex [25]
		Genetic distinctiveness		Number of private alleles (N_P) Number of private haplotypes (N_{PH})	Genalex [25]
		Heterozygosity		Observed heterozygosity (H_O) Expected heterozygoity (H_E)	Genalex [25]
	Quantification	Genetic diversity		Nei´s gene diversity index (h) Nei's haplotypic diversity index (H)	Genalex [25]
				Allelic richness (R)	ADZE [60] FSTAT [61]
Genetic structure	Determination	Individual-based methods	Methods based on distance	Median joining trees	Darwin [62] PopArt [63]
				Haplotype network	Network [64]
			Methods based on models	Bayesian admixture analysis for nuclear data Bayesian mixture analysis for linked cpSSR data	Structure [44] Structure Harvester [65] BAPS [45]
		Subpopulation-based methods	Hierarchical structure using nongenetic criteria	AMOVA using geographic definition of groups	Arlequin [59]
			Hierarchical structure using a genetic criteria	AMOVA using clusters defined by Bayesian analysis	Arlequin [59]
	Quantification	Wright's F_{ST}		Nuclear genetic structure (F_{STnu})	Arlequin [59]

Population genetic measure	Objective of analysis		Analysis	Statistical estimation	Suggested software[a]
				Chloroplast genetic structure (F_{STcp})	
Gene flow	Quantification	Historical	Indirectly estimated from F_{ST}	Gene flow by pollen and seed ($N_e m_{nu}$) Gene flow by seeds ($N_e m_{cp}$)[b]	Arlequin [59]
			From rare alleles	Gene flow by pollen and seed ($N_e m_{nu}$)	Genepop [26]
		Recent	Probability to be a migrant or a recent migrant descendent	Bayesian genetic structure analysis with *a priori* individual's geographical position information	Structure [44]
	Gene flow by pollen versus gene flow by seeds		Indirectly estimated from levels of nuclear and chloroplast genetic structure	Ennos's equation (r)	–
Inbreeding	Quantification		Hierarchical subpopulation-based analyses including within individual level (F_{IS})	AMOVA including within individual levels	Arlequin [59]
			Bayesian inbreeding inference (*f*)	Bayesian analysis	Hickory [52]
			Inbreeding coefficient inference considering null alleles F_{ISnull}	Computer simulations to simultaneous estimation of null alleles by locus and inbreeding coefficient as a multilocus parameter	INEST [53]
Demographic events	Population expansion determination		Neutrality tests	F_S neutrality test (F_S) D_{Tajima} (D_{Tajima})	Arlequin [59]
	Phylogeography		Approximate Bayesian computation (ABC)	Parameter estimation (effective sizes of current and ancestral populations, immigration rates, splitting times, and tree topology) and ancestral model comparison	DiYABC [66]

[a]Free available software.
[b]For angiosperm species.

Table 3. Classification of methods for analysis of microevolutionary processes and demographic events and suggested software.

The differences in the genetic diversity parameters among populations must be statistically significant to arrive at the conclusion of which population is the most diverse. These differences could be tested by permutation, a nonparametric procedure.

5.2. Genetic structure

Population genetic structure is the amount of genetic variability and its distribution within and among local populations and individuals within a species [42]. Given the central role of population genetic structure to microevolutionary processes, additional tools for its measurement and quantification are necessary. In this way, we perform a classification of the several statistical methods to study population genetic structure. However, the researchers must keep in mind the scope and aims of the study to define the analyses of their data.

5.2.1. Individual-based methods

The starting points for these analyses are individual microsatellite's genotypes. The simplest methods are those based on distances, e.g., median joining trees (MJ) and networks (NWK) [43]. These methods are graphical representation of genetic distances among multilocus genotypes (nuSSRs data) or among haplotypes (cpSSRs data). Distance-based methods are usually easy to apply and are often visually appealing. However, the clusters identified may be dependent on both the distance measure and graphical representation chosen, being difficult to assess confidence of clusters obtained [44].

Nowadays, the most popular individual-based methods are those based on models as Bayesian admixture analysis for nuSSRs data [44] and Bayesian mixture analysis for linked loci for cpSSRs data [45]. Methods based on Bayesian theory are extensively used because they give information about the genetic origin of individuals making clusters and assigning individuals to these clusters to infer population structure based on a probabilistic criterion. In addition, these methods include *a priori* information of the geographic origin of individuals to help in the population genetic structure determination [44, 45] and the identification of migrants or descendants of recent immigrants [44]. The results of Bayesian admixture analyses must be analyzed by the Evanno method [46] to determine the most likely level of population subdivision.

5.2.2. Subpopulation-based methods

The starting points of these analyses are groups of individuals. Here these groups are called subpopulations. Different criterion could be considered to grouping individuals: a nongenetic criterion (e.g., geographical groups of individuals, cohort, etc.) or a genetic criterion (e.g., previously identified Bayesian clusters). Subpopulation-based methods are based on the analysis of molecular variance (AMOVA) [47]. This method consists in the analysis of distribution of molecular genetic variation in the previously established different hierarchical levels. Once genetic structure was determined, the strength of genetic structure must to be quantified. The most appropriate way is the estimation of Wright's fixation index (F_{ST}). Sewall Wright [48] devised the fixation index to describe correlations among alleles sampled at hierarchically organized levels of a population. Hence, this index could be estimated from the AMOVA as $F_{ST} = \left(\sigma_a^2 - \sigma_T^2\right)/\sigma_T^2$, where σ_a^2 is the variance among subpopulations and σ_T^2 is the total population variance [49]. Statistical significance estimation of this index could be performed using permutations. F_{ST} index could be estimated among pairwise subpopulations to determinate patterns of genetic differentiation (**Table 3**).

5.3. Gene flow

Genetic exchange between local populations is called gene flow, and it is an evolutionary force that occurs between populations with distinct gene pools [42]. We are going to introduce two ways to estimate levels of gene flow among subpopulations from microsatellite data. The first way is the indirect method based on genetic differentiation among populations [50]. After Wright [48] developed fixation index, he went on to demonstrate that there is a simple relationship between the genetic divergence of two populations, measured as F_{ST}, and the amount of gene flow between them, which is given as $F_{ST} = 1/4 \ \left(N_e m + 1\right)$, where Ne is the effective size of each population and m is the migration rate between populations, and therefore $N_e m$ is the number of breeding adults that are migrants. Hence, for nuSSRs data, the number of migrants could be estimated as $N_e m = \left(1/F_{ST} - 1\right)/4$ and it quantifies the historical gene flow by pollen and seed, while for cpSSRs data, the number of migrants could be estimated as $N_e m = \left(1/F_{ST} - 1\right)/2$ and it quantifies the historical gene flow by seeds in angiosperm species [42]. The second way to estimate gene flow is the method of rare alleles described by Slatkin [51]. He proposed the estimation of Nm from the spatial distribution of rare alleles. He demonstrated that $\log_{10}\left[\bar{p}_{(1)}\right]$, where $\bar{p}_{(1)}$ indicates the average frequency of private alleles, is approximately lineal with $\log_{10}Nm$.

The estimation of relative rates of pollen and seed gene flow could be estimated from an estimator proposed by Ennos [31], which is based on the conception that the effectiveness of pollen and seed in bringing about gene flow depends upon the mode of inheritance of the genetic marker. In most of the angiosperms, gene flow occurs by pollen and seed for nuclear and paternally inherited markers; however, gene flow occurs only by seeds for maternally inherited markers. Consequently, different levels of population differentiation for markers with contrasting modes of inheritance are expected. The relative levels of pollen versus seed gene flow among populations could be estimated as $r = \left[\left(1/F_{STb} - 1\right) - 2 \times \left(1/F_{STm} - 1\right)\right] / \left(1/F_{STm} - 1\right)$, where F_{STb} and F_{STm} are fixation index for nuclear and chloroplast markers for an angiosperm species, respectively.

Finally, Pritchard et al. [43] extended their approach to infer genetic structure including in the algorithm, the geographic position of individuals. In essence, it assumes that each individual originated, with high probability, in the geographical region in which it was sampled, but to allow some small probability that it is an immigrant (or has immigrant ancestry). Immigrants would be individuals whose genetic makeup suggests they were misclassified, and in this way it is possible to quantify recent gene flow (**Table 3**).

5.4. Inbreeding

In its most basic sense, inbreeding is mating between biological relatives [42]. It is not a microevolutionary process because its effect does not change allele frequencies of populations. However, it is important because genotypic composition of populations could be determined by its influence. The presence of inbreeding informs us about reproductive dynamics of the species. Inbreeding coefficient (F_{IS}) could be estimated from AMOVA if the hierarchical level "within individuals" is included in it. Inbreeding could also be estimated using a Bayesian approach (*f*) [52].

Although microsatellites are a very efficient tool for many population genetics applications, they may occasionally produce null alleles, which, when present in high proportion at a particular locus, the observed heterozygosity would be underestimated. As a consequence, the population parameter estimates based on the proportion of heterozygotes could be affected by null alleles. Estimates of Wright's inbreeding coefficient F_{IS} based on microsatellite data could be unclear regarding to the extension of actual level of inbreeding in the studied population and in the degree affected by the presence of null alleles. Population inbreeding model can be applied for simultaneous estimation of null allele frequencies and of the inbreeding coefficient as a multilocus parameter [53] (**Table 3**).

5.5. Demographic events

There has been little focus on the potential of chloroplast microsatellites for demographic inference. Navascués et al. [54] investigated the utility of cpSSRs data for the detection of demographic expansions. The study of historical demography by means of genetic information is based on coalescent theory [55]. One alternative is the development of the F_S neutrality test for determination of population expansion events [56]. This test is based on different expectations for the number of haplotypes when comparing a stationary with expansion demography [56]. Another alternative is the estimation of D_{Tajima} index as $D_{\text{Tajima}} = \pi - (\theta)/\sqrt{V[\pi-(\theta)]}$ where, π is the number of different sites between sequences, V is the numerator variance, and θ is estimated as $\theta = S/a$, where S is the number of polymorphic sites and a is calculated by $a = \sum_{i=1}^{n-1} 1/i$, where i takes values of [1 – (n-1)] and where n is the number of analyzed sequences [57]. Both parameters should be estimated from the distribution of the differences between individuals within a population, and these differences are considered as allelic differences between cpSSRs haplotypes, being this data considered as binary [54].

A new and robust method to examine a species' phylogeography using microsatellite markers is the approximate Bayesian computation (ABC). This model-based method is useful to infer parameters and compare models in population genetics [58] (**Table 3**).

6. Understanding population genetic data analysis results

The challenge in the study of population genetic events based on microsatellite markers is the interpretation of the statistical analysis results from the biological point of view. The aim of this section is to serve as a guide about how to interpret these results in a forest tree species in order to infer which are the forces that determine the distribution of current genetic variation of nuSSRs and cpSSRs?

In the field of population genetics, it is becoming increasingly necessary to focus more attention on understanding the practical limitations of various analyses and applying increased caution when interpreting results generated by molecular markers [24]. Regardless of the question, a molecular marker must fundamentally be selectively neutral and follow Mendelian inheritance in order to be used as a tool for detecting demographic patterns and microevolutionary forces as genetic drift and gene flow [33].

Recombination, selection, and genetic drift affect different genes and regions of the genome in a different way. Consequently, multiple samples of the genome by combining the results from many loci provide a precise and statistically powerful way of comparing populations and individuals [33]. Microsatellites have high mutation rates that generate the high levels of allelic diversity necessary for genetic studies of processes acting on ecological time scales [67, 68]. The new approaches use more of the information in a data set than the summary statistics of traditional approaches (e.g., F_{ST}).

Nowadays, demography and history of populations and relationships of individuals can be described in a detailed manner because the typical data set contains high number of individuals sampled at many loci. Hence, genetic tools allow to address many basic ecological questions for the first time or in new ways [33].

Genetic diversity is essential for the long-term survival of species; without it, species cannot adapt to environmental changes and are more susceptible to extinction. Measuring levels of genetic variation within and among populations is an important first step in evaluating the evolutionary biology and tree improvement potential of a species [1]. Most forest tree species possess considerable genetic variation, much of which can be found within populations, and the expected heterozygosity is approximately 50% higher in a population of forest trees than average heterozygosity expected in populations of annuals and perennials cycle short life species [1].

A number of factors that contribute to the high levels of genetic diversity typically found in forest tree populations are large population size, longevity, high levels of outcrossing, strong gene flow by pollen and seed between populations, and balancing selection [68]. Nuclear DNA is often highly variable, and it is biparentally inherited. Efficient gene flow, in particular, via pollen is the main factor contributing to the high diversity within populations of trees but low differentiation among spatially separated populations [69].

Gene diversity index is the expected heterozygosity averaged over all loci sampled and is the most widely used measure of genetic variation employing genetic markers. Because low-frequency alleles contribute very little to h, it is relatively insensitive to sample size. However, when sampled populations show markedly differences in size, additionally allelic richness (R) could be informed. The observation of variation at nonrecombining chloroplast DNA (cpDNA) is of particular importance for plants. Low mutation rates of cpDNA are responsible for, in general, low variation within species [69]. As a consequence of previous statements, higher levels of genetic diversity with nuSSRs than with cpSSRs are expected.

Populations of forest trees often differ in allele frequencies (especially when they are separated geographically), and it is often of interest to determine the degree to which genetic variation in a region is distributed within and among populations. This information is useful for understanding the degree to which gene flow by pollen and seed counters population subdivision due to selection or genetic drift [70]. It also has practical value when planning seed collections for breeding or gene conservation purposes. Therefore, knowledge of natural patterns of genetic variation and their evolutionary bases also are of great practical significance [1]. The pattern of genotypic variation (heterozygosity vs. homozygosity) among individuals within a subpopulation is highly dependent upon the mating system, whereas the distribution of allelic variation within and among subpopulations is influenced by both gene flow and genetic drift. Because of the opposite effects of gene flow and genetic drift, the balance between them is a primary determinant of the genetic population structure of a species [42]. Total diversity in forest trees is also generally higher than that found in other plants. However, only a small proportion of the total gene diversity in trees is due to differences among populations [1].

Woody species contain more variation within populations but have less variation among them than species with other life forms. Woody species that present large geographic ranges, outcrossing breeding systems, and wind or animal-ingested seed dispersal are more genetically diverse than woody species with other combinations of traits [68]. Hence, from AMOVA results in forest tree species, higher levels of genetic variation is expected in the hierarchical level within populations than the hierarchical level among populations. Genetic differentiation among populations estimated by F_{ST} also varies widely among tree species, ranging from low values in species that have more or less continuous distributions to high values in species with disjunct population distributions [1]. For the interpretation of F_{ST}, the value scale suggested by Wright [71] is a useful tool. The four values are (1) 0–0.05 indicate little genetic differentiation, (2) 0.05–0.15 indicate moderate genetic differentiation, (3) 0.15–0.25 indicate great genetic differentiation and, (4) values above 0.25 indicate very great genetic differentiation. Nuclear F_{ST} in trees is frequently 10% or lower, which is only one-half to one-quarter of the F_{ST} estimates typically found in annuals or other herbaceous species. The lower F_{ST} in trees is most likely because most tree species are outcrossing while a large proportion of annuals and herbaceous plants are either self-pollinated or self-pollination features prominently in their mating system. High levels of self-pollination not only promote inbreeding but also limit pollen gene flow between populations. Both pollen and seed gene flow between populations of forest trees can be extensive [1].

Patterns of seed dispersal shape the composition and genetic structure of plant populations. Species with low levels of gene flow by seeds have high probability to show genetic heterogeneity among subpopulations, whereas species with high levels of gene flow by seeds have low levels of genetic structure [72].

Compared to biparentally inherited and paternally inherited markers, maternally inherited markers detected strong genetic differentiation between populations [69] because normally seeds are distributed to shorter distances than pollen [73]. Moreover, being a haploid genome, effective population size for hermaphrodite outcrossing plants is half that of the corresponding diploid nuclear genome [16]. Hence, gene flow between populations of small size has a lower effective to counteract the effects of genetic drift in loci transmitted maternally [74]. When these occur, F_{ST} values for chloroplast DNA can be markedly higher than those for nuclear genes [75]. Genetic structure of chloroplast genetic variation is also affected by the interaction of seed dispersal with other ecological and genetic processes. Deposition patterns of seeds, pollen dispersal, density of adults, microhabitat selection, and several aspects of the ecology of the species could have significant effects on patterns of genetic variation within species [72]. While both pollen and seed dispersal determines gene flow in plants, seed dispersal is most important because it allows species to colonize habitats and therefore influences the dynamics of populations [76].

Methods based on distance allow grouping individuals according to genetic distance while its graphical representation allows to relate these groups with other information, e.g., the geographical origin of individuals or phenotypic traits [44]. Even though these methods are statistically weak, they still represent a first approach to analyze population genetic structure. Conversely, grouping from methods based on models are statistically powerful and allow to determine the number of clusters using genetic information assigning individuals probabilistically to these clusters even when they require model assumptions (e.g., Hardy-Weinberg equilibrium within populations and complete linkage equilibrium between loci within populations) [44].

Species can become subdivided into genetically distinct subpopulations when gene flow is restricted, leading to variation in the frequency of a gene over space [42]. The number of migrants $N_e m$ represents an estimation of gene flow, and it is important to keep in mind that m is defined in the terms of gene pools, and therefore m represents the amount of exchange of gametes between subpopulations and not necessarily individuals [42]. Most trees species are wind pollinated, and the pollen can be blown from hundreds of miles by the wind. Hence, tree populations that are quite distant can still experience gene flow. Because gene flow requires both movement and reproduction, m is not just the amount of dispersal of individuals between subpopulations but instead m represents a complex interaction between the pattern of dispersal and the mating system [42]. As a consequence of this, in forest tree species, it is really important to know pollen and seed dispersal mechanisms and species matting system to interpret the estimated levels of gene flow from microsatellite data.

The effects of gene flow on genetic variation among and within subpopulations can be summarized as gene flow decreases genetic variation among subpopulations and increases genetic variation within subpopulations. Genetic drift causes an increase in genetic variation among subpopulations and decreases genetic variation within a subpopulation. Hence, the effects of gene flow on genetic variation within and among subpopulations are the opposite of those of genetic drift [42].

For neutral alleles, when gene flow is interrupted, genetic drift is more effective than mutation to produce genetic differentiation among subpopulations [77]. Thereby, gene flow could be a force that maintains species integrated as well as influences the ecologic processes, e.g., determine the persistence and adaptation of local populations, determine pattern of distribution of species, etc. [78]. In this way, studies of gene flow become relevant for the interpretation of microevolutionary patterns and genetic structure of populations [80]. Even a small amount of gene flow can cause two populations to behave effectively as a single evolutionary lineage. One "effective" migrant per generation ($N_em = 1$) defines an inflection point from the relation between F_{ST} and N_em, with increasing effective number of migrants F_{ST} declines only very slowly when $N_em \geq 1$ but with decreasing effective number of migrants F_{ST} rises very rapidly when $N_em \leq 1$. As a consequence of this, $N_em = 1$ marks a transition in the relative evolutionary importance of gene flow to drift. It is impressive that only one or more effective migrants per generation on average are needed to cause gene flow to dominate over genetic drift, leading to great genetic homogeneity among subpopulations [42].

Ennos [31] demonstrated that estimation of the relative rates of pollen and seed migration among plant populations is possible from a simple comparison of F_{ST} values for nuclear and maternally inherited organelle genetic markers. Estimated rates of pollen migration are greater than rates of seed migration for all six species investigated by Ennos [31]; however, differences among species were substantial. The greatest contrast between pollen and seed migration rates was found for oak species, where interpopulation pollen flow is estimated to be 200 times greater than interpopulation seed flow. This result was interpreted by the species reproductive system. Oaks show high rates of interpopulation pollen dispersal because they are outbreeding, wind-pollinated, and disperse pollen from a substantial height. Also, dispersal of acorns by birds and rodents is likely to be restricted [31, 79]. In contrast, lower differences between pollen and seed migration rates were found for wild barley. Gene flow by pollen is estimated to be only four times greater than interpopulation gene flow by seeds. Opportunities for interpopulation pollen dispersal in such a highly self-pollinating species are expected to be rare, and it is not surprising that pollen and seed flow should be of the same order of magnitude for this species [31, 81]. Forest trees species are generally outbreeding, whereby levels of pollen flow versus seed flow (r) may vary according to the potential distances of dispersal related to mechanism of pollen and seed dispersal.

By itself, the mating system does not alter allele frequencies but does affect the relative proportions of different genotypes in populations, which under some circumstances deeply influences the viability and vigor of offspring [1]. Inbreeding coefficient (F_{IS}) measures the fractional reduction in heterozygosity relative to a random mating population with the same allele frequencies. Even though genotypic frequencies in natural populations of forest trees often approximate those expected under random mating, mating systems that depart from random mating do occur and have important implications. Individuals of most temperate forest trees are bisexual and have the capacity for self-fertilization. In addition, nearby trees may be related (e.g., siblings originating from seeds of the same mother tree), providing opportunity for mating between relatives. Therefore, forest trees typically have mixed mating systems, whereby many and perhaps most mates are paired essentially at random.

There is also some mating between genetically related individuals, which occurs more often than expected from random pairings [1]. Inbreeding is of great significance to the genetic makeup of both natural populations and breeding populations of forest trees because it has two major consequences: (1) in comparison to random mating, inbreeding increases the frequency of homozygous offspring at the expense of heterozygotes and (2) mating between close relatives is usually detrimental to the survival and growth of offspring, called inbreeding depression. Therefore, the magnitude of inbreeding among parent trees used to produce seed for reforestation, such as in seed production areas or seed orchards, is of great practical concern [1].

In previous section, we presented three ways to estimate inbreeding coefficient that has different statistical power and assumptions: (1) F_{IS} estimated from AMOVA could be used as first measure of inbreeding for a determinate hierarchical structure, (2) F_{IS} estimated by a Bayesian approximation is a measure statistically more powerful to determine the level of inbreeding in a population, and (3) F_{IS} could be estimated considering null alleles when certain levels of null alleles were determined in the microsatellite loci considered in order to determine the proportion of homozygote genotypes consequence of inbreeding than homozygotes caused by null alleles.

The current distribution and population structure and potential fate in the future are better understood from the knowledge of historical distribution, postglacial phylogeography, and evolution of a species [82]. Regarding to the assessment of demographic history using the F_S neutrality test for population, F_S statistic takes a large negative value within a population affected by expansion due to an excess of rare haplotypes (recent mutations). Significance of the test must to be calculated with data bootstraps. A F_S statistic with $p(F_S) < 0.02$ ($\alpha = 0.05$, due to a particular behavior of this statistics, [56]) is considered as an evidence of population expansion.

Whereas using D_{Tajima} neutrality test, a D_{Tajima} statistic is expected to be close to zero in a population of constant size while statistically significant negative values indicate a sudden expansion of population size and positive values indicate population subdivision or recent bottlenecks. The statistical significance of D_{Tajima} is tested generating random samples using a coalescent simulation algorithm under the hypothesis of population balance. The p-value for D_{Tajima} is obtained by the ratio of random D_{Tajima} less than or equal to the observed D_{Tajima}. Computer-intensive statistical methods have been developed to extract as much information from the data as possible and to provide a flexible framework within which complex models of population history can be handled [83].

Approximate Bayesian computation is a computer-intensive method that has wide applicability, where populations diverge genetically through time, influenced by random genetic drift and migration, ABC uses summary statistics measured from microsatellite loci to make inferences about demographic parameters in different population models. The method can be used to infer effective sizes of current and ancestral populations, immigration rates, splitting times, and tree topology [83].

As a final recommendation, researchers must define which is/are the problem/s and question/s that they would resolve with their study before starting a study with molecular marker in a native forest tree species. This is a founder requisite to determine sampling design, to decide molecular markers to use (keeping in mind the information required and laboratory work to obtain molecular data), and appropriate statistical analysis to obtain the required information. Of course, the researchers must pay attention to biological features of the studied species at the moment to design the study and back to these features at the moment to interpret the results of statistical analyses in a biological context.

7. Conclusion

This chapter helps to researchers that are not familiarizing with statistical methods and population genetics theories to analyze nuclear and chloroplast microsatellite data. Methods allow quantification of genetic variation and genetic structure in native forest species while theories allow knowledge about the past and the present genetic states of populations for making inferences about the future of these populations.

Acknowledgements

M. E. Barrandeguy and M. V. García wishes to thank to Consejo Nacional de Investigaciones Científicas y Técnicas (CONICET). This work has been funded by grant: PICTO UNaM 2011 N°0133 from Agencia Nacional de Promoción Científica y Tecnológica (AGENCIA) and Universidad Nacional de Misiones (UNaM) to M. V. García.

Author details

Maria Eugenia Barrandeguy[1,2,3*] and Maria Victoria Garcia[1,2,3]

*Address all correspondence to: ebarran@fceqyn.unam.edu.ar

1 Departamento de Genética, Facultad de Ciencias Exactas, Químicas y Naturales, Universidad Nacional de Misiones, Argentina

2 Instituto de Biología Subtropical Nodo Posadas (UNaM, CONICET) Posadas, Argentina

3 Consejo Nacional de Investigaciones Científicas y Técnicas (CONICET), Argentina

References

[1] White TW, Adams WT, Neale DB. Forest Genetics. 1st ed. Cambridge, USA: CAB International Publishing; 2007;702 p. DOI: 10.1079/9781845932855.0000

[2] Finkeldey R, Leinemann L, Gailing O. Molecular genetic tools to infer the origin of forest plants and wood. Applied Microbiology Biotechnology. 2010;85:1251–1258. DOI: 10.1007/s00253-009-2328-6

[3] Finkeldey R, Ziehe M. Genetic implications of silvicultural regimes. Forest Ecology Management. 2004;197:231–244. DOI: 10.1016/j.foreco.2004.05.036

[4] Krutovsky KV, Neale DB. Nucleotide diversity and linkage disequilibrium in cold-hardiness- and wood quality-related candidate genes in Douglas fir. Genetics. 2005;171:2029–2041. DOI: 10.1534/genetics.105.044420

[5] Rossetto M. Sourcing SSR markers from related plant species. In: Henry EJ, editor. Plant Genotyping: The DNA Fingerprinting of Plants. 1st ed. Oxon UK: CAB Plant International; 2001;pp. 211–224. DOI: 10.1079/9780851995151.0000

[6] Barbará T, Palma-Silva C, Paggi GM, Bered F, Fay MF, Lexer C. Cross-species transfer of nuclear microsatellite markers: potential and limitations. Molecular Ecology. 2007;16:3759–3767. DOI: 10.1111/j.1365-294X.2007.03439.x

[7] Streiff R, Labbe T, Bacilieri R, Steinkellner H, Glossl J, Kremer A. Within-population genetic structure in *Quercus robur* L. and *Quercus petrea* (Matt.) Liebl. assessed with isozymes and microsatellites. Molecular Ecology. 1998;7:317–328. DOI: 10.1046/j.1365-294X.1998.00360.x

[8] Degen B, Streiff R, Ziegenhagen B. Comparative study of genetic variation and differentiation of two pedunculate oak (*Quercus robur*) stands using microsatellite and allozyme loci. Heredity. 1999;83:597–603. DOI: 10.1038/sj.hdy.6886220

[9] Fernández JF, Sork VL, Gallego G, López J, Bohorques A, Tohme J. Cross-amplification of microsatellite loci in a neotropical *Quercus* species and standardization of DNA extraction from mature leaves dried in silica gel. Plant Molecular Biology Reporter. 2000;18:397a–397e. DOI: 10.1007/BF02825070

[10] Mottura MC, Finkeldey R, Verga AR, Gailing O. Development and characterization of microsatellite markers for *Prosopis chilensis* and *Prosopis flexuosa* and cross-species amplification. Molecular Ecology Notes. 2005;5:487–489. DOI: 10.1111/j.1471-8286.2005.00965.x

[11] Yasodha R, Ghosh M, Sumathi R, Gurumurthi K. Cross-species amplification of eucalyptus SSR markers in Casuarinaceae. Acta Botanica Croatia. 2005;64:115–120.

[12] Moreira PA, Souza SAS, Oliveira EA, Araújo NH, Fernandes GW, Oliviera DA. Charaterization of nine tranferred SSR markers in the tropical tree species *Enterolobium*

contortisiliquum (Fabaceae). Genetics and Molecular Research. 2012;11:2338–2342. DOI: 10.4238/2012

[13] Dayanandan S, Bawa KS, Kesseli R. Conservation of microsatellites among tropical trees (Leguminosae). American Journal of Botany. 1997;84:1658–1663.

[14] Moreno AC, Marchelli P, Vendramin GG, Gallo LA. Cross transferability of SSRs to five species of Araucariaceae: a useful tool for population genetic studies in *Araucaria araucana*. Forest Systems. 2011;20:303–314.

[15] Liu J, Gao LM, Li DZ, Zhang DQ, Möller M. Cross-species amplification and development of new microsatellite loci for *Taxus wallichiana* (Taxaceae). American Journal of Botany. 2011;98:e70–e73. DOI: 10.3732/ajb.1000445

[16] Provan J, Powell W, Hollingsworth PM. Chloroplast microsatellites: new tools for studies in plant ecology and evolution. Trends in Ecology and Evolution. 2001;16:142–147. DOI: 10.1016/S0169-5347(00)02097-8

[17] Weising K, Gardner R. A set of conserved PCR primers for the analysis of simple sequence repeat polymorphism in chloroplast genomes of dicotyledonous. Genome. 1999;42:9–19. DOI: 10.1139/gen-42-1-9

[18] Powell W, Machray GC, Provan J. Polymorphism revealed by simple sequence repeats. Trends in Plant Science. 1996;1:209–245. DOI: 10.1016/1360-1385(96)86898-1

[19] Squirrell J, Hollingsworth PM, Woodhead M, Russell J, Lowe AJ, Gibby M, Powell W. How much effort is required to isolate nuclear microsatellites from plants? Molecular Ecology. 2003;12:1339–1348. DOI: 10.1046/j.1365-294X.2003.01825.x

[20] Barrandeguy ME, Prinz K, García MV, Finkeldey R. Development of microsatellite markers for *Anadenanthera colubrina* var. *cebil* (Fabaceae), a native tree from South America. American Journal of Botany. 2012;99:e372–e374. DOI: 10.3732/ajb.1200078

[21] Fisher D, Bachmann K. Microsatellite enrichment in organisms with large genomes (*Allium cepa* L.). Biotechniques. 1998;24:796–800.

[22] Prinz K, Schie S, Debener T, Hensen I, Weising K. Microsatellite markers for *Spergularia media* (L.) C. Presl. (Caryophyllaceae) and their cross-species transferability. Molecular Ecology Notes. 2009;9:1424–1426. DOI: 10.1111/j.1755-0998.2009.02680.x

[23] Zalapa JE, Cuevas H, Zhu H, Steffan S, Senalik D, Zeldin E, Mccown B, Harbut R, Simon P. Using next-generation sequencing approaches to isolate simple sequence repeat (SSR) loci in the plant sciences. American Journal of Botany. 2012;99:93–208. DOI: 10.3732/ajb.1100394

[24] Putman AI, Carbone I. Challenges in analysis and interpretation of microsatellite data for population genetic studies. Ecology and Evolution. 2014;4:4399–4428. DOI: 10.1002/ece3.1305

[25] Peakall R, Smouse PE. Genalex 6.5: genetic analysis in Excel. Population genetic software for teaching and research—an update. Bioinformatics. 2012;28:2537–2539. DOI: 10.1093/bioinformatics/bts460

[26] Raymond M, Rousset F. GENEPOP (version 1.2): population genetics software for exact test and ecumenicism. Journal of Heredity. 1995;86:248–249.

[27] Van Oosterhout C, Hutchinson WF, Wills DPM, Shipley P. MICRO-CHECKER: software for identifying and correcting genotyping errors in microsatellite data. Molecular Ecology Notes. 2004;4:535–538. DOI: 10.1111/j.1471-8286.2004.00684.x

[28] Avise JC. Molecular Markers, Natural History and Evolution. 2nd ed. Sunderland, Massachusetts: Sinauer Associates; 2004;684 p. DOI: 10.1007/978-1-4615-2381-9

[29] Linhart YB, Grant MC. Evolutionary significance of local genetic differentiation in plants. Annual Review of Ecology and Systematics. 1996;27:237–277. DOI: 10.1146/annurev.ecolsys.27.1.237

[30] Sork VL, Nason J, Campbell DR, Fernandez JF. Landscape approaches to historical and contemporary gene flow in plants. Trends in Ecology and Evolution. 1999;14:219–224. DOI: 10.1016/S0169-5347(98)01585-7

[31] Ennos RA. Estimating the relative rates of pollen and seed migration among plant populations. Heredity. 1994;72:250–259. DOI: 10.1038/hdy.1994.35

[32] Barrandeguy ME, García MV, Prinz K, Rivera Pomar R, Finkeldey R. Genetic structure of disjunct Argentinean populations of the subtropical tree *Anadenanthera colubrina* var. *cebil* (Fabaceae). Plant Systematic and Evolution. 2014;300:1693–1705. DOI: 10.1007/s00606-014-0995-y

[33] Selkoe KA, Toonen RJ. Microsatellites for ecologists: a practical guide to using and evaluating microsatellite markers. Ecology Letters. 2006;9:615–629. DOI: 10.1111/j.1461-0248.2006.00889.x

[34] Kimura M, Crow JF. The number of alleles that can be maintained in a finite population. Genetics. 1964;49:725–738.

[35] Barton NH, Slatkin M. A quasi-equilibrium theory of the distribution of rare alleles in a subdivided population. Heredity. 1986;56:409–415. DOI: 10.1038/hdy.1986.63

[36] Foulley J, Ollivier L. Estimating allelic richness and its diversity. Livestock Science. 2006;101:150–158. DOI: 10.1371/journal.pone.0115203

[37] Nei M. Analysis of gene diversity in subdivided populations. Proceedings of the National Academy of Sciences. 1973;70:3321–3323.

[38] Nagylaki T. Fixation indices in subdivided populations. Genetics. 1998;148:1325–1332.

[39] Nei M. Estimation of average heterozygosity and genetic distance from a small number of individuals. Genetics. 1978;89:583–590.

[40] Nei M. Molecular Evolutionary Genetics. New York: Columbia University Press; 1987;512 p.

[41] Templeton AR. Population Genetics and Microevolutionary Theory. New Jersey: Wiley-Liss Publication; 2006;720 p. DOI: 10.1002/0470047356

[42] Bandelt HJ, Forster P, Rohl A. Median-joining networks for inferring intraspecific phylogenies. Molecular Biology and Evolution. 1999;16:37–48. DOI: 10.1093/oxfordjournals.molbev.a026036

[43] Pritchard JK, Stephens M, Donnelly P. Inference of population structure using multilocus genotype data. Genetics. 2000;155:945–959.

[44] Corander J, Sirén J, Arjas E. Bayesian spatial modelling of genetic population structure. Computational Statistics. 2008;23:111–129. DOI: 10.1007/s00180-007-0072-x

[45] Evanno G, Regnaut S, Goudet J. Detecting the number of clusters of individuals using the software STRUCTURE: a simulation study. Molecular Ecology. 2005;14:2611–2620. DOI: 10.1111/j.1365-294X.2005.02553.x

[46] Excoffier L, Smouse P, Quattro J. Analysis of molecular variance inferred from metric distances among DNA haplotypes: application to human mitochondrial DNA restriction data. Genetics. 1992;131:479–491.

[47] Wright S. The genetical structure of populations. Annals of Eugenetics. 1951;15:323–354.

[48] Weir BS, Cockerham CC. Estimating F-statistics for the analysis of population structure. Evolution. 1984;38:1358–1370.

[49] Freeland JR. Molecular Ecology. 1st ed. England: Wiley-Liss; 2005;388 p.

[50] Slatkin M. Gene flow in natural populations. Annual Review of Ecology and Systematics. 1985;16:393–430.

[51] Holsinger KE, Lewis PO. University of Connecticut, Storrs, Connecticut USA. Hickory: a package for analysis of population genetic data version 1.1. Department of Ecology and Evolutionary Biology [Internet]. 2003. Available from: http://darwin.eeb.uconn.edu/hickory/hickory.html [Accessed: 2013-07-13].

[52] Chybicki IJ, Burczyk J. Simultaneous estimation of null alleles and inbreeding coefficients. Heredity. 2009;100:106–113. DOI: 10.1093/jhered/esn088

[53] Navascués M, Vaxevanidou Z, González-Martínez SC, Climent J, Gil L, Emerson BC. Chloroplast microsatellites reveal colonization and metapopulation dynamics in the

Canary Island pine. Molecular Ecology. 2006;15:2691–2698. DOI: 10.1111/j.1365-294X.2006.02960.x

[54] Emerson BC, Paradis E, Thebaud C. Revealing the demographic histories of species using DNA sequences. Trends in Ecology and Evolution. 2001;16:707–716. DOI: 10.1016/S0169-5347(01)02305-9

[55] Fu YX. Statistical tests of neutrality of mutations against population growth, hitchhiking and background selection. Genetics. 1997;147:915–925.

[56] Pybus OG, Shapiro B. Natural selection and adaptation of molecular sequences. In: Lemey P, Salemi M, Vandamme A, editors. The Phylogenetic Handbook. 2nd ed. Cambridge: Cambridge University Press; 2009;pp. 407–418. DOI: 10.1017/CBO9780511819049.015

[57] Beaumont MA, Nielsen R, Robert C, Hey J, Gaggiotti O, Knowles L, Estoup A, Panchal M, Corander J, Hickerson M, Sisson SA, Fagundes N, Chikhi L, Beerli P, Vitalis R, Cornuet JM, Huelsenbeck J, Foll M, Yang Z, Rousset F, Balding D, Excoffier L. In defence of model-based inference in phylogeography. Molecular Ecology. 2010;19:436–446. DOI: 10.1111/j.1365-294X.2009.04515.x

[58] Excoffier L, Lischer H. Arlequin suite ver 3.5: a new series of programs to perform population genetics analyses under Linux and Windows. Molecular Ecology. 2010;10:564–567. DOI: 10.1111/j.1755-0998.2010.02847.x

[59] Szpiech ZA, Jakobsson M, Rosenberg NA. ADZE: a rarefaction approach for counting alleles private to combinations of populations. Bioinformatics. 2008;24:2498–2504. DOI: 10.1093/bioinformatics/btn478

[60] Goudet J. FSTAT (version 2.9.3.2): a computer program to calculate F statistics. Heredity. 1995;86:485–486.

[61] Perrier X, Jacquemoud-Collet JP. DARwin software [Internet]. 2006. Available from: http://darwin.cirad.fr/ [Accessed: 2016-04-28].

[62] Leigh J, Bryant D. Popart: full-feature software for haplotype network construction. Methods in Ecology and Evolution. 2015;6:1110–1116. DOI: 10.1111/2041-210X.12410

[63] Forster JW, Jones ES, Kolliker R, Drayton CM, Dumsday JL, Dupal MP, Guthridge KM, Mahoney NL, Van Zijll de Jong E, Smith KF. Development and implementation of molecular markers for forage crop improvement. In: Spangenberg G, editor. Molecular Breeding of Forage Crops. Netherlands, Dordrecht: Springer; 2001;pp. 101–133. DOI: 10.1007/978-94-015-9700-5_6

[64] Earl DA, vonHoldt BM. STRUCTURE HARVESTER: a website and program for visualizing structure output and implementing the Evanno method. Conservation Genetics Resources. 2011;4:359–361. DOI: 10.1007/s12686-011-9548-7

[65] Cornuet J, Pudlo P, Veyssier J, Dehne-Garcia A, Gautier M, Leblois R, Marin JM, Estoup A. DIYABC v2.0: a software to make approximate Bayesian computation inferences about population history using single nucleotide polymorphism, DNA sequence and microsatellite data. Bioinformatics. 2014;30:1187–1189. DOI: 10.1093/bioinformatics/btt763

[66] Schlötterer C. Evolutionary dynamics of microsatellite DNA. Chromosoma. 2000;109:365–371.

[67] Hamrick JL, Godt MJW, Sherman-Broyles SL. Factors influencing levels of genetic diversity in woody plant species. New Forests. 1992;6:95–124. DOI: 10.1007/BF00120641

[68] Finkeldey R, Hattemer HH. Tropical Forest Genetics. 1st ed. Heidelberg: Springer; 2007;316 p. DOI: 10.1007/978-3-540-37398-8

[69] Ouborg NJ, Piquot Y, Groenendael MV. Population genetics, molecular markers and the study of dispersal in plants. Journal of Ecology. 1999;87:551–668.

[70] Wright S. Evolution and the Genetics of Population, Variability Within and Among Natural Populations. Chicago: The University of Chicago Press; 1978;590 p.

[71] Hamrick JL, Murawski DA, Nason JD. The influence of seed dispersal mechanisms on the genetic structure of tropical tree populations. Vegetatio. 1993;107:281–297.

[72] Zhan QQ, Wang JF, Gong X, Peng H. Patterns of chloroplast DNA variation in *Cycas debaoensis* (Cycadaceae): conservation implications. Conservation Genetics. 2011;12:959–970. DOI: 10.1007/s10592-011-0198-9

[73] Petit RJ, Duminil J, Fineschi S, Hampe A, Salvini D, Vendramin GG. Comparative organization of chloroplast, mitochondrial and nuclear diversity in plant populations. Molecular Ecology. 2005;14:689–701. DOI: 10.1111/j.1365-294X.2004.02410.x

[74] McCauley DE. The use of chloroplast DNA polymorphism in studies of gene flow in plants. Trends in Ecology and Evolution. 1995;10:198–202.

[75] Ndiade-Bourobou D, Hardy OJ, Favreau B, Moussavou H, Nzengue E, Mignots A, Bouvet JM. Long distance seed and pollen dispersal inferred from spatial genetic structure in the very low-density rainforest tree, *Baillonella toxisperma* Pierre, in Central Africa. Molecular Ecology. 2010;19:4949–4962. DOI: 10.1111/j.1365-294X.2010.04864.x

[76] Slatkin M, Barton NH. A comparison of three indirect methods for estimating average levels of gene flow. Evolution. 1989;43:1349–1368.

[77] Planter EA. Flujo Génico: métodos para estimarlo y marcadores moleculares. In: Eguiarte L, Souza V, Aguirre X, editors. Ecología Molecular. 1st ed. México: INECC; 2007;pp. 49–61.

[78] Bossart DL, Prowell DP. Genetic estimates of population structure and gene flow: limitations, lessons and new directions. Trends in Ecology and Evolution. 1998;13:202–206.

[79] Sork VL. Examination of seed dispersal and survival in red oak, *Quercus Rubra* (Fagaceae), using metal tagged acorns. Ecology. 1984;65:1020–1022.

[80] Brown AHD, Zohary D, Nevo E. Outcrossing rates and heterozygosity in natural populations of *Hordeum spontaneum* Koch in Israel. Heredity. 1978;41:49–62.

[81] Zinck JWR, Rajora OP. Post-glacial phylogeography and evolution of a wide-ranging highly-exploited keystone forest tree, eastern white pine (*Pinus Strobus*) in North America: single refugium, multiple routes. BMC Evolutionary Biology. 2016;16:56. DOI: 10.1186/s12862-016-0624-1

[82] Zinck JWR, Rajora OP. Post-glacial phylogeography and evolution of a wide-ranging highly-exploited keystone forest tree, eastern white pine (Pinus strobus) in North America: single refugium, multiple routes. BMC Evolutionary Biology. 2016; 16 (1): 56. DOI: 10.1186/s12862-016-0624-1.

[83] Beaumont M. Joint determination of topology, divergence time and immigration in population trees. In: Matsumura S, Forster P, Renfrew C, editors. Simulations, Genetics and Human Prehistory. Cambridge: McDonald Institute for Archaeological Research; 2008. p. 134–154.

Chapter 4

Microsatellite Markers Confirm Self-Pollination and Autogamy in Wild Populations of *Vanilla mexicana* Mill. (syn. *V. inodora*) (Orchidaceae) in the Island of Guadeloupe

Rodolphe Laurent Gigant, Narindra Rakotomanga, Chloe Goulié, Denis Da Silva, Nicolas Barre, Gervais Citadelle, Daniel Silvestre, Michel Grisoni and Pascale Besse

Additional information is available at the end of the chapter

http://dx.doi.org/10.5772/64674

Abstract

The study aimed at evaluating the mating system of *Vanilla mexicana* (Orchidaceae) in natural populations in the island of Guadeloupe. A total of 132 *V. mexicana* samples were collected from 12 sites in Guadeloupe (Basse-Terre). Five other samples coming from Martinique and Mexico completed our analyses. Reproductive biology experiments excluding pollinators with bagged flowers revealed 53.9% fruit set, a value identical to the natural fruit set measured in the populations. These results suggested that *V. mexicana,* unlike most *Vanilla* species, was reproducing by self-pollination and autogamy. Due to lack of specific DNA markers for *V. mexicana,* microsatellite markers, previously developed in other *Vanilla* species, were used for the genetic analyses. Only 6 out of the 33 markers tested were transferable and polymorphic in *V. mexicana*. A panel of 51 *V. mexicana* samples genotyped with 3 polymorphic loci was finally retained for Guadeloupe population genetic analyses. A heterozygote deficiency was detected, and the selfing rate was estimated to 74%. These results confirmed the reproductive biology results as self-pollination and autogamy were the most likely explanation for this deficit. Results were compared to those from allogamous wild *Vanilla* species and discussed in the light of suggested existence of a pollinator for *V. mexicana* in other areas (Mexico).

Keywords: autogamy, genetic diversity, Guadeloupe, microsatellites, *Vanilla mexicana*

1. Introduction

Knowledge and management of agricultural genetic resources (AGR) and of their wild relative species [referred to as Crop Wild Relatives (CWR)] are of major importance to ensure the preservation of natural resources, development of sustainable agriculture and food security in a global climate change context. The extremely low genetic diversity in the cultivated vanilla species *V. planifolia* G. Jacks. worldwide has been demonstrated [1–5], and this genetic erosion is a major limit for genetic improvement, particularly with regard to pathogen outbreaks. Vanilla wild relatives can be used for breeding interspecific hybrid varieties. For example, resistance to the virus CymMV was reported for *V. pompona* Schiede [6], and resistance to the fungus *Fusarium* was reported for *V. pompona, V. phaeantha* Rchb. f., *V. barbellata* Rchb. f., *V. aphylla* Blume, *V. andamanica* Rolfe, *V. crenulata* Rolfe, and *V. bahiana* Hoehne [7–10]. As *V. planifolia* wild populations, which are in danger of extinction in Mexico [11], some of the populations of vanilla wild relatives are threatened by deforestation, over-collection, and climate change [12]. This is the case for example for *V. humblotii* Rchb. f., endangered (EN) in Mayotte [13]. Vanilla wild relatives therefore deserve special attention. To date, there is still an important lack of knowledge of genetics and ecology, including breeding systems of vanilla CWR, despite their importance for the improvement of vanilla.

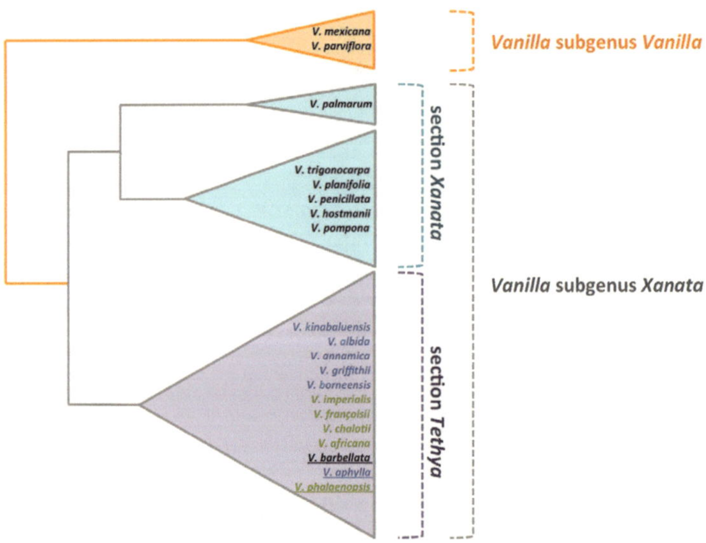

Figure 1. Synthetic representation of the phylogenetic groups in the genus *Vanilla* in relation to the new taxonomic classification proposed by Soto Arenas and Cribb [16]. The 20 species groups defined [16] are also indicated within each clade (without phylogenetic meaning in their order of appearance). American species are in black, African species in green, and Asian species in blue, and aphyllous species are underlined.

Vanilla mexicana Mill. is a distant wild relative of the cultivated vanilla species *Vanilla planifolia*. The *Vanilla* Plum. ex Mill. genus is a primitive lineage in the Orchidaceae family, Vanilloideae subfamily, Vanilleae tribe, and Vanillinae subtribe [14, 15]. In 2010, Soto Arenas and

http://dx.doi.org/10.5772/64674

Cribb [16] proposed a revision of the early taxonomic classification by Portères [17] of the genus *Vanilla*, based on eco-morphological and phylogenetic data, which has been confirmed by other independent studies [18]. This major work proposed taxonomic keys to resolve the 100+ species recognized in the genus into 20 very handy morphological informal species groups, which can in turn be classified phylogenetically into two subgenera, one being the subgenus *Vanilla* including *V. mexicana* (**Figure 1**). The subgenus *Vanilla* comprises two species morphological groups: the *V. parviflora* and *V. mexicana* groups. The *V. mexicana* group includes the species *V. mexicana*, but also *V. costaricensis* Soto Arenas ined, *V. guianensis* Splitg., *V. inodora* Schiede, *V. martinezii* Soto Arenas ined, *V. methonica* Rchb. f. & Warsz., *V. oroana* Dodson, and *V. ovata* Rolfe. These species are distributed in the neotropics from South America, Central America to southern Mexico [16]. Although distinct in this revision [16], but as suggested [17] and confirmed [19], *V. mexicana* and *V. inodora* should be considered as synonymous species.

Geographically, *V. mexicana* is distributed in the northern part of South America (Venezuela, Trinidad, and Tobago), Central America, the Caribbean islands (Cuba, Puerto Rico, Haïti and Guadeloupe), towards Florida in North America [16, 17] (**Figure 2**). Within our current efforts to determine the reproductive biology and genetic diversity in vanilla CWR, which led us so far to study *V. roscheri* Rchb. f. in South Africa [20] and *V. humblotii* in Mayotte [13, 21], we focused on wild populations of *V. mexicana* occurring in the island of Guadeloupe (French west indies) to unravel its mating system.

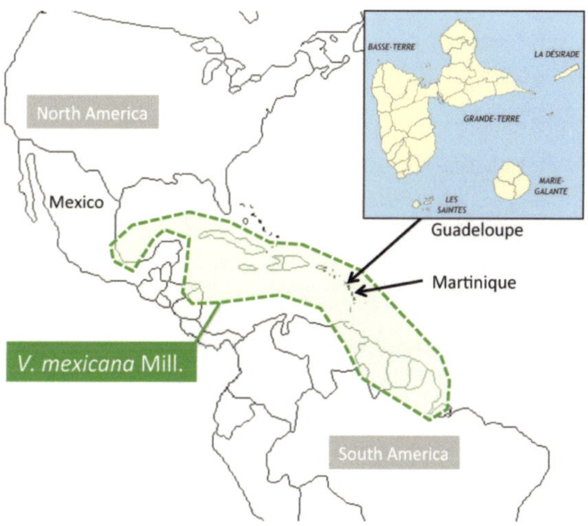

Figure 2. Geographical distribution of *V. mexicana* (from [16, 17]).

The vast majority of *Vanilla* species displays a mixed reproductive mode [1, 4] with both asexual and sexual reproduction. *Vanilla* species are hemi-epiphytic vines, and asexual reproduction is performed by means of natural stem cuttings [1]. It is a very efficient way for the plant to develop settlements and implies that vanilla plants are long-lived as they can indefinitely propagate. In *V. humblotii* in the island of Mayotte, it was shown that 12.5% of the individuals in the Sohoa forest were vegetative clones deriving from vegetative reproduction [13], a similar value to what was observed in Puerto Rico for *V. claviculata* Sw. and *V. barbellata* with 6–25% vegetative clones [22]. Spatial genetic analysis also revealed that vegetative clones showed a phalanx (aggregated) distribution and the average maximal clonal patch size was measured at 4.6 ± 2.7 m in *V. humblotii* [13]. However, these patches can be much bigger as observed in Mexico for *V. planifolia* G. Jackson with the same vegetative clone covering up to 0.2 ha [4, 23].

In *Vanilla* species, sexual mating system is either allogamous or autogamous (**Table 1**), the most common system being allogamous and pollinator-dependent. Allogamous species are, however, self-compatible as demonstrated by manual self-pollination experiments giving up to 100% fruit set in *V. barbellata, V. claviculata, V. dilloniana* Correll, and *V. poitaei* Rchb. f. [24], *V. chamissonis* Klotzsch [25], *V. roscheri* [20], *V. humblotii* [13] and many other species of the genus (our unpublished self-pollination experiments in the shade-houses of BRC Vatel [26]). Manual self-pollination is also the method used to produce fruits in *V. planifolia* cultivation areas in the absence of natural pollinators. Allogamy is only guaranteed because of the floral structure presenting a rostellum, acting as a physical barrier between male and female reproductive organs [4]. Pollinators are needed to ensure pollination of allogamous species. As reviewed in [4], *Vanilla* subgenus *Xanata* section *Xanata* American species are most likely mainly pollinated by Euglossine bees.

Vanilla subgenus	Section	Taxonomic group	Species	Natural fruit set (%)	Mating system
Xanata	*Tethya*	*V. africana*	*V. crenulata*	0.0[a,b]	Allo
		V. barbellata	*V. barbellata*	18.2[c]	Allo
		V. barbellata	*V. claviculata*	17.9[c]	Allo
		V. barbellata	*V. dilloniana*	14.5[c]	Allo
		V. barbellata	*V. poitaei*	6.4[c]	Allo
		V. phalaenopsis	*V. humblotii*	0.8[d]	Allo
		V. phalaenopsis	*V. roscheri*	26.3[e]	Allo
Xanata	*Xanata*	*V. pompona*	*V. chamissonis*	15.0[f]	Allo
		V. pompona	*V. pompona* ssp. *grandiflora*	0.9[g]	Allo
		V. planifolia	*V. cristato-callosa*	6.6[g]	Allo
		V. planifolia	*V. planifolia*	0.1–1.0[c,h,i,j]	Allo
		V. planifolia	*V. ribeiroi*	1.1[g]	Allo
		V. palmarum	*V. bicolor*	42.5[k]–71.0[g]	Auto
		V. palmarum	*V. palmarum*	76.0[h]	Auto
Vanilla		*V. mexicana*	*V. guianensis*	78.0[g]	Auto
		V. mexicana	*V. martinezii*	53.0[m]	Auto
		V. parviflora	*V. edwallii*	15.0[l]	Allo

References cited are: [a]Johansson 1974 as cited in [b][12]; [c][24]; [d][13]; [e][20]; [f][25]; [g][28]; [h][23]; [i][29]; [j][30]; [k][31]; [l][32]; and [m][11].

Table 1. Natural fruit set of some allogamous and autogamous *Vanilla* species (completed from [4]).

In Africa (subgenus *Xanata* section *Tethya* species), it was recently demonstrated that pollinators might be Allodapine bees [13, 20]. On the other hand, some species of the genus, such as *V. palmarum*, *V. bicolor*, *V. guianensis* Splitg., *V. martinezii* Soto Arenas were determined to be autogamous (reviewed in [4] and **Table 1**). *Vanilla* autogamous species are characterized by much higher fruit sets (53.0% for *V. martinezii* to 78.0% for *V. guianensis)* than allogamous species (0.0% for *V. crenulata* to 26.3% for *V. roscheri)* (**Table 1**). These fruit sets are in accordance with known data on tropical orchids showing around 77.0% fruit set for autogamous species and less than 20.0% for allogamous species [24]. *V. savannarum* Britton, *V. griffithii* Rchb. f., and *V. mexicana* were also suggested as autogamous due to the high fruit sets reported [11, 12, 27]. Soto Arenas and Dressler [11], however, also mentioned that in Mexico, besides *V. mexicana* populations with high fruit sets, others have fruit sets as low as 2.5%. *V. mexicana* seems therefore to present also allogamy with potential pollinators supposedly being carpenter bees *Xylocopa* sp. [11, 12]. Measures of natural fruit set in wild populations, in addition to reproductive biology experiments, should therefore give us insights on the mating system of *V. mexicana*.

The use of codominant neutral genetic markers such as microsatellites to perform genetic analyses on natural populations [33, 34] is also a method of choice to estimate mating system parameters such as inbreeding rate [35–38]. As no specific markers were available for *V. mexicana*, we used microsatellite markers previously developed in other *Vanilla* species: the cultivated species *V. planifolia* (an American species from the genus *Vanilla* subgenus *Xanata* section *Xanata*) [2], *V. humblotii* and *V. roscheri* (African species from the genus *Vanilla* subgenus *Xanata* section *Tethya*) [21]. We performed genetic analyses and conducted reproductive biology experiments on *V. mexicana* wild populations from the island of Guadeloupe (French West Indies) to unravel its mating system.

2. *V. mexicana* mating system in Guadeloupe

2.1. Material and methods

2.1.1. Study species

V. mexicana is a vigorous hemi-epiphytic vine with a long stem reaching 10 m. Leaves are longer than internodes (7.5 cm long). Inflorescences are 3–12 cm long racemes bearing 3–5 flowers. Petals and sepals are greenish and very undulate, and labellum is white with a yellow crest. Fruits are nonaromatic, 10–25 cm long and thin [11, 17, 19] (**Figure 3**).

To precisely record morphological descriptors of the studied species, characters were measured to the nearest 0.01 mm using a digital caliper. Floral characters were measured from 11 flowers collected on three sites [Habituée (5), Mazeau (3), and Moreau (3)]: petal and sepal length and width as well as labellum, column and ovary length, width and thickness. The length and diameter of five eight-month-old fruits were also measured from one individual plant (Mazeau). Vegetative characters were assessed (four measures per plant on rank 4–7 leaves and internodes) on 16 plants from four sites [Mazeau- Solitude (6), Moreau (4),

Desbordes (3), and Habituée (3)]: internode length, stem diameter, leaf length, leaf width at 43 mm of the apex, and leaf maximum width (LMW).

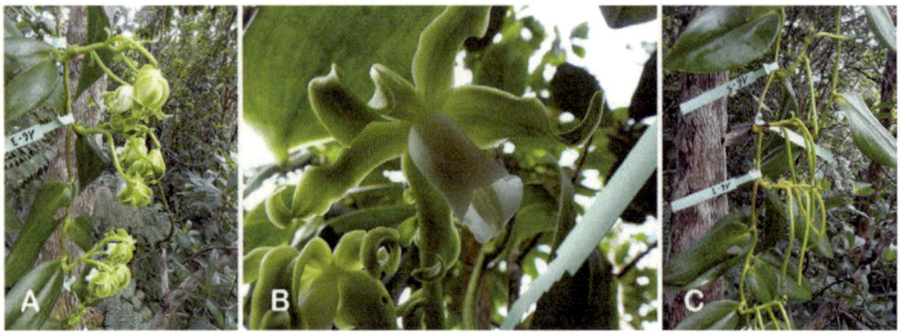

Figure 3. *V. mexicana* inflorescences (A), flower (B), and 1-month-old fruits (C). Photographs by Nicolas Barre.

2.1.2. Study site

Sampling was performed in 2013 by the Association Guadeloupéenne d'Orchidophilie (AGO) mandated by the National Park of Guadeloupe (PNG). According to the inventory of *V. mexicana* in Guadeloupe, based on 22 traces representing 135 km around the Basse-Terre mountain in Guadeloupe [39], *V. mexicana* is mainly found in windward (west) mid-altitude (150–750 m) areas with a preferred altitudinal zone of 300–350 m (**Figure 4**). *V. mexicana* was most frequently found in secondary forests climbing on the following tree species : *Miconia mirabilis, Swietenia macrophylla* (Mahogany), and *Cyathea muricata* (Tree fern). *V. mexicana*

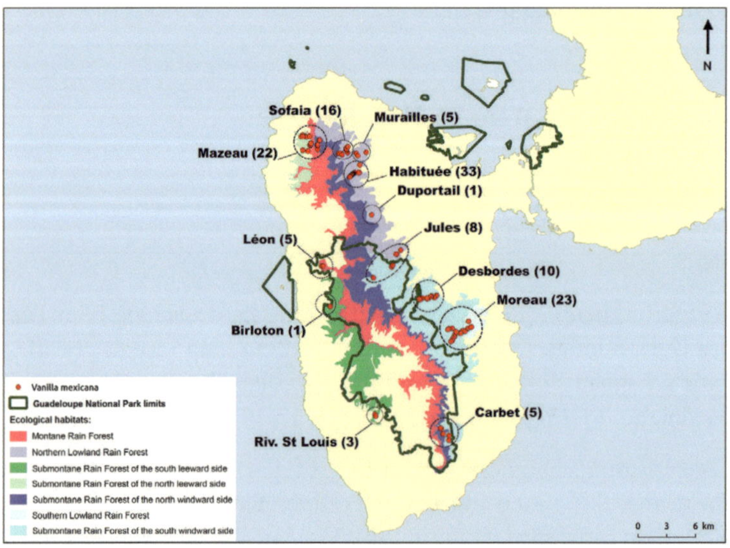

Figure 4. Red dots show the localization of the 132 *V. mexicana* accessions collected from 12 sites in Basse-Terre (Guadeloupe) with numbers of individuals in parenthesis. Ecological habitats [40] and the borders of the National Park of Guadeloupe are indicated.

preferably grows under medium shading (25–50%), and as a consequence, it is found mainly in opened habitats such as along forest tracks [39].

2.1.3. *Plant sampling*

Leaves were sampled from 132 accessions of *V. mexicana* collected from 12 different sites (populations) in Basse-Terre (**Figure 4**). Samples were dehydrated using silica gel for storage. Individual samples were deposited in the Biological Resource Centre (BRC) Vatel vanilla germplasm collection in Réunion Island [26] under accessions number CR2203 to CR2334.

GPS coordinates of each accession were recorded. Populations were named according to the locality (site) where they were collected (**Figure 4**). For the genetic analyses, two other *V. mexicana* accessions from Martinique (CR2352 and CR2353) and three from Mexico (CR2651, CR2658, and CR2665), maintained in the BRC Vatel, were also used.

2.1.4. *Reproductive biology experiments and fruit set measurements*

Flowering rates and season were estimated from June 2014 to June 2015 by surveying on average 96 plants each month in four sites [Habituée (40 plants in mean surveyed per month), Mazeau (22), Moreau (21), and Desbordes (13)]. Plants were checked for the presence of flowers. The lifespan per flower was estimated on 11 flowers from one plant (Desbordes) by measuring the time-laps between flower opening and its wilting.

From June to July 2014, fruit sets were precisely measured from 16 inflorescences (86 flowers in total) on two accessible Mazeau population plants, which were located at about 2 km distance from each other. Eight inflorescences were covered before flower opening by an insect-proof bag to exclude insect visits, while the other eight inflorescences (control) were not bagged. Inflorescences being always at the canopy (10–20 m high), access to flowers had to be performed using a 2 × 8-m-high ladder.

Fruit set was estimated as the ratio of the number of fruits developed at 30 days by the number of flowers at day 0. The natural fruit set (unbagged lowers) was then compared to the spontaneous fruit set observed in bagged flowers using a Student's test with the software *R v. 3.1.1* [41].

Natural fruit set was also assessed globally from June 2015 to June 2016 on 103 inflorescences from 32 plants in four different sites (9 from Habituée, 4 from Desbordes, 8 from Mazeau, and 11 from Moreau), by counting maturing fruits visible using Leica 10 × 40 binoculars. The fruit set was measured as the ratio of the mean number of fruits per inflorescence by the mean number of flowers produced by inflorescence (as determined from the previous Mazeau experiment).

2.1.5. *DNA extraction*

DNA was extracted from each accession from 0.020 to 0.025 g of dehydrated leaf material. Tissues were grinded using a *TissueLyser II* apparatus (Qiagen, Hilden/Germany) and DNA extracted using the DNeasy Plant Mini Kit (Qiagen, Hilden/Germany). DNA was resuspended in 70 µl of elution buffer and its quantity and quality evaluated both on a 2% agarose gel and by Nanodrop V8000 (Thermo Fisher Scientific, Waltham/USA). If the ratio of the OD 260/280 was not in the adequate 1.7–2 range, further purification was performed using the GeneClean® TurboKit (MP Biomedicals, Santa Ana/USA).

2.1.6. Microsatellite analyses

Fourteen microsatellite markers isolated from *V. planifolia* [2] and 19 microsatellite markers isolated from *V. humblotii* and *V. roscheri* [21] were tested in *V. mexicana*. Only six markers (from *V. humblotii* and *V. roscheri*) were transferable to *V. mexicana*, giving readable and repeatable amplifications and were used for subsequent PCR amplifications. These were HU03, HU04, HU06, HU07, HU09, and RO05 using appropriate fluorochrome dyes (see [21] for primer sequences and dyes). PCR volume was 15 µl including 7.5 µl of 2X Qiagen multiplex PCR Master Mix buffer (Qiagen, Hilden/Germany), 0.2 µl of each primer at 20 µM, 5.1 µl HPLC water, and 2 µl DNA (10 ng μl^{-1}). Amplifications were run on a Applied Biosystem GeneAmp® *PCR System 9700* (Thermo Fisher Scientific, Waltham/USA) thermocycler, using the following program: 2 min of predenaturation at 95°C, 45 cycles of 30 s at 95°C, 45 s at 57°C and 1 min at 72°C and a final elongation step for 7 min at 72°C. Amplification success was controlled by migration on a 2% agarose gel (1 h 30 min., at 110 V). PCR products were then diluted (1/10, 1/20, 1/30, or 1/40) depending on the intensity of the bands on the agarose gel. Then, 1 µl of the diluted amplification products were mixed with 10.3 µl formamide and 0.7 µl Gene Scan 500 Liz Size Standard (Applied Biosystems, Foster City/USA) and migrated on a *ABI 3130Xl* (Applied Biosystems, Foster City/USA) sequencer. Microsatellite alleles were visualized using the *GeneMapper v.4* software (Applied Biosystems) and manually scored.

2.1.7. Genetic analyses

An extended dataset comprising all studied accessions from Guadeloupe, Martinique, and Mexico (137 individuals) for the 6 microsatellite loci was used to calculate the total number of alleles for each locus (N_a), the number of private alleles per population (N_p) using the *GenAlex v.6.4* software [42, 43] and to study the levels of polymorphism at the regional scale.

Then, accessions from Martinique and Mexico were excluded from the dataset to calculate for each locus the observed heterozygosity (H_O), expected heterozygosity under Hardy-Weinberg (HW) equilibrium (H_E) and fixation index (F_{IS}) as in [44], using the online version of *Genepop v.4.2* [45]. These parameters and a global fixation index (F_{ST}) as in [44] were also calculated using *Genepop v.4.2* at the population level using a complete dataset (no missing data) with 3 markers (HU03, HU07, and HU09) and 51 individuals (11 populations). The fixation index F_{IS} or inbreeding coefficient is determined by a ratio of H_E and H_O, which indicates a heterozygote deficit or excess in the studied populations. It gives information on the reproduction regime in the populations, and the selfing rates were estimated by hand from F_{IS} using the equation $s = 2 \times F_{IS}/(1 + F_{IS})$ [46]. *Genepop v.4.2* was used to test for deviation from the HW equilibrium using multi-locus exact P-values estimations of the Markov chain method proposed by [47] (with default values).

Linkage disequilibrium between loci was tested using a probability test in *Genepop v.4.2* and Bonferroni correction for multiple comparisons. All loci were also tested for large-allele dropout using *Micro-Checker v. 2.2* [48]. The possible presence of null alleles was assessed with *Micro-Checker v. 2.2* using the Brookfield null estimator 1 [49] with each single locus complete dataset. The occurrence of null alleles was also verified by the program *INEst v.2.0* (Inbreeding/Null allele Estimation) [50], adapted for inbred populations, using the individual inbreeding model (IIM) with 200,000 MCMC iterations, 1000 thinning, and 20,000 burnin. *INEst* uses data from different loci simultaneously, which allows to estimate null allele frequencies at each locus together with the average level of inbreeding. We tested combinations of datasets with no missing data involving 2 to 3 loci of the 4 polymorphic in Guadeloupe and maximizing the number of individuals (35–107 depending on the dataset, datasets with N < 15 were not used).

2.2. Results

2.2.1. Reproductive biology

Morphological character measurements from reproductive and vegetative organs (**Table 2**) fitted the botanical description of *V. mexicana* [11, 17, 19]. The lifespan of a flower (from just-opened to wilted) was estimated to be 6.7 ± 1 days, the flower remaining fully opened for one to three days. Variations in flowering rates assessed on a mean of 96 plants on four sites each month for 1 year revealed that the species flowered almost all year-round, with a peak season in May–July with a maximum flowering rate at the beginning of June where 15.5% of plants were in flowering stage (**Figure 5**). In Guadeloupe, the May–July season is characterized by an increase in temperatures and rainfall.

Organ	Length	Width	Thickness	Diameter
Sepal	44.5 (±6.3)	12.5 (±1.8)		
Petal	44.4 (±5.4)	10.9 (±1.9)		
Labellum	25.8 (±2.0)	11.2 (±0.9)	11.2 (±0.5)	
Column	23.5 (±1.5)	2.4 (±0.3)	2.2 (±0.4)	
Ovary	40.6 (±10.1)	2.6 (±0.4)	2.5 (±0.4)	
Fruit	160 (±18.7)			10.2 (±0.3)
Stem	96.2 (±25.2)^{IL}			4.9 (±1,2)
Leaf	183.4 (±30.4)	48.5 (±8,9)^{LW}		
		82.1 (±21,1)^{LMW}		

The values are the means (±SE) of floral (N = 11), fruit (N = 5), and organ (N = 64) measurements in millimetres. ^{IL}internode length, ^{LW}leaf width at 43 mm from the apex, ^{LMW}leaf maximum width.

Table 2. Flower, fruit, and vegetative organ morphology of *V. mexicana*.

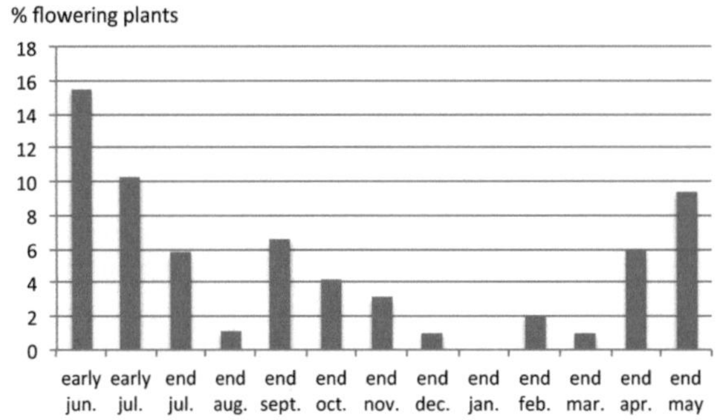

Figure 5. Annual variation in flowering rates in *V. mexicana* in Guadeloupe (June 2014–June 2015).

Results from the reproductive experiments (bagged and unbagged inflorescences) performed on 86 flowers from the Mazeau site are shown in **Table 3**. The mean number of flower per inflorescence in *V. mexicana* was 5.38 ± 0.93. There was no significant difference between the natural fruit set (53.7 ± 21.1%) and the spontaneous selfing rate obtained from bagged flowers (pollinators excluded), which was 53.9 ± 25.3% (**Table 3**). Both values showed important standard errors (SE), witnessing the fact that fruit set ranged from one to maximum six flowers becoming fruits, depending on the inflorescence. The natural fruit set observed in Mazeau was confirmed by visual observations of other 103 inflorescences from four different sites (Habituée, Desbordes, Mazeau, and Moreau), revealing that the mean number of fruits per inflorescence was 2.62 ± 1.72 (again with a high SE). If taking 5.38 as the mean number of flower per inflorescence (as determined in Mazeau), this gave a global natural fruit set estimation of 48.7%.

	Day 0		**Fruit set at day 30 (%)**	
	Control	**Bagged**	**Control**	**Bagged**
Individual	Nb_fl	Nb_fl		
Mazeau 16	6	6	50.0	50.0
	6	5	83.3	80.0
	6	5	66.7	60.0
	6	6	50.0	50.0
Mazeau 4	6	3	33.3	100.0
	5	6	80.0	50.0
	6	4	16.7	25.0
	4	6	50.0	16.7
Total	45	41		
Mean ± SE	5.63 ± 0.7	5.13 ± 1.05	53.7 ± 21.1	53.9 ± 25.3
t test			0.30 (NS)	

Control—inflorescences without protection. Bagged—inflorescence with insect-proof bag, Nb_fl—number of flowers, Mean ± SE—mean number of flower per inflorescence and standard error, mean fruit set value, and standard error, *t* test —*p* value of the Student's test, NS —nonsignificant

Table 3. Mating system of two individuals from *V. mexicana* in Guadeloupe (Mazeau population).

2.2.2. Genetic analyses

A total of 23 alleles were revealed for the 6 loci in the analyses on the complete dataset (**Table 4**), with a mean of 3.67 allele per locus, of which nine were private: four alleles to Mexico (with frequencies >0.1), and one in each of the Guadeloupe populations (with $N \geq 5$) of Desbordes, Habituée, Léon, Moreau, and Sofaia (with frequencies >0.01). The six loci were polymorphic at the regional scale (Guadeloupe, Martinique, Mexico), and only four were polymorphic in Guadeloupe. Eighteen alleles were revealed in Guadeloupe (**Table 4**), with a mean of 3 alleles per locus.

Locus	HU03	HU04	HU06	HU07	HU09	RO05
N_a (Guad)	4(4)	3(1)	4(4)	3(3)	6(5)	3(1)
Size (bp)	119–127	150–161	252–260	165–171	109–203	178–180
Pol_Reg	Yes	Yes	–	Yes	Yes	Yes
Pol_Guad	Yes	No	Yes	Yes	Yes	No
N (Guad)	113(111)	42(40)	43(43)	57(55)	126(125)	48(47)
Guadeloupe						
$Null^{MC}$	0.00	–	0.19	0.34	0.14	–
$Null^{IIM}$	0.01	–	0.12	0.02	0.02	–
H_E	0.333	0.000	0.515	0.525	0.503	0.000
H_O	0.342	0.000	0.227	0.000	0.296	0.000
F_{IS}	-0.026	–	0.559	1.000	0.412	–
HW	NS	–	***	***	***	–

N_a (Guad)—total number of alleles at the regional scale (with total number of alleles in Guadeloupe in parenthesis) per locus. Size (bp)—size range of alleles. Pol_reg—regional polymorphism. Pol_Guad—polymorphism in Guadeloupe. N (Guad)—total number of individuals at the regional scale (total number of individuals in Guadeloupe in parenthesis). Guadeloupe indices: $Null^{MC}$—null allele frequency estimated by *Micro-Checker*. $Null^{IIM}$—mean null allele frequency estimated by *INEst* from various complete multi-locus datasets with $N > 30$, H_E—expected heterozygosity, H_O—observed heterozygosity, F_{IS}—fixation index, HW—Hardy-Weinberg equilibrium deviation, with significant *p* value *<0.05, **<0.01, ***<0.001 and NS (nonsignificant) for *p* value > 0.05.

Table 4. Genetic diversity indices per locus defined by *GenAlex* and *Genepop* on the extended dataset.

Except for HU03, all other 3 polymorphic loci (HU06, HU07, and HU09) deviated significantly from HW expectations due to strong heterozygote deficits in Guadeloupe. The remaining two monomorphic loci (HU04, RO05) were also homozygous in Guadeloupe (**Table 4**), but not in Mexico (data not shown).

The test for genotypic disequilibrium for each pair of locus revealed no significant linkage between loci ($p > 0.05$). No large-allele dropout was detected.

Possible null alleles were detected with *Micro-Checker* for 3 loci (HU06, HU07, and HU09) (**Table 4**), with high frequency (0.14–0.34). However, using *INEst*, which accounts for possible inbreeding, the null allele frequencies calculated became close to zero for HU07 and HU09. For HU06, the frequency was lower than with *Micro-Checker*, but there still remained possibilities of null allele. This marker was therefore excluded from further population genetic analyses.

The analyses per population on the selected complete dataset of 51 individuals for 3 loci (HU03, HU07, and HU09) revealed that the three studied populations with N > 5 individuals (Mazeau, Moreau, and Sofaia) deviated significantly from HW expectations due to a heterozygote deficit (**Table 5**). Deviation from HW expectations was also significant at the scale of Guadeloupe (**Table 5**). Selfing rate was estimated as 79% in Mazeau and 74% in Guadeloupe as a whole (**Table 5**). Global diversity H_E was 0.44 (**Table 5**). F_{ST} value across all populations was calculated as 0.157 using *Genepop*.

Population	N	N_a	A_p	H_E	H_O	F_{IS}	S	HW
Mazeau	14	6	0	0.342	0.119	0.652	0.79	**
Moreau	13	7	0	0.350	0.205	0.415	0.59	**
Sofaia	7	6	0	0.389	0.143	0.633	0.78	**
Guadeloupe	51	9	2	0.438	0.183	0.582	0.74	**

N—number of individuals, N_a—total number of alleles per population for the 3 loci studied, A_p—number of private alleles, H_E—expected heterozygosity, H_O—observed heterozygosity, F_{IS}—fixation index, S—selfing rate, HW—Hardy-Weinberg equilibrium deviation, with significant *p* value *<0.05, **<0.01, ***<0.001 and [S1] NS (nonsignificant) for *p* value > 0.05.

Table 5. Genetic diversity indices per population defined by *Genepop* on the complete dataset for locus HU03, HU07, and HU09 for populations with N > 5 and at the scale of Guadeloupe (51 individuals).

2.3. Discussion

V. mexicana flowers remained opened for 1–3 days, as previously suggested [12]. The flowering season was determined from our measurements to occur between May and July. It allowed to precise previous observations on flowering season, which was described as yearly, but more particularly between May to December [51]. Also in Mexico the species was only described as flowering without a defined period [11]. Reproductive biology experiments were performed during the flowering peak season identified.

Autogamy and self-pollination (53.9% fruit set in bagged inflorescences) explained the totality of the observed natural fructifications (53.7%) for the species *V. mexicana* in the Mazeau site in Guadeloupe. We, therefore, demonstrated that *V. mexicana* is reproducing mainly by autogamy in Mazeau, without the need for a pollinator. The natural fruit set estimated at a larger scale on four sites (but less precisely) was in the same range (48.7%). Both values were in the same order of magnitude of what was observed for autogamous *Vanilla* species (42.5–78%) and tropical orchids [24], therefore, confirming the autogamous mating system proposed for *V. mexicana* in Guadeloupe (**Table 1**). We noticed important standard errors in the mean fruit set estimates, which could be due in part to *Acromyrmex octospinosus* (cassava ant), a neotropical species introduced in Guadeloupe. This insect was observed on many occasions predating some flowers, which can be destroyed in a few hours (N. Barre, personal observation). Natural fruit set may also be underestimated for this reason.

It is noteworthy that it was suspected that *V. mexicana* could not perform asexual reproduction by stem cuttings and was strictly reproducing sexually [1, 11, 27]. This was confirmed by the impossibility to multiply this species by stem cuttings in laboratory conditions (Feldmann and Reyes-Lopez, personal communication, and unpublished observations).

Autogamy is therefore found either in subgenus *Vanilla* (in the *V. mexicana* species group) or in the *V. palmarum* species group of subgenus *Xanata* sect. *Xanata* (**Table 1**, **Figure 1**), two early diverging groups in the phylogeny of the genus. Spontaneous self-pollination is, therefore, an ancestral character in *Vanilla* shared by most, but not all, primitive species. Indeed, *V. edwallii*, from subgenus *Vanilla*, *V. parviflora* group, is not capable of self-pollination and requires a pollinator, supposedly the bee *Epicharis* (*Hoplepicharis*) *affinis* [32]. Autogamy in *V. bicolor* was explained by stigmatic fluids [28, 31], and agamospermy was ruled out [31]. For *V. palmarum*, both a narrow rostellum [4] and stigmatic leak [28] were noted. Our observations under dissecting microscope of *V. mexicana* flowers (data not shown) showed a glandulous and sticky rostellum (which could be due to stigmatic leak) on which the pollinaria are stuck, allowing their contact with the stigmata which they cover entirely (N. Barre, personal communication). Some rare cases of spontaneous self-pollination (6%) in some bagged flower experiments have also been reported for some allogamous species such as *V. planifolia*, *V. chamissonis*, and *V. humblotii* [12, 13, 25], but the mechanisms involved are unknown.

Population genetic parameters indicated a significant deviation from HW equilibrium and/or a homozygote excess for five loci out of six tested (not for HU03) in Guadeloupe vanilla population. Deviation from HW equilibrium was also detected in all the populations with more than five individuals studied, including Mazeau in which reproductive biology experiments were conducted. On the contrary, populations from allogamous species *V. barbellata* and *V. dilloniana* from Puerto Rico did not deviate from HW equilibrium [52] as expected for random mating. Deviation from HW for *V. mexicana* was due to heterozygote deficiency and F_{IS} value at the scale of Guadeloupe (0.582) allowed estimating selfing rate at 74.0%. This result is, as expected, very different from the one detected in the allogamous *V. humblotii* in Mayotte with a F_{IS} of 0.086 [13], which would correspond to a selfing rate of 15.8%. This Mayotte population slightly deviated from HW equilibrium due to limited selfing through geitonogamy between flowers on the same plant or from the same clonal patch [13]. Our genetic results, therefore, confirmed autogamy as the major mating system in *V. mexicana* in Guadeloupe as previously suggested [11, 27].

Deviation from HW equilibrium and homozygote excess could be due not only to homozygosity but also to null alleles, commonly encountered with microsatellite markers. This possibility was therefore also tested. *Micro-Checker* detected possible null alleles with high frequency for loci HU06, HU07, and HU09, but these were the 3 loci that also deviated from HW equilibrium (**Table 3**). This null allele test (like most) is not adapted for populations that do not comply with HW equilibrium, particularly due to inbreeding [53, 54], which is the case in *V. mexicana* populations as demonstrated by the reproductive biology experiments. This often implies overestimation of null allele frequencies in such inbred populations [53, 54]. Van Oosterhout et al. [54] proposed a way to avoid this drawback in *Micro-Checker*, but it requires to have estimated the fixation index values by other markers, which was not possible for the present study. We, therefore, tested the IIM model proposed in the *INEst* software [50] which takes both inbreeding and null alleles into account in a Bayesian multilocus approach and this showed that frequency of null alleles dropped close to zero for the two loci, HU07 and HU09. Homozygote excess in populations of our selected dataset (HU03, HU07, and HU09) was therefore explained by inbreeding, not null alleles.

In autogamous species, only plant seeds ensure efficient gene dispersion whereas pollen also contributes in allogamous species [55, 56]. This has important consequences on the genetic diversity organisation, with autogamous species populations being more strongly differentiated, but less variable than populations from allogamous species [55, 56]. A metadata analysis [55] confirmed that annual or autogamous plants, or with gravity-dispersed fruits, allocate genetic variability among populations rather than within, with therefore high F_{ST} (0.34–0.42) and low H_E (0.41–0.47). On the contrary, long-lived or allogamous taxa, or with wind or ingested dispersed seeds, are more variable within populations than between and show low F_{ST} (0.13–0.22) and high H_E (0.61–0.68). The calculated F_{ST} value in *V. mexicana* (0.157) was, however, similar to the ones revealed in allogamous *Vanilla* species such as *V. humblotii* (F_{ST} = 0.120, [13]), *V. barbellata* (F_{ST} = 0.158) and *V. claviculata* (F_{ST} = 0.123) [52]. These F_{ST} values are moderate and in the range of what would be expected from allogamous species. Between populations differentiation is, therefore, lower than expected in *V. mexicana;* it may be because of a more efficient wind or animal-mediated seed dispersal system, which is still to be elucidated.

Intra-population diversity (H_E) value in *V. mexicana* (H_E = 0.438) was in the range of expected values for self-pollinating species [55], but similar to that of allogamous *V. humblotii* (H_E = 0.450, [13]). H_E values should have been higher for allogamous *V. humblotii*. Most allogamous *Vanilla* species are nevertheless self-compatible, and some degree of selfing can occur by geitonogamy. They are long-lived, thanks to their vegetative propagation capacity. Both factors could diminish intra-population diversity [55], associated in the case of *V. humblotii* with the loss of allelic diversity and the small size of fragmented populations [13]. Counterintuitive situations are not uncommon in *Vanilla* species. *V. roscheri* in South Africa was clearly allogamous with Allodapine pollinators and a relatively high fruit set (20%), but the isolated population near Lake Sibaya showed no diversity and was totally homozygous for the set of microsatellite markers employed, because of its range-edge distribution [20]. *V planifolia,* in the wild in Mexico, although allogamous and requiring pollinators, showed a F_{IS} of 1, witnessing high inbreeding probably through geitonogamy due to large size clonal patches and the scarcity of individual genotypes in the area [23].

It was suggested that *V. mexicana* could, in some populations in Mexico, also be allogamous because of a low fruit set observed [11] and carpenter bees were suggested as pollinators [11, 12]. It is possible that mating systems differ according to the geographical distribution. Evolution towards autogamy of allogamous but self-compatible species is often observed after colonization of isolated islands, a process associated with strong reproductive constraints often due to the absence or scarcity of adapted pollinators or partners [24, 57–60]. This could be the case for *V. mexicana* after colonization of the island of Guadeloupe. This was observed in *Eichhornia paniculata* (Spreng.) Solms (Pontederiaceae), this species was allogamous in Brazil but autogamous in Caribbean islands [61]. Autogamy is predominant also in orchids on islands [24], and this was the case for example for Angraecoideae (Vandeae, Orchidaceae) from Réunion island [59, 62, 63] that colonized the island from Madagascar.

From the set of 14 microsatellites developed from the *Vanilla* subgenus *Xanata* section *Xanata* American species *V. planifolia*, only two (mVplCIR025 and mVplCIR031) were transferable to African species from the subgenus *Xanata* section *Tethya* [2]. Here we demonstrated that none of them were transferable to *Vanilla* subgenus *Vanilla*. On the other hand, the 19 microsatellite markers developed from the *Vanilla* subgenus *Xanata* section *Tethya* African species *V. humblotii* and *V. roscheri* were highly transferable to other species from the same section (18 markers in mean were transferable) as well as to various American species from section *Xanata* (with however a slightly lower mean of 15.7 transferable loci) [21]. We showed that only six of them were transferable to *Vanilla* subgenus *Vanilla*. This reflects the important phylogenetic distance separating the primitive subgenus *Vanilla* from the subgenus *Xanata* species (**Figure 1**) [16, 18]. This preliminary study using these 6 transferable markers allowed the confirmation of the mating system revealed with reproductive biology experiments in *V. mexicana*. However, it is clear that further population genetic studies in *V. mexicana* to resolve more complex questions regarding gene flow, population differentiation, or spatial structuring of the populations will require more numerous loci to be analyzed and will therefore necessitate isolating *V. mexicana*-specific microsatellites through an enriched library construction or NGS (next-generation sequencing). Further studies should also be enlarged to other populations from regions other than Guadeloupe to cover the species distribution range (**Figure 2**) and should include as well reproductive biology experiments and measurements to further unravel *V. mexicana* possibly different mating system in other areas.

3. Conclusion

Our preliminary results obtained with the set of 6 heterologous microsatellite primers allowed the confirmation of the reproductive biology results and showed that *V. mexicana* is mainly reproducing by autogamy via spontaneous self-pollination in Guadeloupe. This trait can be of interest to *V. planifolia* breeding. Indeed, the major constraint to vanilla production is the time-consuming hand pollination. *V. planifolia* flowers are ephemeral and must be self-pollinated by hand every morning during the 2–3 months flowering season. Breeding of self-pollinating vanilla cultivars would first necessitate validating the heritability of the autogamous trait of *V. mexicana*. It could then be envisaged using backcross breeding between *V. mexicana* and *V. planifolia* as recurrent parent (to regain characters associated with fruit quality and aroma lacking in the donor parent). This would be a long, but worthwhile, process (5–7 years between each generation from seed germination to flowering). These results demonstrate the strong interest in pursuing the effort of characterization of wild vanilla populations.

Acknowledgements

This work was funded under the VaBiome project by ANR # 11-EBIM-005-06 to Parc National de Guadeloupe, ANR # 11-EBIM-005-01 and Réunion Regional Council # DGADD/PE/20120590 to UMR 53 PVBMT Réunion, as part of the EU Era-Net NetBiome call for projects. The authors thank Alain Ferchal (PNG, Parc National de Guadeloupe) for drawing the map in **Figure 4**; Alain Rousteau (UAG, University of Antilles Guyane) for the help in habitat names translation; Céline Lesponne (PNG) for support to Chloé Goulié mapping work during her Master 2 thesis; Monique Citadelle and Marie-France Barre (AGO) for their participation in field work; Danièle Roques (Cirad Guadeloupe) for her participation in flowering monitoring; Philippe Feldmann (Cirad), Thierry Guillon and Pascal Segrétier (PNG), and Claudine and Pierre Guezennec for precious information given on *V. mexicana* populations.

Author details

Rodolphe Laurent Gigant[1], Narindra Rakotomanga[1], Chloe Goulié[2], Denis Da Silva[1], Nicolas Barre[3], Gervais Citadelle[3], Daniel Silvestre[2], Michel Grisoni[4] and Pascale Besse[1*]

*Address all correspondence to: pascale.besse@univ-reunion.fr

1 University of La Réunion, UMR PVBMT, Saint Pierre, La Réunion, France

2 National Park of Guadeloupe, Saint Claude, Guadeloupe, France

3 AGO Association Guadeloupéenne d'Orchidophilie, Jarry, Guadeloupe, France

4 CIRAD, UMR PVBMT, Saint Pierre, La Réunion, France

References

[1] Bory S, Brown S, Duval M-F, Besse P. Evolutionary Processes and Diversification in the Genus *Vanilla*. In: Grisoni M, Odoux E, editors. Vanilla: Taylor and Francis Group; 2010. p. 15–28

[2] Bory S, Da Silva D, Risterucci A-M, Grisoni M, Besse P, Duval M-F. Development of microsatellite markers in cultivated vanilla: polymorphism and transferability to other vanilla species. Scientia Horticulturae. 2008;115:420–425. doi:10.1016/j.scienta.2007.10.020

[3] Bory S, Lubinsky P, Risterucci AM, Noyer JL, Grisoni M, Duval M-F, et al. Patterns of introduction and diversification of *Vanilla planifolia* (Orchidaceae) in Reunion island (Indian ocean). American Journal of Botany. 2008;95(7):805-815. doi:10.3732/ajb.2007332

[4] Gigant RL, Bory S, Grisoni M, Besse P. Biodiversity and Evolution in the *Vanilla* Genus. In: Oscar G, Gianfranco V, editors. The Dynamical Processes of Biodiversity: Case Studies of Evolution and Spatial Distribution. Rijeka: Intechopen; 2011. p. 1–26

[5] Lubinsky P, Bory S, Hernandez JH, Kim S-C, Gomez-Pompa A. Origins and dispersal of cultivated vanilla (*Vanilla planifolia* Jacks. [Orchidaceae]). Economic Botany. 2008;62:127–138. doi:10.1007/s12231-008-9014-y

[6] Grisoni M, Pearson MN, Farreyrol K. Virus diseases of *Vanilla*. Vanilla. Boca Raton, FL (USA): CRC Press; 2010

[7] Divakaran M, Nirmal Babu K, Ravindran PN, Peter K. Interspecific hybridization in vanilla and molecular characterization of hybrids and selfed progenies using RAPD and AFLP markers. Scientia Horticulturae. 2006;108(4):414–422. doi:10.1016/j.scienta.2006.02.018

[8] Knudson L. Germination of seeds of *Vanilla*. American Journal of Botony. 1950;37:241–247. doi:10.2307/2437909

[9] Koyyappurath S, Conejero G, Dijoux J-B, Montes-Lapeyre F, Jade K, Chiroleu F, et al. Differential responses of vanilla accessions to root and stem rot and colonization by *Fusarium oxysporum f.* sp. *radicis-vanillae*. Frontiers in Plant Science. 2015. doi: 10.3389/fpls.2015.01125

[10] Theis T, Jimenez FA. A *Vanilla* hybrid resistant to *Fusarium* root rot. Phytopathology. 1957;47:578–581

[11] Soto Arenas MA, Dressler RL. A revision of the mexican and central american species of *Vanilla* Plumier ex. Miller with a characterization of their ITS region of the nuclear ribosomal DNA. Lankesteriana. 2010;9:285–354. doi:10.15517/lank.v0i0.12065

[12] Soto Arenas MA, Cameron KN. *Vanilla*. In: Pridgeon AM, Cribb PJ, Chase MW, Rasmussen FN, editors. Genera Orchidacearum: Orchidoideae. USA: Oxford University Press; 2003. p. 321–334

[13] Gigant RL, De Bruyn A, M'sa T, V G, Viscardi G, Gigord L, et al. Combining pollination ecology and fine-scale spatial genetic structure analysis to unravel the reproductive strategy of an insular threatened orchid. South African Journal of Botany. 2016;105:25–35. doi:10.1016/j.sajb.2016.02.205

[14] Cameron KM. Utility of plastid *psa*B gene sequences for investigating intrafamilial relationships within Orchidaceae. Molecular Phylogenetics and Evolution. 2004;31(3):1157–1180

[15] Cameron KM, editor. Recent Advances in the Systematic Biology of *Vanilla* and Related Orchids (Orchidaceae: subfamily Vanilloideae). First International Congress; Princeton, NJ, USA; 2005:11–12 Nov 2003

[16] Soto Arenas MA, Cribb P. A new infrageneric classification and synopsis of the genus *Vanilla* Plum. ex Mill. (Orchidaceae: Vanillinae). Lankesteriana. 2010;9:355–398. doi: 10.15517/lank.v0i0.12071

[17] Portères R. Le genre *Vanilla* et ses espèces. In: Lechevalier P, editor. Le vanillier et la vanille dans le monde. Paris; 1954. p. 94–290

[18] Bouétard A, Lefeuvre P, Gigant R, Bory S, Pignal M, Besse P, et al. Evidence of transoceanic dispersion of the genus *Vanilla* based on plastid DNA phylogenetic analysis. Molecular Phylogenetics and Evolution. 2010;55:621–630. doi:10.1016/j.ympev.2010.01.021

[19] Fournet J. Flore illustrée des phanérogames de Guadeloupe et de Martinique: Cirad, Gondwana éditions; 2002

[20] Gigant RL, De Bruyn A, Church B, Humeau L, Gauvin-Bialecki A, Pailler T, et al. Active sexual reproduction but no sign of genetic diversity in range-edge populations of *Vanilla roscheri* Rchb. f. (Orchidaceae) in South Africa. Conservation Genetics. 2014;15:1403–1415. doi:10.1007/s10592-014-0626-8

[21] Gigant RL, Brugel A, De Bruyn A, Risterucci A-M, Guiot V, Viscardi G, et al. Nineteen polymorphic microsatellite markers from two african *Vanilla* species: across-species transferability and diversity in a wild population of *V. humblotii* from Mayotte. Conservation Genetics Resources. 2012;4(1):121–125. doi: 10.1007/s12686-011-9489-1

[22] Nielsen RL. Natural hybridization between *Vanilla claviculata* (W.Wright) Sw. and *V. barbellata* Rchb.f. (Orchidaceae): genetic, morphological, and pollination experimental data. Botanical Journal of the Linnean Society. 2000;133(3):285–302. doi:10.1006/boj1.2000.0336

[23] Soto Arenas MA. Filogeografia y recursos genéticos de las vainillas de México. México, 102 p.: Herbario de la Asociación Mexicana de Orquideología [Internet] 1999. Available from: http://www.conabio.gob.mx/institucion/proyectos/resultados/InfJ101.pdf [Accessed: 2016-06-14]

[24] Tremblay RL, Ackerman JD, Zimmerman JK, Calvo RN. Variation in sexual reproduction in orchids and its evolutionary consequences: a spasmodic journey to diversification. Botanical Journal of the Linnean Society. 2005;84:1–54

[25] Macedo Reis CA. Biologia reprodutiva e propagacao vegetativa de *Vanilla chamissonis* Klotzsch: subsidios para manejo sustentado [thesis]. Luiz de Queiroz, Piracicaba, Sao Paulo, Brasil, Piracicaba, SP – Brasil: Escola Superior de Agric; 2000

[26] Grisoni M, Moles M, Besse P, Bory S, Duval M-F, Kahane R. Towards an international plant collection to maintain and characterize the endangered genetic resources of vanilla. Acta Horticulturae (ISHS). 2007;760:83–91. doi:10.17660/ActaHortic.2007.760.9

[27] Cameron KN. Vanilloid orchids. In: Odoux E, Grisoni M, editors. Vanilla: CRC Press Taylor and Francis Group; 2010

[28] Householder E, Janovec J, Balarezo Mozambite A, Huinga Maceda J, Wells J, Valega R. Diversity, natural history, and conservation of *Vanilla* (Orchidaceae) in amazonian wetlands of Madre De Dios, Peru. Journal of the Botanical Research Institute of Texas. 2010;4:227–243

[29] Childers NF, Cibes HR. Vanilla culture in Puerto Rico, Circular N°28. Washington DC: Federal Experiment Station in Puerto Rico of the United States Department of Agriculture; 1948

[30] Weiss EA. Chapter 7: Orchidaceae. Spice Crops. Wallington, UK: CABI Publishing; 2002. p. 136–154

[31] Van Dam AR, Householder JE, Lubinsky P. *Vanilla bicolor* Lindl. (Orchidaceae) from the Peruvian Amazon: auto-fertilization in *Vanilla* and notes on floral phenology. Genetic Resources and Crop Evolution. 2010;57:473–480. doi:10.1007/s10722-010-9540-1

[32] Pansarin ER, Aguiar JMRBV, Pansarin LM. Floral biology and histochemical analysis of *Vanilla edwallii* Hoehne (Orchidaceae: Vanilloideae): an orchid pollinated by *Epicharis* (Apidae: Centridini). Plant Species Biology. 2014;29:242–252. doi:10.1111/1442-1984.12014

[33] Jarne P, Lagoda PJL. Microsatellites, from molecules to populations and back. TREE. 1996;11(10):424–429. doi:10.1016/0169-5347(96)10049-5

[34] Powell W, Machray GC, Provan J. Polymorphism revealed by simple sequence repeat. Trends in Plant Science. 1996;1(7):215–222. doi:10.1016/s1360-1385(96)86898-0

[35] Alexander JM, Poll M, Dietz H, Edwards PJ. Contrasting patterns of genetic variation and structure in plant invasions of mountains. Diversity and Distributions. 2009;15:502–512. doi:10.1111/j.1472-4642.2008.00555.x

[36] Bentley KE, Berryman KR, Hopper M, Hoffberg SL, Myhre KE, Iwao K, et al. Eleven microsatellites in an emerging invader, *Phytolacca americana* (Phytolaccaceae), from its native and introduced ranges. Applications in Plant Sciences. 2015;3(3):1500002. doi: 10.3732/apps.1500002

[37] Blouin MS. DNA-based methods for pedigree reconstruction and kinship analysis in natural populations. Trends in Ecology and Evolution. 2003;18:503–511. doi:10.1016/s0169-5347(03)00225-8

[38] Van Glabeke S, Coart E, Honnay O, Roldán-Ruiz I. Isolation and characterization of polymorphic microsatellite markers in *Anthyllis vulneraria*. Molecular Ecology Notes. 2007;7:477–479. doi:10.1111/j.1471-8286.2006.01625.x

[39] Goulié C. Répartition et écologie de *Vanilla mexicana* en Guadeloupe [thesis]. Pointe à Pitre: Université des Antilles et de la Guyane; 2014

[40] Rousteau A, Portecop J, Rollet B. Carte écologique de la Guadeloupe. Jarry, Guadeloupe: ONF, UAG, PNG, CGG; 1996

[41] R Core Team. R: A language and environment for statistical computing. Vienna, Austria.: R Foundation for Statistical Computing; 2014

[42] Peakall R, Smouse PE. GENALEX 6: genetic analysis in Excel. Population genetic software for teaching and research. Molecular Ecology Notes. 2006;6:288–295. doi: 10.1111/j.1471-8286.2005.01155

[43] Peakall R, Smouse PE. GenAlEx 6.5: genetic analysis in Excel. Population genetic software for teaching and research – an updat. Bioinformatics. 2012;28:2537–2539. doi: 10.1093/bioinformatics/bts460

[44] Weir BS, Cockerham CC. Estimating F-statistics for the analysis of population structure. Evolution. 1984;38:1358–1370. doi:10.2307/2408641

[45] Raymond M, Rousset F. Genepop version 1.2: population genetics software for exact tests and ecumenicism. Journal of Heredity. 1995;86:248–249

[46] Rousset F. Equilibrium values of measures of population subdivision for stepwise mutation processes. Genetics. 1996;142:1357–1362

[47] Guo SW, Thompson EA. Performing the exact test of Hardy-Weinberg proportion for multiple alleles. Biometrics. 1992:361–372. doi:10.2307/2532296

[48] Van Oosterhout, C, Hutchinson WF, Wills DPM, Shipley P. Micro-checker: software for identifying and correcting genotyping errors in microsatellite data. Molecular Ecology Notes. 2004;4:535–538. doi:10.1111/j.1471-8286.2004.00684.x

[49] Brookfield JFY. A simple new method for estimating null allele frequency from heterozygote deficiency. Molecular Ecology Notes. 1996;5:453–455. doi:10.1046/j.1365-294x.1996.00098.x

[50] Chybicki IJ, Burczyk J. Simultaneous estimation of null alleles and inbreeding coefficients. Journal of Heredity. 2009;100:106–113. doi:10.1093/jhered/esn088

[51] Feldmann P, Barré N. Atlas des Orchidées Sauvages de la Guadeloupe. Paris: Cirad-M.N.H.N.; 2001

[52] Nielsen RL, Siegismund HR. Interspecific differentiation and hybridization in *Vanilla* species (Orchidaceae). Heredity. 1999;83(5):560–567. doi:10.1038/sj.hdy.6885880

[53] Campagne P, Smouse PE, Varouchas G, Silvain J-F, Leru B. Comparing the van Oosterhout and Chybicki-Burczyk methods of estimating null allele frequencies for inbred populations. Molecular Ecology Resources. 2012;12:975–982. doi:10.1111/1755-0998.12015

[54] Van Oosterhout C, Weetman D, Hutchinson WF. Estimation and adjustment of microsatellite null alleles in nonequilibrium populations. Molecular Ecology Notes. 2006;5:255–256. doi:10.1111/j.1471-8286.2005.01082.x

[55] Nybom H. Comparison of different nuclear DNA markers for estimating intraspecific genetic diversity in plants. Molecular Ecology. 2004;13:1143–1155. doi:10.1111/j.1365-294x.2004.02141.x

[56] Ronfort J, Jenczewski E, Muller M. Les flux de gènes et leur impact sur la structure de la diversité génétique. Le cas des prairies: Génétique et prairies. Fourrages (Versailles). 2005;182:275–286

[57] Baker HG. Reproductive methods as factors in speciation in flowering plants. Cold Spring Harbor Symposia on Quantitative Biology. 1959;24:177–190. doi:10.1101/sqb.1959.024.01.019

[58] Baker HG. Evolutionary mechanisms in pollination biology. Science. 1963;139:877–883. doi:10.1126/science.139.3558.877

[59] Micheneau C, Carlsward BS, Fay MF, Bytebier B, Pailler T, Chase MW. Phylogenetics and biogeography of Mascarene angraecoid orchids (Vandeae, Orchidaceae). Molecular Phylogenetics and Evolution. 2008;46:908–922. doi:10.1016/j.ympev.2007.12.001

[60] Stebbins GL. Adaptive radiation of reproductive characteristics in angiosperms, I: pollination mechanisms. Annual Review of Ecology and Systematics. 1970;1:307–326. doi:10.1146/annurev.es.01.110170.001515

[61] Barrett SCH. The evolution of plant reproductive systems: how often are transitions irreversible? Proceedings of the Royal Society B. 2013;280:20130913. doi:10.1098/rspb.2013.0913

[62] Jacquemyn H, Micheneau C, Roberts DL, Pailler T. Elevation gradients of species diversity, breeding system and floral traits of orchid species on Réunion Island. Journal of Biogeography. 2005;32:1751–1761. doi:10.1111/j.1365-2699.2005.01307.x

[63] Micheneau C. Systématique moléculaire de la sous-tribu des Angraecinae: perspectives taxonomiques et implications de la relation plantes-pollinisateurs dans l'évolution des formes florales [thesis]. Saint Denis: Université de La Réunion; 2005

Chapter 5

Microsatellite Markers in Analysis of Forest-Tree Populations

Justyna Anna Nowakowska

Additional information is available at the end of the chapter

http://dx.doi.org/10.5772/64867

Abstract

The present state of knowledge regarding the genetic diversity of forest tree species has been greatly improved with the development of the powerful research tool that the microsatellite markers represent. These noncoding sequences are considered to be neutral, highly polymorphic, and species specific. The usefulness of the microsatellite markers was recently proven by the determination of differentiation at inter- and intrapopulation level, gene flow in natural forest-tree populations, heritability processes, and sustainable management of forest genetic resources in many natural forest stands. In this chapter, I aim to describe the practical approach of microsatellite markers, used in determination of genetic structure of 14 Scots pine populations from North-eastern Poland. Investigated pine populations exhibited high genetic parameter variation, for example, mean PIC = 79.3, Shannon Index I = 2.488, observed (H_O = 0.778) and expected (H_E = 0.849) heterozygosity. Low level of F_{st} = 0.031 demonstrated that studied populations are more differentiated within than among stands, which were grouped into one cluster of genetic similarity. In conclusion, the present distribution of genetically related populations of Scots pine in North-eastern Poland seems to reflect the historical events such as postglacial colonization of Poland from different European refugia and/or human management carried out in the past.

Keywords: cpSSR, genetic distance, genetic variation and differentiation, heterozygosity level, *Pinus sylvestris* L., SSR markers

1. Introduction

The sustainable management of forest genetic resources requires a good knowledge of the genetic diversity of species. Because of their longevity and wide geographic distribution, forest-tree species have developed a high level of genomic heterogeneity as a genetic potential through which they adapt to the specific environmental factors of a given habitat [1, 2]. Human industrial activities and changing environmental conditions have exposed many species to the threat of extinction, and, with a view to the appropriate gene-conservation measures being taken, many governments are aware of the need for forest management to maintain the biodiversity of locally adapted species. Equally, not only endangered forest-tree species but also economically important ones should be protected in a specific conservation programs based on valuable genetic data [3].

If the conservation of forest-tree genetic resources is to be pursued, molecular markers such as DNA sequences would seem suitable where the study of the genetic variation among trees is concerned [4–6]. Appropriate marker systems can facilitate investigation of the genetic relationships between forest-tree stands and the mapping of gene positions on chromosomes. For these purposes, several methods of DNA diversity assessment are commonly used, for example, RAPD (random-amplified polymorphic DNA), AFLP (amplified fragment length polymorphism), RFLP (restriction fragment length polymorphism), STS (sequence-tagged site), and microsatellites [4, 5, 7–12].

1.1. Characterization of microsatellite markers

Since the early 1990s, a powerful molecular marker has emerged in the shape of the microsatellite sequences discovered in the genomes of all living organisms. Microsatellites (or SSRs—simple sequence repeats) comprise tandem repeats of short DNA sequences from one to six base-pair motifs, largely distributed over the entire genome. They are considered to be highly polymorphic DNA markers with codominant inheritance and selectively neutral behavior [4, 5, 13]. SSR sequences are present in all living organisms, including protists, prokaryotes, eukaryotes, and fungi. In many species, the majority (48–67%) of tandem repeats are dinucleotides, mostly localized in noncoding regions of the genome [14]. Mononucleotide repeats are considered to be the most abundant class of microsatellites in primates, while tri-, tetra-, and hexanucleotide SSR repeats are reported in other organisms. Exposed to high incidences of mutation ranging from 10^{-2} to 10^{-6} nucleotide per locus and per generation, microsatellites are characterized by considerable polymorphism and species specificity [4, 14].

Despite the neutrality assigned to microsatellite markers, the SSR sequences seem to serve some function in different eukaryotic organisms [15]. So far, no evident role for the abundant tandem-repeated sequences has been found, though the SSRs are presumably involved in chromatin organization in the nucleus, DNA replication, regulation of gene expression, and (putatively) in the mismatch-repair system [4, 16]. Tandem-repeated sequences located in the introns of genes could trigger the disruption of the triplet-reading code. The new reading frame may be lethal, or present some advantage from the evolutionary point of view. In fact, the microsatellite triplets are more often subjected to polymerase slippage during the replication and transcription of genes. Long trinucleotide repeats, for example, CAG, CTG, CGG, and CCG, may also form secondary structures of DNA strands and influence recombination [4, 5]. Many promoters contain repeated cis-acting DNA fragments, while microsatellites may also be involved in the regulation of gene expression.

1.2. Advantages and weak points of SSR markers

The precise identification of biological samples based on microsatellite loci remains a fundamental for population genetics study [17, 18]. These markers present many advantages, for example, locus specificity, the small amount of DNA required, the almost absolute sizing of alleles, and fast detection [4, 5, 19]. The SSR fragments (also called alleles) are screened by their length expressed in base pairs, and the differences in allele sizing among individuals of one species are caused by varying numbers of repeats in microsatellite motifs.

From practical point of view, an unexpected allele sizing of microsatellite sequences sometimes occurs. In many genomes, the microsatellites mutate by errors in replication or unequal crossing over during recombination process [20]. Moreover, homoplasy, null alleles, and short allele dominance may cause problems during microsatellite scoring [5, 14, 21, 22].

Homoplasy concerns the alleles of the same size but presenting different base-pair composition. Null alleles mean the lack of polymerase chain reaction (PCR) amplification of allele caused by nucleotide mutation in primer-binding sites. The short allele dominance is observed when large allele size dropout occurs. The amplification of nonexpected allele size often results from polymerase slippage during PCR. First of all, long and nonperfect motif repeats of microsatellite loci, especially with polyA tracks in the internal sequence, may enhance polymerase slippage [23]. Furthermore, some fluorescent dyes such as Ned, 6-Fam, and Hex in ABI sequencer 3500 Genetic Analyzer (Life Technologies™) or Well-Red D2, D3, and D4 dyes in CEQ™ 8000 Genetic Analysis System (Beckman Coulter, Fullerton, CA) used to label the primers can modify the mobility of the PCR products on the gel [24], and generate nonstandard scoring of alleles. The various lengths of SSR-flanking regions should also be taken into consideration as a putative source of nonstandard allele polymorphism [24]. Sometimes, the microsatellite allele sizes alone are insufficient to determine species biogeography for organisms with predominant asexual mode of reproduction [25].

2. Need for SSR markers and appropriate methodologies

In conifers, mostly di-, tri-, and tetranucleotide repeats are present in high proportion in the genome [19, 26]. In the case of *Pinus sylvestris* (L.), only a few nuclear microsatellite loci have so far been distinguished, for example, SPAC 3.7 (Genbank code AJ223769), SPAG 7.14 (AJ223771), SPAC 11.4 (AJ223766), SPAC 11.5 (AJ223768), SPAC 11.6 (AJ223767), SPAC 11.8 (AJ223770), and SPAC 12.5 (AJ223772), mentioned by Soranzo et al. [9] and available on the websites [27–29]. More Scots pine nuclear microsatellite loci can also be found in the Kostia et al. [30] and Chagné et al. [31] publications.

The transferability of the microsatellite loci between conifers is generally difficult. Many microsatellites need to be isolated *de novo* because the specificity of flanking SSR regions is high [32, 33]. This is partly due to the high rate of nucleotide substitution in noncoding regions of the genome. Moreover, conifers exhibit larger genome size (between 21×10^9 and 134×10^9 megabases) and higher genome complexity than deciduous trees [34]. Transferability of SSR sequences between *P. taeda, P. radiate,* and *P. pinaster* has been reported, for example, by Chagné et al. [31] and González-Martínez et al. [33]. In Scots pine, most SSR investigations are based on microsatellite loci transferred from *P. taeda* or *P. pinaster* [35, 36].

The structure of the Scots pine genome is complex. Nevertheless, some studies of microsatellites in European Scots pine populations reveal a low level of genetic differentiation [9, 37–39]. These data are concordant with the low genetic variation in polymorphism frequencies of Scots pine stands assessed with isozyme markers in Europe [40]. The main reason for this limited genetic variation in Scots pine populations lies in the transfer of seed material in the past, as enhanced by the long-distance gene flow occurring among Scots pine stands in Europe [41].

The microsatellite markers in forest-tree species are analyzed following the general pathway composed by four general steps: (1) isolation of genomic DNA from plant tissue, (2) DNA amplification by polymerase chain reaction, (3) fragment length sizing and allele determination of the obtained PCR products performed using a capillary electrophoresis in automatic sequencer, and (4) statistical analyses of population genetic variation and differentiation.

2.1. Isolation of genomic DNA

Many methods of genomic DNA extraction from plant tissue have been proposed, for example, cetyltrimethylammonium bromide (CTAB) method-based isolation described by Doyle and Doyle [42], DNeasy Plant Mini Kit (Qiagen®), MagAttract 96 DNA Plant Core Kit (Qiagen®) [43], and NucleoSpin Plant II (Macherey-Nagel®) [43]. The mentioned methods yield c.a. 1–2 μg of DNA per 50–100 mg of plant tissue, which is sufficient for nuclear and organelle DNA amplification. According to the tissue type, that is, cambium, sapwood, or hardwood, a different yield of the DNA may be obtained, in favor of cambial cells in *P. radiata* [44] and *Quercus robur* [45]). Good quantity and quality DNAs were also obtained by Asif and Cannon [46] and Tibbits et al. [44], who supplemented the classical CTAB method with buffer containing NaCl and BSA effectively removing co-extracted contaminants. The main difficulty in DNA-based analyses remains in proper DNA extraction method from wood tissues because of the high amount of polysaccharides and polyphenolic compounds residuals which inhibit the Taq polymerase during the PCR [44]. The removal of contaminants guarantees the success of further amplification and accurateness of DNA fragment (allele or gene) detection during the capillary electrophoresis performed in automated sequencer.

Sometimes, the genomic DNA isolation step may be overcome by a direct PCR performed on fresh plant tissue with Phire® Plant Direct PCR kit (Finnzymes®, Vantaa, Finland), as demonstrated for silver fir samples [43].

2.2. DNA amplification by polymerase chain reaction

Prior to amplification, the quality of DNA is checked by electrophoresis or with NanoDrop® ND-1000 spectrophotometer (Wilmington, USA). The first method relies on classical gel-based separation in the electric field of DNA fragments in c.a. 1% agarose gel or on chip-based electrophoresis in Bioanalyzer apparatus using Agilent DNA 1000 kit (Agilent Techn. Wald-

http://dx.doi.org/10.5772/64867

bronn, Germany). Good quality and sufficient quantity of DNA molecules guarantee high yield of further amplification by polymerase chain reaction. Developed in 1983 [47], the PCR consists in three major steps: (1) initial denaturation of double-stranded DNA matrix generally in temperature of 94–98°C for 30 s, to 1 mi; (2) annealing of primers in temperature of 50–60°C for 20–30 s; and (3) extension and elongation step in 72°C. The time and the temperature of each step strongly depend on primer structure and polymerase used in the reaction [48]. All steps are repeated 30–40 times in a thermal cycler, for example, Veriti 96 Thermal Cycler (Life Technologies™, USA), T1000 Touch™ Thermal Cycler (Bio-Rad Laboratories, Inc., USA), or TPersonal Thermocycler (Biometra®, Germany). At the end, several thousands of copies of initial DNA matrix are generated.

2.3. Fragment length sizing and allele determination of the obtained PCR products performed using a capillary electrophoresis in automatic sequencer

The PCR products are generally analyzed with capillary sequencer, for example, CEQ8000™ (Beckman-Coulter®, USA) or 3500 Genetic Analyzer (Life Technologies™, USA) using appropriate software for data collection. The typical programs are: CEQ™8000 Genetic Analysis System version 9.0 (Beckman Coulter®) in the case of the CEQ8000 apparatus, and 3500 Data Collection Software and GeneMapper® v. 5 in the case of the 3500 Genetic Analyzer (Life Technologies™, USA).

2.4. Statistical analyses of population genetic variation and differentiation

In general, statistical analyses of population genetic variation and differentiation comprise the parameters describing population genetic variation and differentiation, that is, observed and expected number of alleles (n_a, n_e, respectively), observed and expected heterozygosity (H_O, H_E), Shannon diversity index (I), and fixation index/inbreeding coefficient of F-statistics (F_{is}, F_{st}). The significant deviations from Hardy-Weinberg equilibrium (HWE) per each locus, analysis of null alleles (commonly found in SSR loci), and polymorphism information content (*PIC*) are also computed [21, 49–51]. The statistical methods, used in the study of population genetics, should be applied according to the defined objective. Many genotype-distribution methods are based on data for allele/gene frequencies, distograms of genetic dissimilarity, or mapping of gene position. The spatial patterns depend on many factors such as isolation by distance, and factors of environmental selection, migration, and human activity [52]. Several items of software can be applied in this field (e.g., GeneAlEx, PopGen, SPAGeDi, etc.). Those programs take into account Hardy-Weinberg equilibrium, multiple allele and loci inheritance, natural selection, genetic drift, migration, mutation, and inbreeding analyses [51, 53].

All statistical methods should consider the effect of interaction between genotype and the environment, in order to precise the estimation values of observed genotype in given conditions. Forest-genetic field experiments are based on tests of adjustment for local environmental factors and on the estimation of breeding values. The multi-trait selection measures attempt to predict trees' response to the selection effect. The assessment of valuable quantitative trait loci (QTL) mapping, gene-expression analysis, or the long-term response of evolutionary selection makes use of several programs, for example, analysis of variance (ANOVA), statistical analysis system (SAS, restricted maximum likelihood (RML), and S-Plus [38].

In order to illustrate the genetic similarity between studied populations, usually the dendrogram based on the distance matrix is constructed. To this end, very often the UPGMA (unweighted pair group method with arithmetic mean) method is applied [50, 53]. To produce a dendrogram of genetic similarity, the UPGMA method employs a sequential clustering algorithm. For instance, the DendroUPGMA software is a good tool for computing the clustering from the sets of variables [49, 54], with several factors such as Pearson coefficient, Jaccard similarity coefficient, and Dice coefficient.

The resulting tree (dendrogram) of genetic similarity gathers the populations in branches defined by, for example, 100-bootstrap replicates, which give an estimation of probability for particular node. The calculation of the CoPhenetic correlation coefficient (*CP*), which values are comprised between 0 and 1, gives a measure of distance accurateness of the dendrogram.

3. Genetic variability of forest stands assessed with microsatellite markers: a case study of *P. sylvestris* (L.) in North-eastern Poland

3.1. Object of the study

Scots pine (*P. sylvestris* L.) is the most widely distributed coniferous species in Europe. The species enjoys major economic relevance, especially in Northern and Eastern European countries. In Poland, *P. sylvestris* accounts for 69.4% of total forest area, in Finland 64.9%, and in Lithuania 36.5% [55–57]. The present genetic structure to the Scots pine stands in Europe has been largely influenced by climatic and environmental factors [58]. Above all, the recolonization of the continent after the last glaciation period contributed to the rapid expansion of Scots pine populations from their South-European and Central Russian refuges to the North of the continent [40, 59–61]. Second, the distribution of many Scots pine stands in the European landscape reflects the present situation and socioeconomic changes, for example, privatization, the increased demand for wood, deforestation, and reforestation [58]. Due to the high level of anthropogenic pressure, the genetic resources of many forest-tree species in Europe have frequently been impoverished. Moreover, the transfer of genetic material across European countries has modified the natural gene pools in many forest-tree stands [58].

Recent advances in regard to the genetic diversity *P. sylvestris* have highlighted the usefulness of nuclear SSR markers in forest-tree genetics, focusing especially on genotyping of the Scots pine populations in Poland. In the present study, 14 natural or seminatural, 110-year-old Scots pine populations, located in North-eastern part of Poland were investigated (**Table 1**).

3.2. Methodology of Polish case study

The extraction of total DNA from the 100 mg of needles was performed using Qiagen DNeasy Plant Mini kit according to the manufacturer's instruction (Qiagen® Hilden, Germany). The quality and purity of DNA were analyzed by absorption in 230, 260, and 280 nm in NanoDrop® spectrophotometer (Wilmington, USA). Four nuclear microsatellite DNA markers were amplified, that is, SPAG 7.14, SPAC 12.5, PtTX3025, and SsrPt-ctg4363 [9, 31, 38]. For all loci, Well-Red labeled primers were synthetized by Sigma-Aldrich Company (St Louis, USA). The PtTX primers were originally designed for *P. taeda* but they were proved to be as useful as markers developed for *P. sylvestris*. The obtained PCR amplicons were analyzed using DNA capillary electrophoresis in CEQ8000 Beckman Coulter® sequencer, and analyzed using the software CEQ™8000 Genetic Analysis System v 9.0 (Fullerton, USA).

Population (Forest Directorate, Forest stand)	**Location**	N	n_a	n_e	I	H_O	H_E	h **Nei**
1. Czarna Białostocka, Polanki	53°18′N, 22°25′E	50	16.500	10.211	2.163	0.710	0.795	0.785
2. Czarna Białostocka, Budzisk	53°17′N, 23°18′E	48	16.750	10.250	2.175	0.798	0.802	0.793
3. Dojlidy	53°05′N, 23°11′E	50	15.500	8.630	2.115	0.741	0.800	0.791
4. Supraśl	53°17′N, 23°30′E	50	16.250	9.726	2.217	0.832	0.824	0.815
5. Waliły	53°12′N, 23°39′E	48	16.750	9.325	2.235	0.750	0.833	0.823
6. Żednia, Nowa Wola	52°59′N, 23°33′E	50	16.750	9.540	2.210	0.815	0.819	0.810
7. Żednia, Borsukowina	53°15′N, 23°38′E	50	16.750	9.715	2.223	0.828	0.831	0.822
8. Hajnówka	54°15′N, 23°05′E	50	19.250	11.499	2.278	0.776	0.802	0.793
9. Browsk	52°55′N, 23°36′E	48	18.500	10.532	2.250	0.789	0.811	0.802
10. Bielsk	52°36′N, 23°23′E	50	17.000	8.750	2.231	0.751	0.828	0.818
11. Rudka	52°54′N, 22°52′E	50	16.250	8.974	2.124	0.785	0.782	0.774
12. Knyszyn, Szelągówka	53°20′N, 22°41′E	50	17.000	10.269	2.244	0.783	0.824	0.815
13. Knyszyn, Kopisk	53°17′N, 23°04′E	50	17.000	10.028	2.161	0.733	0.804	0.796
14. Augustów	53°46′N, 23°10′E	50	17.750	9.315	2.228	0.780	0.818	0.810
Total		1260	30.750	12.400	2.488	0.778**	0.849**	$H_T = 0.848$
								$F_{st} = 0.031$

N, numbers of sampled trees; n_a, observed number of alleles; n_e, effective allele number; I, Shannon index; H_O and H_E, observed and expected heterozygosity; h, mean heterozygosity [46]; H_T, genetic diversity among populations; F_{ST}, coefficient of genetic differentiation of populations [49]. Test of heterozygote deficiency in Hardy-Weinberg equilibrium: $^{**}p < 0.01$

Table 1. Genetic differentiation level of microsatellite nSSR loci in studied Scots pine populations.

Parameters of genetic diversity (H_O, H_E, H_T), differentiation (F-statistics), and genetic distance matrix were computed according to Nei [49,50] in GenALEx v. 6 software [53]. The mean polymorphism information content values were established for each set of markers in MolKin 2.0 software [62].

The dendrogram of genetic distances between studied populations was constructed using DendroUPGMA software [63], validated by *CP* computing. Moreover, Bayesian clustering using Markov Chain Monte Carlo (MCMC) algorithm was performed in BAPS 2.0 program, with randomization = 100,000, burning = 50,000, for $p = 0.02$ [64].

3.3. Results of the Polish case study

3.3.1. Quality and quantity of the analyzed DNA

Spectrophotometrical assessment of the genomic DNA isolated from Scots pine samples yielded good quantity and quality of the nucleic acids (**Figure 1**). For all samples, the mean DNA purity ($A_{260/280} = 1.67$ and $A_{260/230} = 1.82$) and the mean DNA concentration (148.89 ng/μl ± 11 S.E.) were suitable for further amplification of microsatellite loci in PCR.

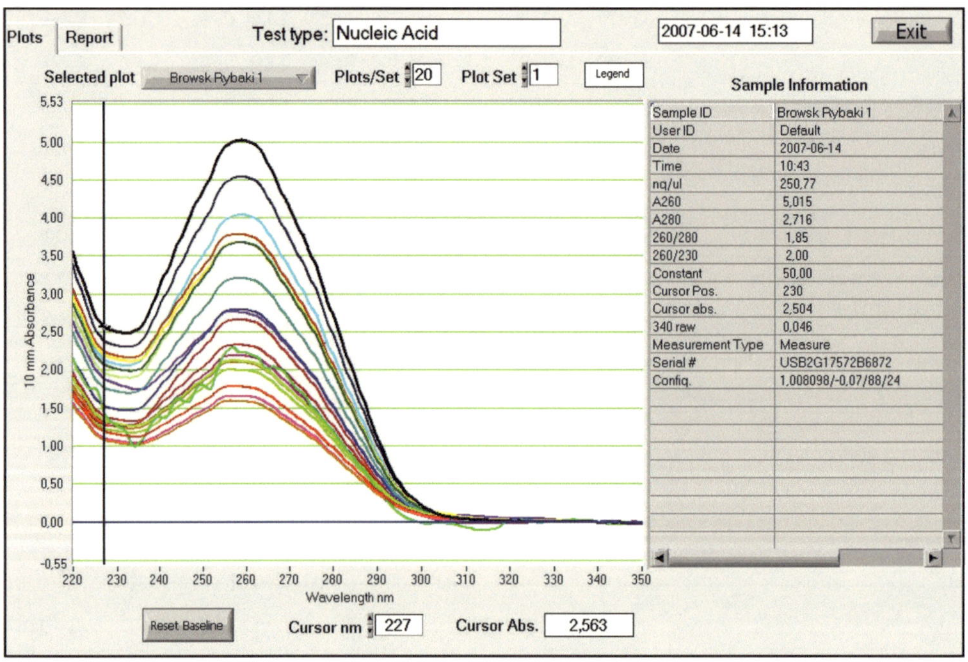

Figure 1. Spectrophotometrical assessment of the DNA extracts from Scots pine leaf samples population Browsk, in the spectrophotometer NanoDrop® ND-1000 (TK-Biotech, USA).

3.3.2. Genetic differentiation level

The studied trees harbored both heterozygotes and homozygotes in four microsatellite loci as illustrated in **Figure 2**. All loci were very polymorphic (mean *PIC* = 79.3), with highest values for loci SPAG 7.14 (*PIC* = 95.4) and SPAC 12.5 (*PIC* = 94.5). Total allele frequency distribution revealed 50 different alleles in SPAG 7.14 locus (**Figure 3**), 48 alleles in SPAC 12.5 (**Figure 4**), 31 alleles in PtTX3025 (**Figure 5**), and 18 alleles in SsrPt-ctg4363 locus (**Figure 6**). The allele

http://dx.doi.org/10.5772/64867

sizing was corrected in all loci because consecutive polymerase slippage was denoted. Null allele content was minor (2.3%) for all microsatellite loci.

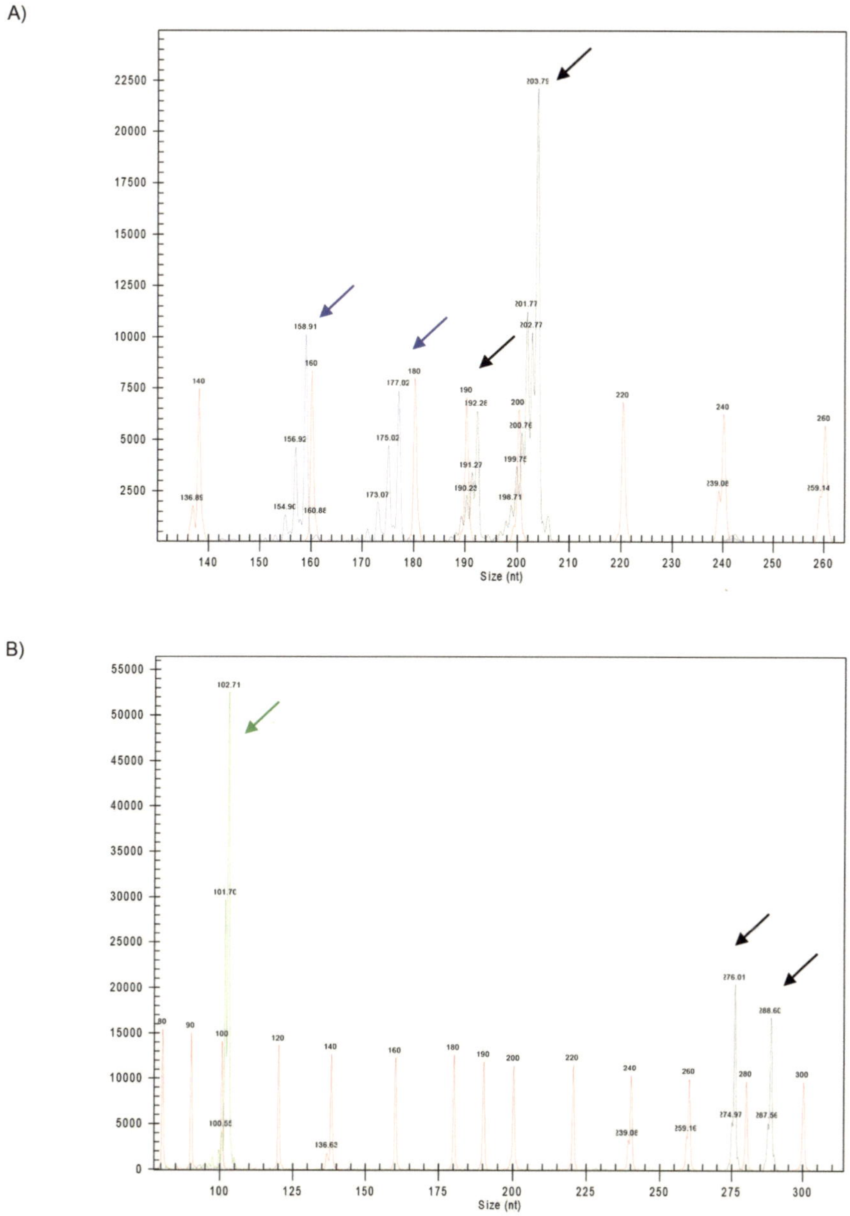

Figure 2. Example of microsatellite nuclear DNA analysis in Scots pine populations from North-eastern Poland: two alleles 159 and 177 base pairs in locus SPAG 7.14 (blue color) and two alleles 192 and 204 bp in locus SPAC 12.5 (black color) (A), one allele 102 bp in locus SsrPt-ctg4363 (green color) and two alleles 276 and 288 bp in locus PtTX3025 (black color) (B). Obtained from DNA capillary electrophoresis after Beckman Coulter® software CEQ™ 8000 Genetic Analysis System v 9.0 (Fullerton, USA).

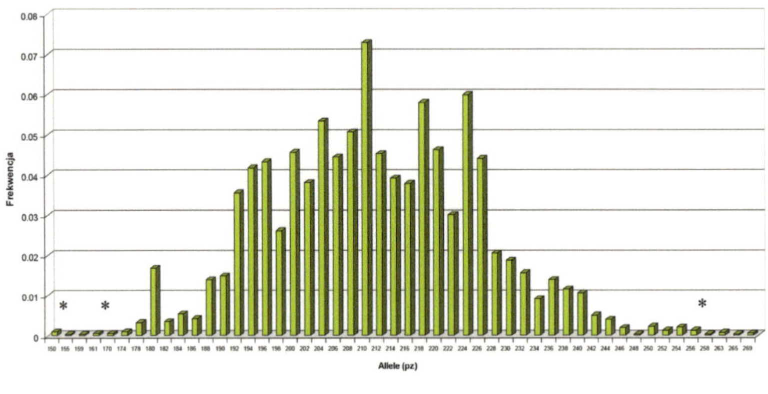

Figure 3. Total allele frequency distribution of SPAG 7.14 locus among studied Scots pine populations. *Polymerase slippage.

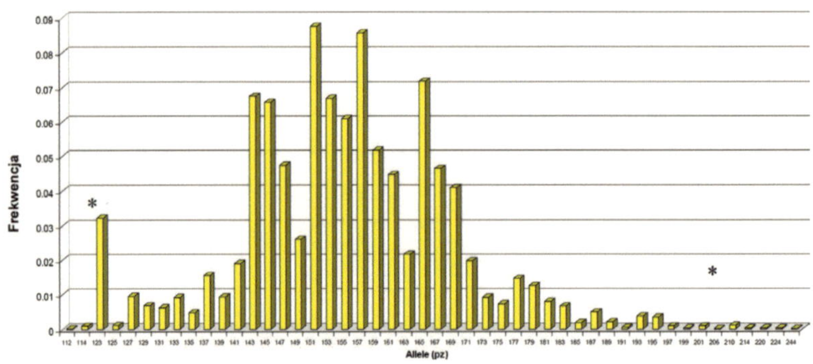

Figure 4. All allele frequency distribution according to their size for SPAC 12.5 locus among studied Scots pine populations. *Polymerase slippage.

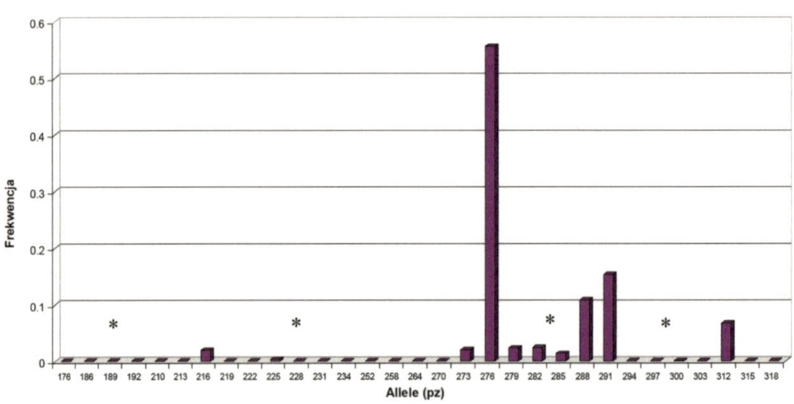

Figure 5. All alleles distribution according to their size of PtTX3025 microsatellite locus in Scots pine stands. *Polymerase slippage.

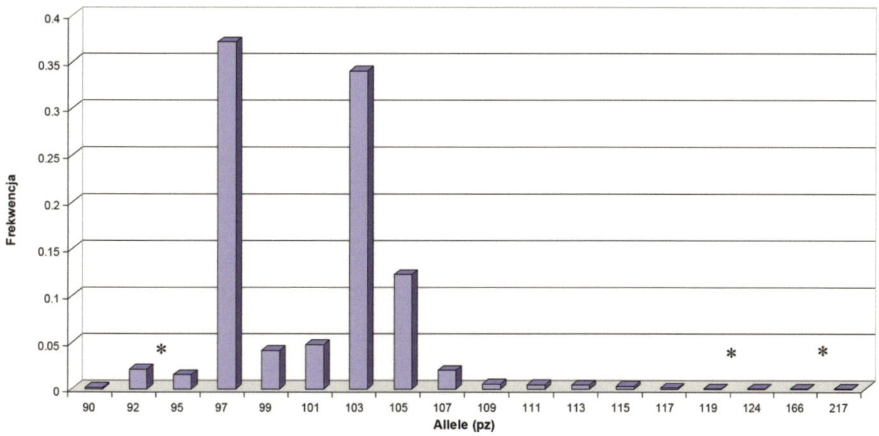

Figure 6. Total allele frequency distribution of SsrPt-ctg4363 locus among studied Scots pine populations. *Polymerase slippage

	pop1	pop2	pop3	pop4	pop5	pop6	pop7	pop8	pop9	pop10	pop11	pop12	pop13	pop14
pop1	0	1.262	0.062	0.090	0.085	0.051	0.076	0.030	0.039	0.073	0.048	0.073	1.173	0.067
pop2		0	1.393	1.434	1.175	1.245	1.189	1.372	1.383	1.069	1.347	1.264	0.037	1.111
pop3			0	0.086	0.058	0.054	0.042	0.061	0.043	0.084	0.059	0.068	1.354	0.070
pop4				0	0.115	0.094	0.094	0.085	0.091	0.156	0.116	0.062	1.391	0.111
pop5					0	0.074	0.062	0.091	0.063	0.091	0.074	0.089	1.113	0.113
pop6						0	0.061	0.045	0.056	0.081	0.066	0.057	1.191	0.056
pop7							0	0.071	0.057	0.079	0.062	0.056	1.165	0.052
pop8								0	0.046	0.066	0.045	0.062	1.283	0.062
pop9									0	0.086	0.041	0.056	1.309	0.062
pop10										0	0.072	0.109	0.996	0.086
pop11											0	0.087	1.329	0.084
pop12												0	1.240	0.053
pop13													0	1.100
pop14														0

Table 2. Distance matrix based on SSR marker frequencies in studied Scots pine populations.

Genetic differentiation level of microsatellite nSSR loci in studied Scots pine populations has been resumed and is listed in **Table 1**. All populations exhibited high genetic parameter variation, with total mean observed (n_a = 30.750) and effective (n_e = 12.400) allele number per locus, Shannon Index I = 2.488, observed (H_O = 0.778), and expected (H_E = 0.849) heterozygosity. The highest h Nei heterozygosity values (h = 0.832 and 0.822) were found in Waliły and Żednia

Borsukowina stands, respectively. The lowest (H = 0.774) was observed in Rudka stand. Total genetic diversity among populations was high (H_T = 0.848). Low level of F_{st} = 0.031 proved that the studied Scots pines are more differentiated within than among examined stands (**Table 1**).

3.3.3. *Genetic distance* (D_N)

The dendrogram built on the distance matrix based on SSR markers frequencies (**Table 2**) revealed two main clusters of populations (**Figure 7**). Two populations from the first group of dendrogram (number 2, Czarna Białostocka Budzisk, and 13, Knyszyn Kopisk) were separated by a distance of 0.612 from the second group. Moreover, two populations from the first group were closely located one to another in North-eastern Poland (**Figure 8**). Nevertheless, the robust MCMC analysis revealed only one cluster of population genetic grouping, proved also by CoPhenetic Correlation Coefficient value close to 1 (*CP* = 0.993).

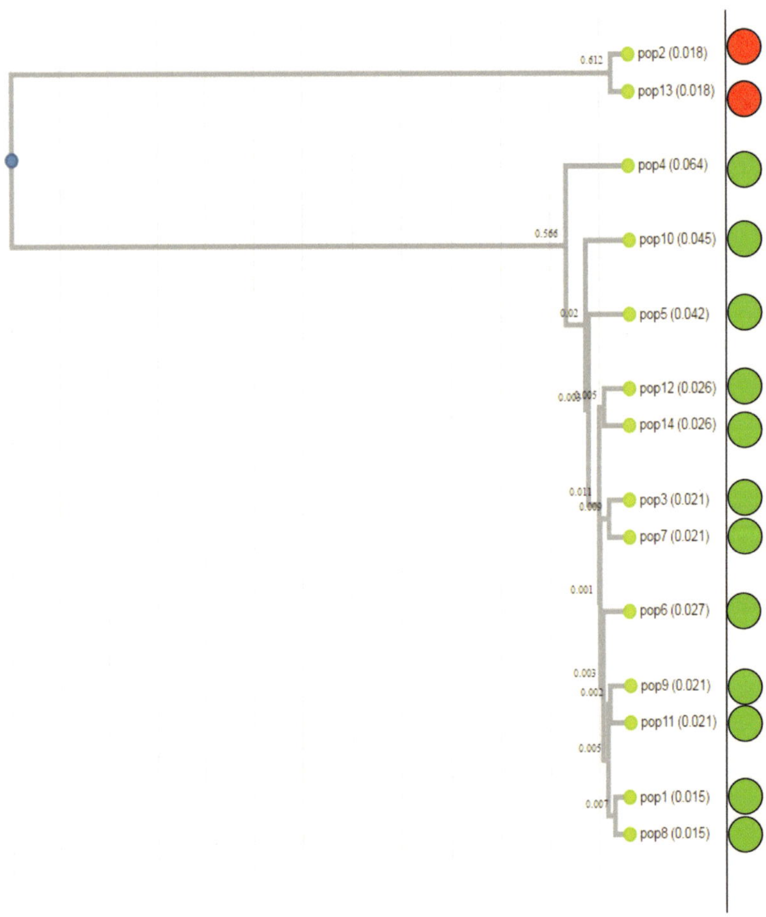

Figure 7. Dendrogram of genetic distances of Nei [49] based on microsatellite loci in studied Scots pine populations. Number of populations following **Table 1**.

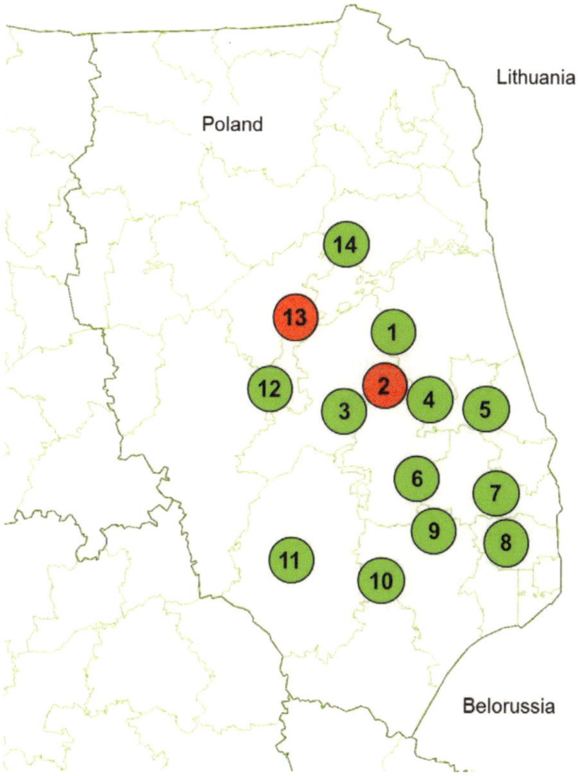

Figure 8. Geographical distribution of two genetically related groups of populations of Scots pine from North-eastern Poland, according to the dendrogram of genetic distances (**Figure 7**). Pop1, Czarna Białostocka Polanki; pop2, Czarna Białostocka Budzisk; Pop3, Dojlidy; pop4, Supraśl; pop5, Waliły; pop6, Żednia Nowa Wola; pop7, Żednia Borsukowina; pop8, Hajnówka; pop9, Browsk; pop10, Bielsk; pop11, Rudka; pop12, Knyszyn Szelągówka; pop13, Knyszyn Kopisk; pop14, Augustów. Map source: [82]

4. Discussion

The development of an appropriate genetic conservation strategy for native Scots pine populations in European countries seems to be a very relevant priority. Numerous nuclear microsatellite markers have already been described for different conifer species, for example, fir, larch, pine, and spruce (for review, see [9, 14, 19, 31, 33, 65–69]). Some DNA markers have also been used to characterize the genetic variation of *P. sylvestris* populations, for example, RAPD [12, 70], RFLP [59], STS [10], and microsatellites [6, 9, 30, 31, 36, 39, 71, 72].

In Poland, Scots pine resources are classified by reference to 26 seed regions, based on the boundary delineation of physicogeographical features, for example, a homogeneous climate and geographic conditions [12]. Programs for the *in situ* conservation of valuable Scots pine provenances are put in place with regard to the distribution of seed regions, as well as the location of what are known as natural-forest regions. The present rules for the transfer of Scots pine genetic resources in Europe are mainly founded upon such provenance tests, with only a few investigations being based on molecular markers [12, 40, 73].

In the present study, low genetic differentiation level of 14 Scots pine stands from the North-eastern Poland was determined thanks to the DNA profiles established on a basis of four microsatellite nuclear DNA loci (SPAG 7.14, SPAC 12.5, PtTX3025, and SsrPt-ctg4363). These data support previous investigations of the genetic structure performed using four nuclear microsatellite markers on 42 Scots pine populations located in different regions in Poland [38]. Pine trees from 42 stands were characterized by high polymorphism level (PIC = 80.0%), and low level of interpopulation differences (F_{st} = 0.033). The Baltic, Śląska, and Wielkopolsko-Pomorska Regions revealed the highest genetic differentiation (F_{st} = 0.036, H_S = 0.323, and H_S = 0.207, respectively). The UPGMA analysis performed with nuclear microsatellite markers in 42 populations generated two main groups of populations with a very weak probability of clustering. The geographical distribution of the genotypes emerging from dendrogram was scattered across the country. Moreover, no spatial correlation between the gene diversity and the geographical locations of stands was found [38]. In this regard, data obtained for 14 Scots pine populations from North-eastern Poland (present study) reflect similar level of the genetic variation (F_{st} = 0.031), and no spatial correlation between stand location and genetic distance was found. Such a situation is often described for many forest-tree species natural populations, and reflects forest-tree characteristics, such as longevity, long-distance pollen dispersion, and great potential for adaptation to various climatic changes [1, 2, 6, 26, 41, 60, 61].

Scattered distribution of genetically related populations of Scots pine seems to reflect the historical events such as colonization of Poland by this species from different postglacial refugia and/or by significant human management practiced in the past. These data were supported by mitochondrial gene study, which have a maternal mode of transmission, and non-recombinational nature in conifers was used in the study of maternal lineages and the postglacial migration of *P. sylvestris* across Europe [10].

Another type of microsatellite sequences located in chloroplast genome (cpSSR) could also present an interesting tool to which the genetic diversity and gene flow among *Pinus* populations could be analyzed. Since the chloroplast and mitochondrial genomes are uniparentally inherited in conifers, these markers are not exposed to the recombination process [74]. CpSSR loci present some advantages, for example, they are less variable than nuclear SSR, express low mutation rate, and high species specificity [37]. Most of the cpSSR analyses have been reported for different *Pinus* species, for example, *P. leucodermis* [66], *P. halepensis* [75], *P. pinaster* [11,33,76], *P. resinosa* [67], *P. brutia* [77], *P. torreyana* [37], *P. cembra*, *P. sibirica*, and *P. pumila* [78], and *P. echinata* [79]. In most cases, the cpSSR markers have been successfully used in paternity analysis, in the monitoring of the gene flow between populations and in the study of population history following the postglacial migration of pine species.

Recently, investigation focusing on nuclear and chloroplast microsatellite DNA markers in wood tissue identification is an efficient method to be used for forensic purposes. The present methodology helps to compare detailed DNA patterns of Scots pine (*P. sylvestris*), Norway spruce (*P. abies* L. Karst.), European silver fir (*A. alba* L.), and European larch (*L. decidua* Mill.), with high probability of identity (c.a. of 99.99%) [43].

Both adaptive and neutral markers (e.g., microsatellites) present many advantages in modern forest genetics [60, 65, 75, 78, 80]. In order to find the genetic basis of the neutral or adaptive diversity of natural populations, simulations based on adaptive traits, quantitative trait loci, and neutral markers are performed [81].

5. Conclusions

The conservation of genetic variability is a major focus in forest-tree selection and sustainable forest management (SFM). The preservation of genetic diversity in different forest-tree species facing changes of environmental conditions and increasing human industrial activity is still the great challenge for researchers involved in adaptive and evolutionary genetics. Genetic variation may be investigated by means of several molecular techniques using DNA markers. Among them, the microsatellites are the most powerful and suitable tool in the identification and characterization of the genetic resources in forest. Because of their relatively high mutation rate, microsatellites are often used to study genetic variation and population structure. The SSR markers constitute an effective tool by which the European Scots pine populations have been studied on the basis of nuclear and chloroplast DNA. In this context, stress is placed on the accurateness of the chosen marker for a given purpose, as well as the statistical methods of calculation.

The nuclear SSRs are mainly used in studying genomic differentiation. The discriminatory power of nuclear SSR markers points out their applicability to the study of various forest-tree populations. The comparative study of dominant and codominant nuclear markers in forest-tree genetics shows that even a few microsatellite loci can be used in the high-accuracy prediction levels of genetic diversity. It is supposed that the populations with low level of genetic variation are generally less genetically stable and more vulnerable to pathogenic infections and harmful changes of environmental conditions [1, 39, 41]. The researchers involved in the field of forestry foresee the need for further analysis using molecular genetic tools.

Particular attention should be drawn to the avoidance of some errors occurring during the scoring of microsatellite allele (in Scots pine or other organisms, we can meet null allele, short allele dominance, and polymerase slippage). The use of the specialized genotyping software is therefore strongly advised.

Many approaches to the conservation of genetic diversity, the exploration of plant-genetic resources, and the design of plant-improvement programs require a specific knowledge on the amount and distribution of genetic diversity within investigated species. The genetic information contained in DNA, particularly in microsatellite sequences, offers valuable input when it comes to the *in situ* and *ex situ* conservation of forest-genetic resources. Notwithstanding the intensive use and management of the species, very little is still known about the genetic variability of Scots pines in Europe. The present chapter attempted to give an introduction to the practical side of microsatellite analysis and the interpretation of genomic data obtained for Scots pine (*P. sylvestris*) populations in Poland.

Acknowledgements

The results mentioned in this chapter are parts of the research funded by the General Directorate of State Forests (grant BLP-309). Many thanks are expressed to colleagues from the Forest Research Institute IBL Poland, especially Jolanta Bieniek, Małgorzata Borys, M.Sc., Dr Anna Zawadzka, Dr Jan Kowalczyk, Michał Zawadzki, M.Sc., and Jerzy Przyborowski involved in plant material collection and laboratory DNA analyses.

Author details

Justyna Anna Nowakowska

Address all correspondence to: J.Nowakowska@ibles.waw.pl

Forest Research Institute, Laboratory of Molecular Biology, Sękocin Stary, Raszyn, Poland

References

[1] Hamrick JL. Response of forest trees to global environmental changes. For. Ecol. Manag. 2004;197:323–335. DOI:10.1016/j.foreco.2004.05.023.

[2] Ahuja MR, Neale DB. Evolution of genome size in conifers. Silvae Genet. 2005;54:126–137.

[3] Lexer C, Heinze B, Alia R, Rieseberg LH. Hybrid zones as a tool for identifying adaptive genetic variation in outbreeding forest trees: lessons from wild annual sunflowers (*Helianthus* ssp.). For. Ecol. Manag. 2004;197:49–64. DOI: 10.1016/j.foreco.2004.05.004.

[4] Li Y-C, Korol AB, Fahima T, Beiles A, Nevo E. Microsatellites: genomic distribution, putative functions and mutational mechanisms: a review. Mol. Ecol. 2002;11:2453–2465. DOI: 10.1046/j.1365-294X.2002.01643.x.

[5] Zhang DX, Hewitt GM. Nuclear DNA analysis in genetic studies of populations: practice, problems and prospects. Mol. Ecol. 2003;12:563–584. DOI: 10.1046/j.1365-294X.2003.01773.x.

[6] Robledo-Arnuncio JJ, Smouse PE, Gil L, Alía R. Pollen movement under alternative silvicultural practices in native populations of Scots pine (*Pinus sylvestris* L.) in central Spain. For. Ecol. Manag. 2004;197:245–255. DOI:10.1016/j.foreco.2004.05.016.

[7] Neale DB, Devey ME, Jermstad KD, Ahuja MR, Alosi MC, Marshall KA. Use of DNA markers in forest tree improvement research. New For. 1992;6:391–407. DOI: 10.1007/BF00120654.

[8] DeVerno LL, Mosseler A. Genetic variation in red pine (*Pinus resinosa*) revealed by RAPD and RAPD-RFLP analysis. Can. J. For. Res. 1997;27:1316–1320. DOI: 10.1139/x97-090.

[9] Soranzo N, Provan J, Powell W. Characterization of microsatellite loci in *Pinus sylvestris* L. Mol. Ecol. 1998;7(9):1260–1261.

[10] Soranzo N, Alía R, Provan J, Powell W. Patterns of variation at a mitochondrial sequence-tagged-site locus provides new insights into the postglacial history of European *Pinus sylvestris* populations. Mol. Ecol. 2000;9:1205–1211. DOI: 10.1046/j.1365-294x.2000.00994.x.

[11] Ribeiro MM, Mariette S, Vendramin GG, Szmidt E, Plomion C, Kremer A. Comparison of genetic diversity estimates within and among populations of maritime pine using chloroplast simple-sequence repeat and amplified fragment length polymorphism data. Mol. Ecol. 2002;11:869–877. DOI: 10.1046/j.1365-294X.2002.01490.x.

[12] Nowakowska J. Genetic diversity of Scots pine (*Pinus sylvestris* L.) Polish provenances based on RAPD analysis. Sylwan. 2003;11:26–37.

[13] Lefort F, Echt C, Streiff R, Vendramin GG. Microsatellite sequences: a new generation of molecular markers for forest genetics. For. Genet. 1999;6(1):15–20.

[14] Wang Z, Weber JL, Zhong G, Tanksley SD. Survey of plant short tandem DNA repeats. Theor. Appl. Genet. 1994;88:1–6. DOI: 10.1007/BF00222386.

[15] Kashi Y, Soller M. Functional roles of microsatellites and minisatellites. Microsatellites: Evolution and Applications. Goldstein DB, Schlötterer C, Eds., Oxford University Press, Oxford, Great Britain; 1999. p. 10–23. ISBN: 9780198504078.

[16] Gur-Arie R, Cohen CJ, Eitan Y, Shelef L, Halleman EM, Kashi Y. Simple sequence repeats in *Escherichia coli*: abundance, distribution, composition, and polymorphism. Gen. Res. 2000;10:62–71. doi: 10.1101/gr.10.1.62.

[17] Schmidt A, Doudrick RL, Heslop-Harrison JS, Shmidt T. The contribution of short repeats of low sequence complexity to large conifer genomes. Theor. Appl. Genet. 2000;101:7–14.

[18] Karhu A, Dieterich JH, Savolainen O. Rapid expansion of microsatellite sequences in pines. Mol. Biol. Evol. 2000;17:259–265. ISSN: 0737-4038.

[19] Echt CS, MayMarquardt P. Survey of microsatellite DNA in pine. Genome. 1997;40:9–17.

[20] Buschiazzo E, Gemmell NJ. The rise, fall and renaissance of microsatellites in eukaryote genomes. BioEssays. 2006;28:1040–1050. DOI: 10.1002/bies.20470.

[21] Pemberton JM, Slate J, Bancroft DR, Barrett JA. Non-amplifying alleles at microsatellites loci: a caution for parentage and population studies. Mol. Ecol. 1995;4:249–252. DOI: 10.1111/j.1365-294X.1995.tb00214.x.

[22] Navascués M, Emerson BC. Chloroplast microsatellites: measures of genetic diversity and the effect of homoplasy. Mol. Ecol. 2005;14:1333–1341. DOI: 10.1111/j.1365-294X.2005.02504.x.

[23] Deforce DLD, Millecamps REM, Van Hoofstat D, Van den Eeckhout EG. Comparison of slab gel electrophoresis and capillary electrophoresis for the detection of the fluorescently labeled polymerase chain reaction products of short tandem repeat fragments. J. Chromatogr. A. 1998;806:149–155. DOI: 10.1016/S0021-9673(97)00394-4.

[24] Delmotte F, Leterme N, Simon JC. Microsatellite allele sizing: difference between automated capillary electrophoresis and manual technique. BioTechniques. 2001;31:810–818.

[25] Howells EJ, Willis BL, Bay LK, Van Oppen MJH. Microsatellite allele sizes alone are insufficient to delineate species boundaries in Symbiodinium. Mol. Ecol. 2016. DOI: 10.1111/mec.13631.

[26] Scotti I, Vendramin GG, Matteotti LS, Scarponi C, Sari-Gorla M, Binelli G. Postglacial recolonization routes for *Picea abies* K. in Italy as suggested by the analysis of sequence-characterized amplified region (SCAR) markers. Mol. Ecol. 2000;9:699–708. DOI: 10.1046/j.1365-294x.2000.00911.x.

[27] The European Bioinformatics Institute [Internet]. 2016. Available from: http://www.ebi.ac.uk [Accessed from 2016-07-05].

[28] National Center for Biotechnology Information [Internet]. 2016. Available from: http://www.ncbi.nlm.nih.gov [Accessed from 2016-07-05].

[29] Wiley Online Library [Internet]. 2016. Available from: http://www.blackwell-synergy.com [Accessed from 2016-07-05].

[30] Kostia S, Varvio SL, Vakkari P, Pulkkinen P. Microsatellite sequences in a conifer, *Pinus sylvestris*. Genome. 1995;38:1244–1248. DOI: 10.1139/g95-163.

[31] Chagné D, Chaumeil P, Ramboer A, Collada C, Guevara A, Cervera MT, Vendramin GG, Garcia V, Frigerio J-M, Echt C, Richardson T, Plomion C. Cross-species transferability and mapping of genomic and cDNA SSRs in pines. Theor. Appl. Genet. 2004;109:1204–1214. DOI: 10.1007/s00122-004-1683-z.

[32] Zane L, Bargelloni L, Patarnello T. Strategies for microsatellite isolation: a review. Mol. Ecol. 2002;11:1–16. DOI: 10.1046/j.0962-1083.2001.01418.x.

[33] González-Martínez SC, Robledo-Arnuncio JJ, Collada C, Díaz A, Williams CG, Alía R, Cervera MT. Cross-amplification and sequence variation of microsatellite loci in Eurasian hard pines. Theor. Appl. Genet. 2004;109:103–111. DOI: 10.1007/s00122-004-1596-x.

[34] Leitch IJ, Hanson L, Winfield M, Parker J, Bennet MD. Nuclear DNA C-values complete familial representation in Gymnosperms. Ann. Bot. 2001;88:843–849. DOI: 10.1006/anbo.2001.1521.

[35] Mariette S, Chagné D, Decroocq S, Vendramin GG, Lalanne C, Madur D, Plomion C. Microsatellite markers for *Pinus pinaster* Ait. Ann. For. Sci. 2001;58:203–206.

[36] García-Gil MR, Floran V, Östlund L, Mullin TJ, Andersson Gull B. Genetic diversity and inbreeding in natural and managed populations of Scots pine. Tree Gen. Gen. 2015;11(28). DOI: 10.1007/s11295-015-0850-5.

[37] Provan J, Soranzo N, Wilson NJ, Goldstein DB, Powell W. A low mutation rate for chloroplast microsatellites. Genetics. 1999;153:943–947.

[38] Nowakowska JA. Genetic variation of Polish Scots pine (*Pinus sylvestris* L.) populations assessed with DNA polymorphism markers. Habilitation dissert. Instytut Badawczy Leśnictwa Ed., Sękocin Stary; 2007. 118 p. ISBN 978-83-878647-70-4 (in Polish, with abstract, summary, tables and figures in English.)

[39] Belletti P, Ferrazzini D, Piotti A, Monteleone I, Ducci F. Genetic variation and divergence in Scots pine (*Pinus sylvestris* L.) within its natural range in Italy. Eur. J. Forest Res. 2012;131:1127–1138. DOI: 10.1007/s10342-011-0584-3.

[40] Prus-Głowacki W, Stephan BR. Genetic variation of *Pinus sylvestris* from Spain in relation to other European populations. Silvae Gen. 1994;43:7–14.

[41] Kremer A, Ronce O, Robledo-Arnuncio JJ, Guillaume F, Bohrer G, Nathan R, Bridle JR, Gomulkiewicz R, Klein EK, Ritland K, Kuparinen A, Gerber S, Schueler S. Long-distance gene flow and adaptation of forest trees to rapid climate change. Ecol. Lett. 2012;15:378–392. DOI: 10.1111/j.1461-0248.2012.01746.x.

[42] Doyle JJ, Doyle JL. Isolation of plant DNA from fresh tissue. BRL Focus. 1990;12:13–15.

[43] Nowakowska JA, Oszako T, Tereba A, Konecka A. Forest Tree Species Traced with a DNA-Based Proof for Illegal Logging Case in Poland. Evolutionary Biology: Biodiversification from Genotype to Phenotype, Pierre Pontarotti, Ed., Springer Publisher, vol. 19, 2015. p. 373–388. ISBN 978-3-319-19931-3.

[44] Tibbits JFG, McManus LJ, Spokevicius AV, Bossinger G. A rapid method for tissue collection and high throughput isolation of genomic DNA from mature trees. Plant Mol. Biol. Rep. 2006;24: 81–91. DOI:10.1007/BF02914048.

[45] Nowakowska JA. Application of DNA markers against illegal logging as a new tool for the forest guard service. Folia For. Pol. Series A. 2011;53(2):142–149.

[46] Asif MJ, Cannon CH. DNA extraction from processed wood: a case study for the identification of an endangered timber species (*Gonystylus bancanus*). Plant Mol. Biol. Rep. 2005;23:185–192. DOI: 10.1007/BF02772709.

[47] Bartlett JMS, Stirling D. A Short History of the Polymerase Chain Reaction. PCR Protocols. Methods in Molecular Biology 226 (2nd ed.) Humana Press Inc., Totowa, NJ. 2003. pp. 3–6. DOI: 10.1385/1-59259-384-4:3. ISBN 1-59259-384-4.

[48] Sambrook J, Russell DW. Molecular Cloning. A Laboratory Manual. Cold Spring Harbor Laboratory Press, Cold Spring Harbor, New York, NY, USA, 2001. Vol. 2. ISBN 0-87969-577-3.

[49] Nei M. Analysis of gene diversity in subdivided populations. Proc. Natl. Acad. Sci. USA. 1973;70(12):3321–3323.

[50] Nei M. Estimation of average heterozygosity and genetic distance from a small number of individuals. Genetics. 1978;89:583–590.

[51] Nowakowska JA, Sułkowska M. Capillary electrophoresis as useful tool in analysis *Fagus sylvatica* population genetic dynamics. Electrophoresis Book, Kiumars Ghowsi, Ed., Open Science INTECH, Croatia. p. 49–68. ISBN 978-953-51-2025-4.

[52] Gömöry D, Paule L, Brus R, Tomović Z, Gračan J. Genetic differentiation and phylogeny of beech on the Balkan peninsula. J. Evol. Biol. 1999;12(4):746–754. DOI: 10.1046/j.1420-9101.1999.00076.x.

[53] Peakall R, Smouse PE. GenAlEx 6.5: genetic analysis in Excel. Population genetic software for teaching and research—an update. Bioinformatics. 2012;28:2537-2539. DOI: 10.1093/bioinformatics/bts460.

[54] Garcia-Vallvé S, Palau J, Romeu R. Horizontal gene transfer in glycosyl hydrolases inferred from codon usage in *Escherichia coli* and *Bacillus subtilis*. Mol. Biol. Evol. 1999;16(9):1125–1134.

[55] Poland—The State Forests in figures 2013 [Internet]. 2013. Available from: www.lasy.gov.pl/publikacje/in-english/the-state-forests-in-figures-2013 [Accessed: 07-07-2016].

[56] Forest Finland in brief 2003. Y. Sevola, Ed. The Finnish Forest Research Institute, Forest Statistics Information Service, Helsinki, Finland. p. 33.

[57] Pivoriunas A. Cooperation of private forest owners: case study in Lithuania. Miskininkyste. 2004;2(56):69–77.

[58] Bradshaw RHW. Past anthropogenic influence on European forest and some possible genetic consequences. For. Ecol. Manag. 2004;197:203–212. DOI: 10.1016/j.foreco.2004.05.025.

[59] Sinclair WT, Morman JD, Ennos RA. The postglacial history of Scots pine (*Pinus sylvestris* L.) in western Europe: evidence from mitochondrial DNA variation. Mol. Ecol. 1999;8:83–88. DOI: 10.1046/j.1365-294X.1999.00527.x.

[60] Kremer A, Reviron MP. Dynamics and conservation of genetic diversity in forest ecosystems. For. Ecol. Manag. 2004;197:1–2. DOI: 10.1016/j.foreco.2004.05.001.

[61] Petit RJ, Bialozyt R, Garnier-Géré P, Hampe A. Ecology and genetics of tree invasion: from recent introductions to quaternary migrations. For. Ecol. Manag. 2004;197:117–137. DOI: 10.1016/j.foreco.2004.05.009.

[62] Gutiérez JP, Royo LJ, Álvarez I, Goyache F. MolKin v2.0: a computer program for genetic analysis of populations using molecular coancestry information. J. Heredity. 2005;96(6): 718–721. DOI: 10.1093/jhered/esi118.

[63] DendroUPGMA: A dendrogram construction utility [Internet]. 2016. Available from: http://genomes.urv.cat/UPGMA/index.php [Accessed from 2016-07-05].

[64] Corander J, Waldmann P, Sillanpää MJ. Bayesian analysis of genetic differentiation between populations. Genetics. 2003;163:367–374.

[65] Amarasinghe V, Carlson JE. The development of microsatellite DNA markers for genetic analysis in Douglas-fir. Can. J. For. Res. 2002;32:1904–1915. DOI: 10.1139/x02-110.

[66] Powel W, Morgante M, McDevitt R, Vendramin GG, Rafalski JA. Polymorphic simple sequence repeat regions in chloroplast genomes: applications to the population genetics of pines. Proc. Natl. Acad. Sci. USA. 1995;92:7759–7763.

[67] Echt CS, Vendramin GG, Nelson CD, Marquardt P. Microsatellite DNA as shared genetic markers among conifer species. Can J. For. Res. 1999;29:365–371. DOI: 10.1139/cjfr-29-3-365.

[68] Shepherd M, Cross M, Maguire TL, Dieters MJ, Williams CG, Henry RJ. Transpecific microsatellites for hard pines. Theor. Appl. Genet. 2002;104:819–827. DOI 10.1007/s00122-001-0794-z.

[69] Besnard G, Achere V, Faivre Rampant P, Favre JM, Jeandroz S. A set of cross-species amplifying microsatellite markers developed from DNA sequence databanks in *Picea* (*Pinaceae*). Mol. Ecol. Notes. 2003;3:380–383. DOI: 10.1046/j.1471-8286.2003.00456.x.

[70] Žvingila D, Verbylaite R, Abraitis R, Kuusiene S., Ozolinčius R. Assessment of genetic diversity in plus tree clones of *Pinus sylvestris* L. using RAPD markers. Baltic For. 2002;8(2):2–7.

[71] Auckland L, Bui T, Zhou Y, Shepherd M, Williams C. Conifer Microsatellite Handbook. Texas A&M University, College Station, TX, USA; 2002. 57 p.

[72] Komulainen P, Brown GR, Mikkonen M, Karhu A, García-Gil MR, O'Malley D, Lee B, Neale DB, Savolainen O. Comparing EST-based genetic maps between *Pinus sylvestris* and *Pinus taeda*. Theor. Appl. Genet. 2003;107:667–678. DOI: 10.1007/s00122-003-1312-2.

[73] Giertych M. Provenance Variation. Biology of Scots Pine. Sorus PAN Ed Poznań-Kórnik; 1993. p. 325–339.

[74] Sperisen C, Büchler, Mátyás G, Anzidei M, Madaghiele A, Skrøppa T, Vendramin GG. Polymorphic tandem repeats in the chloroplast and mitochondrial genomes of Norway

spruce. Genetics and breeding of Norway spruce. Skrøppa T, Paule L, Gömöry D, Eds., Arbora Publisher, Zvolen, Slovakia; 1998: p. 15–24.

[75] Morgante M, Felice N, Vendramin GG. Analysis of hypervariable chloroplast microsatellites in *Pinus halepensis* reveals a dramatic genetic bottleneck. Molecular tools for screening biodiversity: plants and animals. Karp A, Isaac PG, Ingram DS, Eds., Chapman and Hall, London, UK; 1997. p. 407–412. DOI: 10.1007/978-94-009-0019-6_73.

[76] Vendramin GG, Lelli L, Rossi P, Morgante M. A set of primers for the amplification of 20 chloroplast microsatellites in Pinaceae. Mol. Ecol. 1996;5(4):595–598. DOI: 10.1111/j.1365-294X.1996.tb00353.x.

[77] Bucci G, Anzidei M, Madaghiele A, Vendramin GG. Detection of haplotypic variation and natural hybridisation in *halepensis*-complex pine species using chloroplast SSR markers. Mol. Ecol. 1998;7:1633–1643. DOI: 10.1046/j.1365-294x.1998.00466.x.

[78] Gugerli F, Senn J, Anzidei M, Madaghiele A, Büchler U, Sperisen C, Vendramin GG. Chloroplast microsatellites and mitochondrial *nad*1 intron 2 sequences indicate congruent phylogenetic relationships among Swiss stone pine (*Pinus cembra*), Siberian stone pine (*Pinus sibirica*), and Siberian dwarf pine (*Pinus pumila*). Mol. Ecol. 2001;10:1489–1497. DOI: 10.1046/j.1365-294X.2001.01285.x.

[79] Dyer RJ, Sork VL. Pollen pool heterogeneity in shortleaf pine, *Pinus echinata* Mill. Mol. Ecol. 2001;10:859–866. DOI: 10.1046/j.1365-294X.2001.01251.x.

[80] Ouborg NJ, Piquot Y, Van Groenendael JM. Population genetics, molecular markers and the study of dispersal in plants. J. Ecol. 1999;87(4):551–568. DOI: 10.1046/j.1365-2745.1999.00389.x.

[81] Slate J. Quantitative trait locus mapping in natural populations: progress, caveats and future directions. Mol. Ecol. 2005;14(2):363–79. DOI: 10.1111/j.1365-294X.2004.02378.x.

[82] Lasy na mapach—Bank Danych o Lasach [Internet]. 2016. Available from: www.bdl.lasy.gov.pl/portal/mapy [Accessed from 05-07-2016].

Chapter 6

Application of Microsatellites in Genetic Diversity Analysis and Heterotic Grouping of Sorghum and Maize

Beyene Amelework, Demissew Abakemal,
Hussein Shimelis and Mark Laing

Additional information is available at the end of the chapter

http://dx.doi.org/10.5772/65078

Abstract

Sorghum and maize are major cereal crops worldwide and key food security crops in Sub-Saharan Africa. The difference in the mating systems, maize as predominantly a cross-fertilizer and sorghum as a self-fertilizer is reflected in differences in visible phenotypic and genotypic variations. The reproductive differences dictate the level of genetic variation present in the two crops. Conventionally, a heterotic group assignment is made based on phenotypic values estimated through combining ability and heterosis analyses. However, phenotypic evaluation methods have their limitation due to the influence of the environment and may not reflect the heterotic pattern of the lines accurately. Therefore, more effective and complementary methods have been proposed for heterotic grouping of candidate lines. Estimation of molecular-based genetic distance has proven to be a useful tool to describe existing heterotic groups, to identify new heterotic groups, and to assign inbreds into heterotic groups. Among the molecular markers, microsatellites markers have proved to be a powerful tool for analyzing genetic diversity and for classifying inbred lines into heterotic groups. Therefore, the aim of this chapter was to elucidate the use of microsatellite markers in genetic diversity analysis and heterotic grouping of sorghum and maize.

Keywords: genetic diversity analysis, heterotic grouping, maize, microsatellites, simple sequence repeats, sorghum

1. Introduction

Maize and sorghum have been more widely evaluated in genetic and cytogenetic studies than other cereal crops. Maize is one of the domesticated crop species with the highest level of molecular polymorphism. Nucleotide diversity of more than 5% has been reported at some loci of the maize genome [1], and this has been confirmed by high genetic variability in maize. The molecular diversity of maize is approximately 3- to 10-fold higher than any other domesticated grass species [2]. Several factors have been suggested as reasons for the diversity in maize including: (1) differences in the growing environments, cultivation geared toward various production systems and varied consumption preferences [3] that influenced breeding of maize varieties to severe diverse human needs worldwide; (2) high level of cross-fertilization and independent assortment of genes that led to considerable gene transfer between populations, including wild relatives; (3) presence of duplications and recombination of genes leading to creation of mutations and ultimate phenotypic variability [4]; and (4) existence of transposons and retro-transposable genetic elements leading to marked genetic variation among maize populations [5].

Similarly, sorghum is one of the most genetically diverse self-fertilizing crops. Early domestication and selection of sorghum in response to environmental factors and human needs resulted in the wide variability. The environmental factors included day length, altitude, temperature, rainfall, and soil characteristics. Humans usually required a large panicle, a nonshattering habit, large grain, tall plant height, and early maturity. The greater genetic diversity is, therefore, partly due to the diverse physical environments and partly due to the interaction of man with the environment [6]. As a result, the new and stable sorghum biotypes that have emerged can be attributed to selection, adaptation, intercrossing, and the movement of plant material from place to place. Introduction of new genotypes that have evolved in other places may result in intercrossing with the native genetic resources leading to the development of new biotypes. This movement and evolution of germplasm gave rise to five major sorghum races: bicolor, caudatum, guinea, kafir, and durra [7].

Morpho-agronomic characters of crop plants have traditionally been used for assessment of genetic variability. These characters reflect genetic variations that are manifested as visible morphological traits [8]. However, assessments based on these characters are not efficient or reliable because they are strongly affected by environmental factors. Other genetic variations are compositional or chemicals that require various tests for evaluation [9]. Isozymes [10] and seed storage proteins [11] were the most widely used biochemical markers. Since the late 1980s, analyses using various electrophoretic [12] and reversed-phase high-performance liquid chromatography (RP-HPLC) [13] of seed storage proteins have been developed and are considered effective methods for cultivar identification. Often, the importance of these types of markers is inherently impeded by low polymorphism.

The application of DNA molecular markers as compared to morphological and biochemical markers overcomes the problem of low polymorphism. DNA markers are highly informative and have facilitated the identification of agronomic traits in wild, traditional, and improved germplasm through the dissection of quantitative traits [14]. DNA-based molecular markers are independent to environmental factors. DNA markers are fast, efficient, and robust providing clear genetic differences than phenotypic markers [15] . Several DNA marker technologies are available for determining genetic variations. Nevertheless, selection of the best marker system depends on the target species, the aim of the marker analysis, and the resource capacity [14]. PCR-based markers are widely preferred for genotype characterization in diverse crop species, including sorghum and maize, as they are relatively simple to use, nondistractive, and require small quantity of DNA, thus permitting many reactions from a single sample [16]. In addition, genetic distance (GD) estimates using molecular markers are reportedly helpful to identify the best parent combinations for new pedigree starts and to assign lines into heterotic groups [17, 18].

Molecular markers, such as restricted fragment length polymorphisms (RFLPs), random amplified polymorphic DNA (RAPD), amplified fragment length polymorphism (AFLPs), and simple sequence repeats (SSRs) or microsatellites, have been proposed as tools not only to evaluate breeding lines and hybrids and cultivars [19] but also to facilitate the monitoring of introgression, mapping of quantitative trait loci (QTLs), and the assessment of genetic diversity [20, 21] in various crops, including sorghum and maize. SSR markers have been widely applied for the assessment of genetic diversity and characterization of germplasm [22–24], identification and fingerprinting of genotypes [14], and estimation of genetic distances between and within populations [22] and to assign inbred lines into heterotic groups [25, 26]. SSR data from a number of loci have the potential to provide unique allelic profiles or DNA fingerprints for precisely establishing genotypic identity. They also have greater discriminatory power than restricted fragment length polymorphisms markers and can exhibit genetic relations that are reflective of the pedigree of the inbred lines [27]. Genotyping of inbred lines using SSRs is a reliable way of germplasm characterization which, together with morphological descriptions, leads to unambiguous differentiation of genotypes that can be utilized for a hybrid breeding program [28]. Therefore, SSR markers are the efficient marker of choice due to their ability to provide informative multiallelic loci, highly reproducible test with great powers of genotypic differentiation, which are relatively simple to use [29].

Classification of the available complementary inbreds into distinct heterotic groups is crucial to the development of superior hybrids and in developing genetic pools and breeding populations for designed breeding and genetic analyses. Exploitation of heterosis, utilization of heterotic groups, and their patterns is well established and developed in maize [30]. However, efforts to determine heterotic groups in sorghum have not been successful in clearly delineating any patterns [31]. The phenomenon of heterosis between genetically distant or unrelated genotypes has been widely reported. A heterotic group is a group of related or unrelated genotypes displaying similar combining ability effects and providing a heterotic response when crossed to other genetically distinct and complementary group [32]. Classification of inbred lines into heterotic groups based on phenotypic values could be inaccurate due to the influence of the environment and may not truly reflect the heterotic pattern of the lines. Therefore, more effective methods have been proposed for genetic grouping of candidate lines, including the use of molecular markers, line by tester analysis, and diallel crosses, among others. Recently, the use of genetic distance as indices of genetic relatedness and as a tool for defining potential heterotic groups has been used in numerous crop plants. Simple sequence repeats (SSRs) have proved to be a powerful tool for analyzing genetic diversity and for classifying inbred lines. Therefore, the aim of this chapter was to elucidate the use of SSR markers in the heterotic grouping of the two model crops using experimental data.

2. Use of SSR markers in assessing genetic diversity and heterotic grouping

2.1. Determination of genetic diversity using SSRs in sorghum

Assessment of genetic variability in crops has a strong impact on crop improvement programs and conservation of genetic resources [33]. SSR markers appear to be particularly useful for measuring diversity, for assigning genotypes to heterotic groups, and for genetic fingerprinting [34]. The study reported by our group [26], involving 36 sorghum lines, provided clear genetic differentiation using the 30 SSR markers (**Table 1**).

No.	Sorghum			Maize			
	Name	Origin	Type	Name	Origin	Heterotic group[a]	Type
1	72472	Ethiopia	Restorer	142-1-eQ	Ethiopia	Ecuador	QPM
2	72482	Ethiopia	Restorer	CML144	CIMMYT	Ecuador	QPM
3	72572	Ethiopia	Restorer	CML176	CIMMYT	Unknown	QPM
4	73059	Ethiopia	Restorer	CML491	CIMMYT	A	QPM
5	75454	Ethiopia	Restorer	F7215Q	Ethiopia	Kitale	QPM
6	200538	Ethiopia	Restorer	FS111	CIMMYT	Ecuador	QPM
7	200654	Ethiopia	Restorer	FS112	CIMMYT	Unknown	QPM
8	214855	Ethiopia	Restorer	FS151-3SR	CIMMYT	Pool 9A	QPM
9	237260	Ethiopia	Restorer	FS170N	CIMMYT	Unknown	Non-QPM
10	239156	Ethiopia	Restorer	FS170Q	CIMMYT	Unknown	QPM
11	239175	Ethiopia	Restorer	FS211-1SR	CIMMYT	Kitale	QPM
12	239208	Ethiopia	Restorer	FS232N	CIMMYT	Pool 9A	Non-QPM
13	242036	Ethiopia	Restorer	FS232Q	CIMMYT	Pool 9A	QPM
14	242047	Ethiopia	Restorer	FS2-3SR	CIMMYT	Unknown	QPM
15	244712	Ethiopia	Restorer	FS4-3SR	CIMMYT	Unknown	QPM
16	244715	Ethiopia	Restorer	FS45	CIMMYT	Ecuador	QPM
17	244727	Ethiopia	Restorer	FS48	CIMMYT	Kitale	QPM
18	244733	Ethiopia	Restorer	FS48-1SR	CIMMYT	Kitale	QPM
19	211239B	Ethiopia	Restorer	FS59-2	CIMMYT	Kitale	QPM
20	214838A	Ethiopia	Restorer	FS59-4N	CIMMYT	Ecuador	Non-QPM

No.	Sorghum			Maize			
	Name	Origin	Type	Name	Origin	Heterotic group[a]	Type
21	214838B	Ethiopia	Restorer	FS59-4Q	CIMMYT	Ecuador	QPM
22	239167A	Ethiopia	Restorer	FS60	CIMMYT	Pool 9A	QPM
23	242039B	Ethiopia	Restorer	FS67(BC1)	CIMMYT	Kitale	QPM
24	242049A	Ethiopia	Restorer	FS67(BC2)	CIMMYT	Kitale	QPM
25	242050B	Ethiopia	Restorer	FS67-N	CIMMYT	Kitale	Non-QPM
26	244725A	Ethiopia	Restorer	FS68(BC1)	CIMMYT	Kitale	QPM
27	244725B	Ethiopia	Restorer	FS68(BC2)	CIMMYT	Kitale	QPM
28	244735A	Ethiopia	Restorer	KIT12	CIMMYT	Ecuador	QPM
29	69286A	Ethiopia	Restorer	KIT29	CIMMYT	Unknown	QPM
30	71160A	Ethiopia	Restorer	KIT31	CIMMYT	Unknown	QPM
31	72578A	Ethiopia	Restorer	KIT32N	CIMMYT	Ecuador	Non-QPM
32	73056A	Ethiopia	Restorer	KIT32Q	CIMMYT	Ecuador	QPM
33	ICSA 101	ICRISAT	A1-CMS	KIT34	CIMMYT	Ecuador	QPM
34	ICSA 743	ICRISAT	A2-CMS	SRSYN20N	CIMMYT	Pool 9A	Non-QPM
35	ICSA 749	ICRISAT	A3-CMS	SRSYN20Q	CIMMYT	Pool 9A	QPM
36	ICSA 756	ICRISAT	A4-CMS	SRSYN48	CIMMYT	Ecuador	QPM

[a] Putative heterotic grouping based on phenotypic data of the non-QPM counterparts before conversion to QPM.

Table 1. Description of the 36 sorghum and maize genotypes.

The 32 lowland sorghum lines from Ethiopia were crossed with the four cytoplasmic male-sterile (CMS) lines using a line x tester mating design. The 128 single-cross hybrids, along with the parental genotypes plus four checks, were evaluated under rainfed and irrigated conditions. A 12 × 14 incomplete block design (alpha lattice), with three replications, was used for the evaluation of the hybrids and check varieties. To determine the magnitude of heterosis and combining ability effects, the maintainer lines were used in place of their male sterile counterparts. An interrow spacing was 0.75 m and intrarow spacing of 0.30 m. Each genotype was planted in three rows of 3 m long. A 1 m pathway was used to separate between plots. Two sorghum seeds were planted per hill, and two weeks after emergence the seedlings were thinned keeping one healthy and vigorous plant.

Performance data on 128 F1 hybrids generated from these parents were used for this study. Grain yield data were recorded on both rainfed and irrigated plots. Best linear unbiased estimates (BLUEs) were made from the grain yield performance of 128 hybrids. The BLUEs of hybrid performance were calculated using trial data from two environments (rainfed and irrigated) using Genstat for Windows 17th Edition [35]. The BLUEs were then used to calculate general combining ability (GCA), specific combining ability (SCA) effects, and the level of heterosis. Heterotic group's specific and general combining ability (HSGCA) was computed as the sum of GCA and SCA. A phylogenetic tree was constructed from the genetic distance matrix and HSGCA value using the neighbor-joining method implemented in DARwin software ver 5.0 [36].

This study detected a total of 203 putative alleles and the number of alleles per locus detected was highly variable ranging from 2 (mSbCIR223, Xcup61, and Xtxp040) to 15 (Xtxp145), with a mean of 6.8 per locus (**Table 2**). Our results were slightly higher than Folkertsma et al. [37] and Ganapathy et al. [25] but lower than Wang et al. [38] and Mutegi et al. [34]. The higher level of allelic diversity of the SSR loci examined in this study was probably associated with the wide range of genetic diversity represented in sorghum R lines sampled. The results of a χ^2 test showed significant differences in major allele frequencies with a mean major allele frequency of 0.50. This result is in congruence with the results of Wang et al. [38]. A total of 60 rare alleles, those occurring at a frequency of ≤5%, were detected by the 30 SSR markers. The detection of a significant number of rare alleles could be attributed to the high genetic diversity within the sorghum lines. Polymorphism information content (PIC) values ranged from 0.15 (mSbCIR223) to 0.90 (Xtxp145) with a mean of 0.63 (**Table 2**). High PIC values have been reported by others [22, 39]. Among the tested SSRs, 26 markers (87%) revealed PIC values of greater than 0.5, indicating their usefulness in discriminating between the genotypes. Observed heterozygosity (*Ho*) ranged from 0.0 to 0.03, with a mean of 0.01, indicating that the test lines used in the present study were genetically pure lines, which were maintained by continued self-fertilization. The mean expected heterozygosity (*He*) was observed to be 0.64 with maximum and minimum *He* values recorded by SSR markers, Xtxp145 (0.91) and mSbCIR223 (0.15), respectively. Expected heterozygosity was higher for test materials, suggesting that 64% of individuals are expected to be heterozygous at a given locus under random mating conditions. This can be explained by the higher outcrossing rate (5%–50%) observed in sorghum [40]. The genetic distance between the lines ranged from 0.40 to 0.80, with overall mean of 0.63 [26].

Locus	LG	Genetic parameter				
		N	*A*	*Ho*	*He*	PIC
gpsb067	H (8)	6	0.49	0.03	0.68	0.67
gpsb123	H (8)	3	0.47	0.00	0.58	0.57
mSbCIR223	B (2)	2	0.92	0.00	0.15	0.15
mSbCIR240	H(8)	10	0.46	0.03	0.76	0.75
mSbCIR276	C (3)	3	0.64	0.00	0.53	0.52
mSbCIR283	G (10)	10	0.42	0.00	0.79	0.78
mSbCIR286	A (1)	7	0.67	0.00	0.54	0.53
mSbCIR306	A (1)	3	0.50	0.00	0.56	0.55
SbAGB02	E (7)	7	0.36	0.00	0.79	0.78
Xcup02	F (9)	3	0.56	0.00	0.54	0.54

http://dx.doi.org/10.5772/65078

Locus	LG	Genetic parameter				
		N	*A*	*Ho*	*He*	PIC
Xcup14	C (3)	3	0.81	0.00	0.33	0.33
Xcup53	A (1)	3	0.67	0.00	0.51	0.50
Xcup61	C (3)	2	0.51	0.03	0.51	0.50
Xgap206	F (9)	10	0.17	0.03	0.89	0.88
Xgap72	I (6)	7	0.44	0.00	0.69	0.68
Xgap84	B (2)	10	0.33	0.00	0.81	0.80
Xtxp010	F (9)	5	0.67	0.00	0.52	0.51
Xtxp012	D (4)	9	0.24	0.03	0.84	0.83
Xtxp015	J (5)	10	0.49	0.00	0.73	0.72
Xtxp021	D (4)	6	0.60	0.03	0.61	0.60
Xtxp040	E (7)	2	0.81	0.00	0.32	0.31
Xtxp057	I (6)	6	0.44	0.00	0.73	0.72
Xtxp114	C (3)	3	0.81	0.00	0.33	0.33
Xtxp141	G (10)	11	0.29	0.03	0.84	0.83
Xtxp145	I (6)	15	0.19	0.00	0.91	0.90
Xtxp265	I (6)	8	0.28	0.00	0.81	0.80
Xtxp273	H (8)	12	0.22	0.00	0.87	0.86
Xtxp278	E (7)	4	0.68	0.03	0.51	0.50
Xtxp320	A (1)	11	0.42	0.00	0.79	0.78
Xtxp321	H (8)	12	0.42	0.00	0.79	0.78
Mean		6.77	0.50	0.01	0.64	0.63
SE		0.68	0.04	0.00	0.04	0.03

N = number of alleles, *A* = major allele frequency, *Ho* = observed heterozygosity, *He* = expected heterozygosity, PIC = polymorphism information content.

Table 2. Summary statistics for the 30 SSR loci screened across 36 sorghum genotypes.

2.2. Determination of genetic diversity using SSRs in maize

Comparing two marker systems (SSRs and RAPDs), researchers [23] reported that the RAPDs produced several polymorphic bands, although the resolution power of the agarose gel electrophoresis was not good enough to allow the bands of both marker systems to be seen clearly. In the study by Demissew et al. [23], the 25 RAPD markers yielded a total of 31 alleles, with an average of 1.24 alleles per locus. Only 7.5% of the RAPD primers exhibited polymorphic bands, while the majority of the markers were monomorphic. The results were consistent with the findings of Asif et al. [41]. The application of a given marker in characterizing genotypes can be determined by the level of polymorphism it can detect and its discriminatory potential to distinguish individuals. Higher PIC value was observed for the SSR markers as compared to RAPD, reflecting the better discriminating power of SSR markers over RAPDs that makes them ideal for use in fingerprinting of maize lines as was reported by Liu et al. [42]. Garcia et al. [43] also found that the RFLP and SSR polymorphism information content means were higher than the RAPD and AFLP means.

Marker	**Chrom.**	**RPL**	*N*	*Ho*	*A*	**PIC**
nc130	5	3	3	0.000	0.333	0.404
nc133	2	5	3	0.000	0.343	0.454
phi029	3	4	3	0.029	0.443	0.410
phi046	3	4	3	0.000	0.472	0.412
phi056	1	3	4	0.030	0.561	0.633
phi065	9	5	4	0.056	0.611	0.604
phi072	4	4	4	0.056	0.306	0.401
phi075	6	2	3	0.028	0.236	0.354
phi076	4	6	6	0.143	0.600	0.663
phi079	4	5	5	0.028	0.625	0.690
phi084	10	3	2	0.056	0.333	0.346
phi102228	3	4	3	0.000	0.222	0.337
phi114	7	4	4	0.000	0.515	0.524
phi123	6	4	3	0.000	0.417	0.505
phi299852	6	3	7	0.028	0.681	0.735
phi308707	1	3	3	0.000	0.528	0.541
phi331888	5	3	4	0.028	0.458	0.512
phi374118	3	3	4	0.000	0.417	0.542
phi96100	2	4	4	0.083	0.597	0.659
umc1161	8	6	8	0.091	0.409	0.577
umc1304	8	4	3	0.143	0.386	0.380
umc1367	10	3	4	0.000	0.194	0.303
umc1545	7	4	5	0.000	0.314	0.423
umc1917	1	3	4	0.029	0.357	0.497
umc2250	2	3	2	1.000	0.500	0.375
Mean			3.9	0.073	0.434	0.491

N = number of alleles, *A* = minor allele frequency, *Ho* = observed heterozygosity, PIC = polymorphism information content.

Table 3. Summary statistics for the 25 SSR loci screened across 36 maize genotypes.

In another study, a total of 98 alleles, with a mean of 3.9 alleles per marker, were detected across 30 quality protein maize (QPM) and 6 non-QPM maize inbred lines using 25 SSR markers [24] (**Table 3**). The number of alleles detected in this study was in agreement with other studies [44]. Beyene et al. [45] genotyped 62 traditional Ethiopian highland maize accessions with 20 SSRs and reported a total of 98 alleles and a mean of 4.9 alleles per marker. Legesse et al. [20] reported an average of 3.9 alleles per marker by genotyping 56 highland and mid-altitude non-QPM inbred lines using 27 SSRs. Krishna et al. [15] reported a mean of 4.1 alleles using 48 SSR loci and 63 QPM inbred lines. The mean number of alleles in these studies were, however, lower than the 5.4 and 6.4 alleles previously reported by Wu et al. [46] and Yao et al. [47], respectively, but higher than the 3.3 alleles reported by Kassahun and Prasanna [48] and the 2.4–3.4 alleles reported by Babu et al. [49, 50]. The differences in mean numbers of alleles among different studies could be attributed to the type of germplasm, sample size, and repeat length of the SSRs used [24].

Demissew et al. [24] reported PIC values ranging from 0.30 (less discriminative marker, umc1367) to 0.735 (highly discriminative marker, phi299852) with a mean of 0.491 (**Table 3**). According to Botstein et al. [51] PIC guideline, 14 markers from Demissew et al. [24] were reasonably informative (0.30 < PIC < 0.50) and the remaining 11 markers were highly informative (PIC > 0.50). The values were comparable with previous reports by Dhliwayo et al. [52] and Mahar et al. [53] but lower than those of reported by Krishna et al. [15] . Smaller PIC values may have been due to the presence of relatively few dinucleotide repeat SSR markers [24] as opposed to a greater number of dinucleotides used in other studies [49, 50] or the presence of little genetic variability among the genotypes used in that particular study [52].

3. Use of SSR markers in population structure analysis and heterotic grouping

3.1. Population structure and heterotic grouping in sorghum

In sorghum, a predominantly self-pollinated crop, the exploitation of heterosis began in the USA in the 1950s. There have been few studies on the mechanism of heterosis, heterotic grouping, and the use of molecular markers as selection criteria for parents in sorghum when compared to other crops such as maize [54]. Heterosis in sorghum has been reported in the form of increased grain, hastened flowering and maturity, increased height, and larger stems and panicles [54]. Enhanced grain yield was reported by Kambal and Webster [55] to be a product of an increased number of seeds per panicle and increased seed weight. Hybrid sorghum cultivars have been demonstrated to be more productive than pure line varieties [56]. Significant heterosis for grain yield and other agronomic traits has been reported in sorghum [57]. It has also been reported that F_1 hybrids have superior buffering capacity across variable environments than pure lines in sorghum [58]. Consequently, breeding for hybrid cultivars is a better option than pure line varieties while improving sorghum grain yield.

SSR marker data have frequently been used as a tool to examine the dynamics of differentiation and population structures within germplasm collections [34, 38]. Cluster analysis using neighbor-joining tree analysis and structure analysis can estimate the number of subpopulations and the genetic relatedness among assessed genotypes. The study by Amelework et al. [22] investigated the extent of genetic differentiation, population structure, and patterns of relationship among 200 sorghum landraces collected from lowland agro-ecology. The results obtained from both model-based population structure analysis and neighbor-joining tree analysis revealed that two group patterns existed. The two distinct subgroups resulted from farmers' selection for adaptation for the two main seasons. The results obtained from these two separate analyses support each other, with small discrepancy between groupings. Out of the 200 landraces, 32 genotypes were selected based on prior study on the basis of their relatively better yield performance and better adaptability in a moisture stress environment. They were kept homogenous through continued selfing and selection.

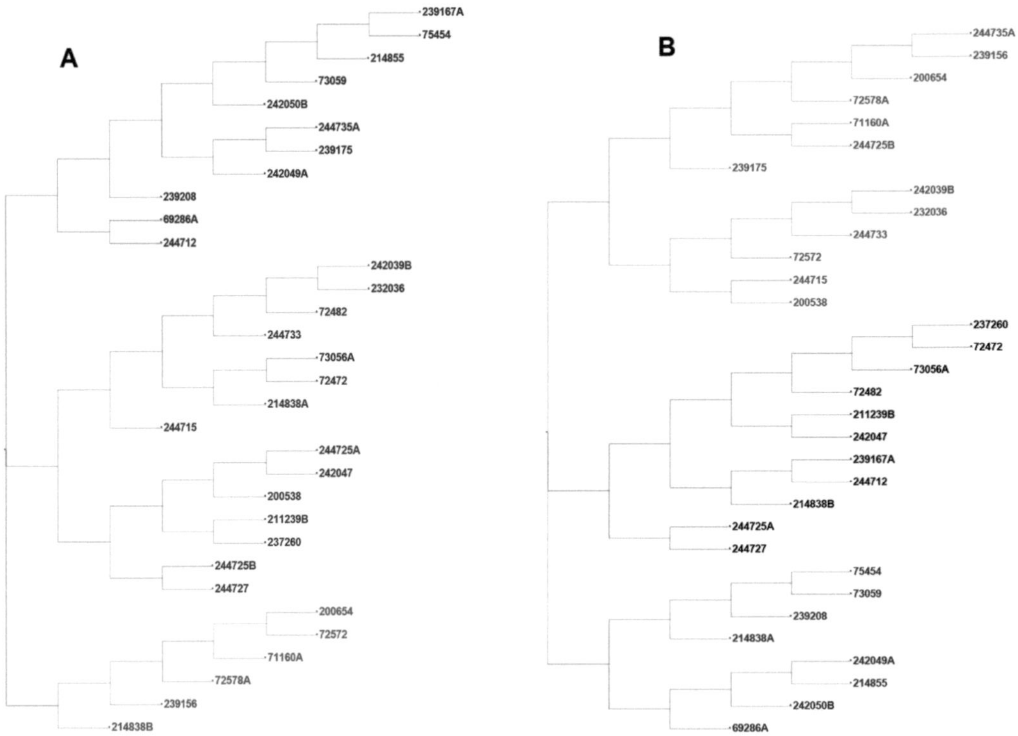

Figure 1. Dendograms using neighbor-joining based on UPGMA depicting genetic relationship between 32 sorghum lines: (A) genetic relationship based on HSGCA value under irrigated conditions. (B) Genetic relationship based on HSGCA value under rainfed conditions. The different groups identified by specific colors (blue for lines that revealed high and positive HSGCA with ICSA 743, red for ICSA 756, purple for ICSA 749, and black ICSA 101).

Estimation of molecular-based genetic distance have been proven to be a useful way to describe existing heterotic groups, to identify new heterotic groups, and to assign inbreds of unknown genetic origin to established heterotic groups [25]. The cluster analysis carried out on the 32 lines and 4 A/B female lines, based on SSR markers, revealed three distinct groups among the 36 parental genotypes [26]. Cluster I consisted of a large number of landraces (15 genotypes).

This cluster consisted of R lines such as 242039B, 244733, 242036, 244735A, 73059, and 214855 that showed highest significant HSGCA in cross-combination with ICSA 749 and ICSA 756. This group was dominated by late flowering and high biomass lines. The high biomass was, in turn, expressed as large numbers of leaf and larger leaf width per plant. The second cluster was composed of 11 landraces and 1 CMS line. All the R lines clustered in this group except 244727, revealing positive HSGCA in cross-combination with ICSA 756. Cluster II was dominated by early flowering with small panicle and high 100 seed weight genotypes. It was reported that heterosis in sorghum is expressed as a high plant or crop growth rate as compared with the parents [59]. The third cluster (III) composed of six landraces and three CMS. This cluster consisted of three R lines (75454, 239208, and 242049A) with high and positive HSGCA in cross-combination with ICSA 743 and ICSA 756.

Heterotic groups comprise sets of genotypes that perform well when crossed with genotypes from a different heterotic group [30]. Heterotic groups in sorghum have been defined by the milo-kafir cytoplasmic genetic male-sterility system where lines are grouped either as A/B-lines or R-lines [25]. The independent cluster analysis carried out based on HSGCA value for grain yield under irrigation and rainfed condition revealed three heterotic patterns based on the distribution of the 32 lines across environments (**Figure 1A** and **B**). In this study, R and B lines did not show distinct heterotic grouping. The groupings that appeared were mainly based on the female parents. For example, in **Figure 1A**, the genotypes assigned to the first cluster (blue) had high and positive HSGCA value in a cross-combination with ICSA 743. The second group (purple) composed of 15 genotypes that showed positive HSGCA values in a cross-combination with ICSA 749. The third group (blue) was mainly represented by genotypes that revealed positive HSGCA values in a cross-combination with ICSA 756.

The extent of genetic diversity between the two parents has been proposed as a possible measure of the prediction of heterosis [60]. Although it has been suggested that the genetic distance between parents is positively correlated with heterosis of F_1 hybrids, strong association has rarely been observed between heterosis and genetic distance between parents [61]. However, studies in different crops have shown moderate to strong correlation between combining ability and *per se* performance [62]. Even though this method is extensively used for prediction of heterosis, it is hypothetical and relies heavily on field evaluation. In the study of Amelework et al. [26], it was found that there were significant variations for grain yield, SCA, HSGCA, mid-, and better-parent heterosis among the 128 F_1 hybrids and 36 parental lines for grain yield. However, the results of the correlation analysis revealed that SSR-based genetic distance had no significant association with any of the grouping methods across environments (**Table 4**). Better-parent heterosis (BPH) under irrigated conditions had no significant correlation with SCA and HSGCA under both irrigated and rainfed conditions. On the contrary, both mid- and better-heterosis under rainfed conditions showed significant association with SCA, HSGCA, mid-parent heterosis (MPH) under irrigation, and across the two environments. The lack of significant association between genetic distance and other hybrid performance indicator in this study is also supported by other studies. In studies on rice [63], wheat [64], and grain sorghum [65], there were also nonsignificant relationships between whole genome-based genetic distance and hybrid performance. However, Boppenmaier et al.

[66] and Mosar and Lee [67] reported significant genetic relationships between genetic distance and hybrid performance of maize and oats, respectively. The prediction power of genetic distance has been inconsistent in many studies using different species and different germplasm [68]. This may be because of the peculiarities of many agronomic traits and lack of common phenotypic assaying methods across environments.

	SCA_C	SCA_I	SCA_R	HSGC A_C	HSGC A_I	HSGC A_R	MPH_C	MPH_I	MPH_R	BPH_C	BPH _I	BPH _R
GD	−0.07ns	−0.04ns	−0.13ns	−0.07ns	−0.05ns	−0.11ns	−0.07ns	−0.00ns	−0.09ns	−0.09ns	0.10ns	−0.14ns
SCA_C		0.89**	0.78**	0.93**	0.84**	0.74**	0.67**	0.66**	0.51**	0.61**	0.03ns	0.36**
SCA_I			0.49**	0.82**	0.93**	0.48**	0.62**	0.70**	0.36**	0.58**9	0.10ns	0.23*
SCA_R				0.74**	0.51**	0.91**	0.55**	0.45**	0.53**	0.46**	0.12ns	0.35**
HSGCA_C					0.90**	0.79**	0.80**	0.78**	0.59**	0.71**	0.11ns	0.43**
HSGCA_I						0.54**	0.72**	0.83**	0.41**	0.65**	0.21*	0.29*
HSGCA_R							0.68**	0.53**	0.70**	0.58**	0.11ns	0.50**
MPH_C								0.88**	0.78**	0.95**	0.38**	0.70**
MPH_I									0.48**	0.83**	0.56**	0.41**
MPH_R										0.75**	0.11ns	0.92**
BPH_C											0.40**	0.73**
BPH_I												0.16ns
BPH_R												

GD = SSR-based genetic distance; SCA_C = specific combining ability effects across irrigation and rainfed conditions; SCA-I = specific combining ability effects under irrigated condition; SCA_R = specific combining ability effects under rainfed conditions; HSGCA_C = general plus specific combining ability effects across irrigated and rainfed conditions; HSGCA_I = general plus specific combining ability effects under irrigated conditions; HSGCA_R = general plus specific combining ability effects under rainfed conditions; MPH_C = mid-parent heterosis across irrigated and rainfed conditions; MPH_I = mid-parent heterosis under irrigated conditions; MPH_R = mid-parent heterosis under rainfed conditions; BPH_C = better-parent heterosis across irrigated and rainfed conditions; BPH_I = better-parent heterosis under irrigated conditions; BPH_R = better-parent heterosis under rainfed conditions; ns, nonsignificant.

* Significant at 5% level of probability.

** Significant at 1% level of probability.

Table 4. Correlation matrix of the methods of heterotic grouping of the128 hybrids yield performance under irrigated and rainfed conditions.

3.2. Use of SSR markers in delineation of maize population structures and heterotic groups

Genetic distance estimates are indicators of the presence or absence of relationships among genotypes. The estimates can be made using various types of molecular markers. Heterotic group assignment is often made through combining ability experiments. Also, several authors suggested the use of molecular markers in heterotic grouping [17, 18]. A comparison of SSRs and SNPs markers were carried out by Hamblin et al. [69] to characterize maize inbred lines,

http://dx.doi.org/10.5772/65078

to elucidate the population structure, and the genetic relationships among individuals. The authors reported that the SSRs were markers of choice than SNPs by clustering the test germplasm into populations and providing more resolution in measuring genetic distance.

A study by Demissew et al. [24] indicated the extent of genetic differentiation, population structure, and patterns of relationship among 36 maize inbred lines developed from CIMMYT source germplasm (**Table 1**). This study used 25 SSRs and applied a model-based population structure, neighbor-joining cluster, and principal coordinate analyses. All these different multivariate methods revealed the presence of two to three primary cluster groups, which was in general agreement with prior pedigree information and partly with the putative heterotic groups. The model-based population structure analysis in the same study assigned about half of the inbred lines into their putative heterotic group previously defined by breeders. There were 17, 14, and 5 inbred lines in cluster groups I, II, and III, respectively (**Figure 2**). Cluster Group I was dominated by six lines from the Ecuador heterotic group, four from the Kitale group, two from the Pool 9A group, three from previously uncategorized lines, and two CMLs (CML144 and CML491). Out of the 17 lines in Group 1, 8 of them were converted to QPM using CML176 as donor, whereas only 3 lines out of 17 were converted to QPM using CML144 as donor.

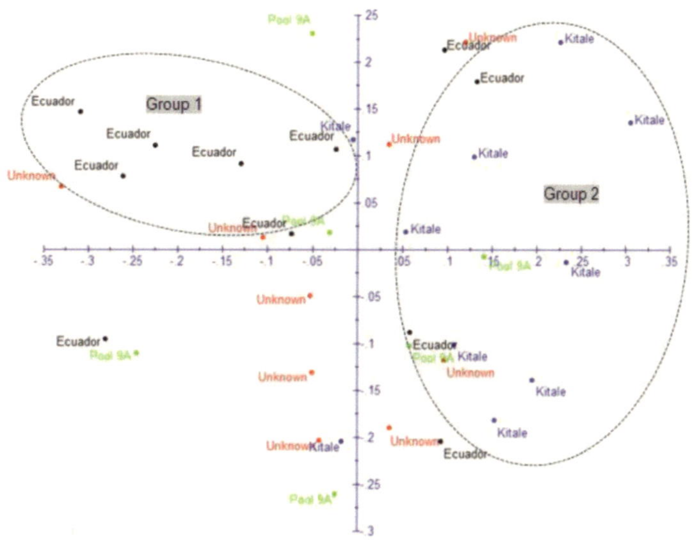

Figure 2. Plot of PC1 (13.0%) and PC2 (10.5%) from principal coordinate analysis of 36 inbred lines genotyped using 25 SSR markers. Lines that belong to the same heterotic group are indicated with the same color (Ecuador = black; Pool9A = green; Kitale = blue and unknown = red). *Source*: Demissew et al. [24].

Three lines in Group I were non-QPM counterparts. A mid-altitude line (F7215Q), which was converted into QPM using CML159 as donor parent, was also found in this group. Similarly, the cluster in Group II was dominated by five lines extracted from the Kitale heterotic group, four from Ecuador, four Pool9A, and one previously uncategorized line. Six lines in Group II were converted to QPM using CML144. Five lines were converted using CML176 and the remaining three lines were again non-QPM counterparts. The other mid-altitude line (142–1eQ) which was converted into QPM using CML176 as donor parent was also found in this group. As regards cluster Group III, it included two previously uncategorized lines with CML144 being used for their conversion to QPM, one from Kitale with CML144 again used as the QPM donor, one from Pool9A where CML176 was the QPM donor, and CML176 itself. However, in the report of Bantte and Prasanna [70], it was noted that CML176 and CML144 were categorized together into one cluster group. Such incongruities with the results of other investigators in assigning inbred lines into heterotic groups may occur due to error in seed handling or pollination [71]. It may also be caused by differential selection of the different lines in different environments or genetic drift and mutation [27].

The inconsistent results in identifying heterotic pools following phenotypic evaluations during the initial phase of development of the inbred lines might have contributed to the failure of the SSR markers to categorize the remaining 50% of the inbred lines into the known heterotic groups [24]. Partial or unclear heterotic patterns were previously reported by Semagn et al. [72] in tropical and subtropical CIMMYT maize inbred lines. It was also noted from the present study that prior conversions of conventional maize inbred lines into QPM counterparts were not done systematically leading to disruption of the original heterotic system. The inbred lines from the three known heterotic groups (Kitale, Ecuador, and Pool 9A) were spread throughout the three genetic clusters (**Figure 2**).

The conversions had been done using phenotypic selections without monitoring the genetic backgrounds using molecular markers. Consequently, recombinants were selected and only a small portion of the genome of the recurrent parent was recovered. This suggested the need to use marker-assisted backcrossing (MAB) or marker-assisted selection (MAS) in the development of QPM lines through backcross procedures. Marker-assisted breeding and/or MAS can be used to facilitate background selection and to avoid disruption of newly established heterotic groups. Furthermore, earlier phenotypic selection methods used by CIMMYT could have contributed for the lack of genetic information and the partial success of the SSR markers to recognize all the available heterotic groups. In the early 1990s, broad-based genetic pools and populations were utilized by CIMMYT breeders to develop inbred lines and open pollinated varieties (OPV). Consequently, the classification of CIMMYT populations and inbred lines into heterotic groups through various mating designs has been intensified to exploit hybrid technologies using different representative testers. However, it is not easy to cluster inbred lines into their respective heterotic groups if they are extracted from similar genetic pool or source population without considering origin or heterotic pattern of inbred lines [73]. Therefore, many generations of reciprocal recurrent selection may be necessary before the lines from each heterotic group begin to significantly diverge [74].

3.3. Genetic purity analysis of maize lines using SSRs and implications for heterotic grouping

In a previous study Demissew et al. [23], the genetic variability of quality protein maize (QPM) inbred lines were investigated using SSR and RAPD markers. A single SSR amplification product (allele) per locus was expected from all the inbred lines given the high level of expected homozygosity. However, "double bands" were detected using SSR markers, which could have been masked should RAPD markers were only used in that study. The "double bands" or SSR heterozygosity indicated that some of the QPM inbred lines were not homozygous at the specific locus. This genetic background is not expected for inbred lines given that these individuals are a product of continuous and controlled selfing yielding high levels of homozygosity. The SSR markers used in the present study facilitated differentiation of homozygotic and heterozygotic alleles in the tested inbred lines sourced from the same genetic pool. The SSR profile observed in this study concurs with the reports of Bantte and Prasanna [70]. A study by Shehata et al. [75] used SSRs and analyzed the molecular diversity and heterozygosity. The authors reported that different seed sources of the same inbreeds were important source of genetic variations. Also, there is a limited genetic variability that can be expected within inbred lines sourced from the same genetic sources suggesting the danger of ignoring this during sampling of inbred lines yet evolved through continued selfing. This is not uncommon in cross-fertilizing crops such as maize where a wide range of genetic variability is expected due to random crosses or mutational events over time [76].

In a related study conducted by Demissew et al. [24], the genetic purity and classification of maize inbred lines were tested using SSR markers. The authors reported 4.0–16.7% heterozygosity present among the tested inbred lines showing higher than the expected value after four generations of continuous selfing. In another study (B. Tadesse, unpublished), a total of 88 maize inbred lines were genotyped using a subset of 191 SNPs, identified for a routine quality control analysis [77]. This result showed that nearly 78% of the inbred lines showed high levels of heterozygosity. Factors such as seed admixture, pollen contamination, mislabeling of seed sources, and mixing of different seed stocks for planting are reported to be the source of heterozygous-inbred lines (K. Semagn, unpublished). The study by Warburton et al. [73] reported that bulking during maintenance breeding, seed regeneration, and contamination with seeds or pollen of other samples could possibly cause small changes in allelic frequencies. However, high levels of heterozygosity can significantly change phenotypic uniformity, heterotic patterns, and hence performance of hybrids. These may result in the distribution of mixed hybrids lacking proper genetic identity. Consequently, additional generations of selfing for all lines with high levels of heterozygosity are essential. The levels of homozygosity should be monitored frequently, especially in QPM materials, because opaque2 is a recessive gene that is liable to contamination. For new pedigree starts, such problems could be minimized by implementing a routine quality control genotyping using a subset of informative markers at different stages in a breeding program [77].

4. Conclusions

SSRs have been proved to be a valuable tool for diversity analysis and to assign inbred lines into heterotic groups in both sorghum and maize [22–24, 26]. SSR have greater discriminatory power than RAPDs markers, and can identify genetic relations that are reflective of the pedigree of the inbred lines. SSR markers were also found to be useful in studying the genetic purity and the level of heterozygosity in inbred lines. Genotyping of inbred lines using SSRs is a reliable way of germplasm characterization which, together with morphological descriptions, leads to unambiguous differentiation of genotypes that can be utilized for hybrid breeding programs.

Heterotic groups in sorghum have been defined either as A/B-lines or R-lines. However, recent molecular marker-based diversity studies that utilize more detailed analyses have indicated the existence of a more complex system of genetic relationships among elite parental lines. In this study, although nonsignificant association between genetic distance and hybrid performance was observed, some patterns were detected in the distribution of sorghum genotypes. The challenges of using SSR markers as a tool for heterotic grouping in sorghum is that the genetic distance estimates can be affected by several factors such as the distribution of markers in the genome, the number of markers used, and the nature of the evolutionary mechanism underlying the variation measured. Additionally, the basic assumption for molecular diversity to predict hybrid performance is the existence of high levels of gametic phase linkage disequilibrium between yield quantitative trait loci and marker alleles. QTLs influencing heterosis in grain yield are located in certain chromosomal regions, which are unevenly distributed over the genome. Therefore, future research should focus on combined use of field-based progeny tests for yield and yield components, and molecular-based distance measurements to improve breeding efficiency. To improve prediction efficiency of molecular markers, dissecting the diversity of individual linkage groups will be exploited.

Author details

Beyene Amelework[1*], Demissew Abakemal[1,2], Hussein Shimelis[1] and Mark Laing[1]

*Address all correspondence to: amele_g@yahoo.com

1 African Center for Crop Improvement, University of KwaZulu-Natal, Pietermaritzburg, South Africa

2 Ethiopian Institute of Agricultural Research, Ambo-PPRC, Ethiopia, Ambo, Ethiopia

References

[1] Henry AM, Damerval C. High rates of polymorphism and recombination at the opaque-2 locus in cultivated maize. Molecular and General Genetic. 1997;256:147–157.

[2] Buckler ES, Thornsberry JM, Kresovich S. Molecular diversity, structure and domestication of grasses. Genetic Resources. 2001;77:213–218.

[3] Gomez JAA, Bellon MR, Smale M. A regional analysis of maize biological diversity in South-Eastern Guanajuato, Mexico. Economic Botany. 2000;54:60–72.

[4] Helentjaris T, Weber D, Wright S. Identification of genomic locations of duplicate nucleotide sequences in maize by analysis of restriction fragment length polymorphisms. Genetics. 1998;118:353–363.

[5] Bennetzen JL, Jianxin MA, Devos KM. Mechanisms of recent genome size variation in flowering plants. Annals of Botany. 2005;95:127–132.

[6] Rao NGP, Murty UR, Rana BS. Sorghum. In: Chapra VL, Prakash S, editors. Evolution and Adaptation of Cereal Crops. Science Publishers Inc., Enfield, USA; 2002. pp. 213–238. DOI: 10.1093/AOB/MCG049

[7] Rooney WL, Smith CW. Techniques for developing new cultivars. In: Smith CY, Fredericksen RA, editors. Sorghum, History, Technology, and Production. Wiley, New York; 2000. pp. 329–347.

[8] Ayana A, Bekele E. Multivariate analysis of morphological variation in sorghum (*Sorghum bicolor* (L.) Moench) germplasm from Ethiopia and Eritrea. Genetic Resource and Crop Evolution. 1999;46:378–384.

[9] Shechter Y. Biochemical systematic study in *Sorghum bicolor*. Bulletin of the Torry Botanical Club. 1975;102:334–339.

[10] Zong JD, Gouyon PH, Sarr A, Sandmeier M. Genetic diversity and phylogenetic relations among Sahelian sorghum accessions. Genetic Resources and Crop Evolution. 2005;52:869–878.

[11] Gepts P. Genetic diversity of seed storage proteins in plants. In: Brown AHD, Clegg MT, Kahler AL, Weir BS, editors. Plant Population Genetic, Breeding and Genetics Resources. Sinauer Associates, Inc., USA; 1990. pp. 98–115.

[12] Tkachuk R, Mellish VJ. Wheat cultivar identification by high voltage electrophoresis. Annals of Technology in Agriculture. 1980;29:207–212.

[13] Scanlon MG, Sapirstein HD, Bushuk W. Computerized wheat varietal identification by high-performance liquid chromatography. Cereal Chemistry. 1989;66:439–443.

[14] Lorz H, Wenzel G. Biotechnology in Agriculture and Forestry: Molecular Marker Systems in Plant Breeding and Crop Improvement. Vol. 55. Springer-Verlag, Berlin; 2008. DOI: 10.1007/b137756.

[15] Krishna MSR, Reddy SS, Naik VCB. Assessment of genetic diversity in quality protein maize (QPM) lines using simple sequence repeat (SSR) markers. African Journal of Biotechnology. 2012;11:16427–16433.

[16] Soleimani VD, Baum BR, Johnson DA. Identification of Canadian durum wheat [*Triticum turgidum* L. subsp. durum (Desf.) Husn.] cultivars using AFLP and their STS markers. Canadian Journal Plant Sciences 2002;82:35–41.

[17] Flint-Garcia SA, Buckler ES, Tiffin P, Ersoz E, Springer NM. Heterosis is prevalent for multiple traits in diverse maize germplasm. PLoS One 2009;4:e7433.

[18] Lu Y, Yan J, Guimaraes C, Taba S, Hao Z, Gao S, Chen S, Li J, Zhang S, Vivek B, Magorokosho C, Mugo S, Makumbi D, Parentoni S, Shah T, Rong T, Crouch J, Xu Y. Molecular characterization of global maize breeding germplasm based on genome-wide single nucleotide polymorphisms. Theoretical and Applied Genetics. 2009;120:93–115.

[19] Mohanty A, Martin JP, Aguinagalde I. Chloroplast DNA study in wild populations and some cultivars of *Prunus avium* L. Theoretical and Applied Genetic. 2001;103:112–117.

[20] Legesse BW, Myburg AA, Pixley KV, Botha AM. Genetic diversity of African maize inbred lines revealed by SSR markers. Hereditas. 2007;144:10–17.

[21] Pooja D, Singh NK. Heterosis, molecular diversity, combining ability and their inter-relationships in short duration maize (*Zea mays* L.) across the environments. Euphytica. 2011;178:71–81.

[22] Amelework B, Shimelis H, Tongoona P, Laing M, Mengistu F. Genetic variation in lowland sorghum (*Sorghum bicolor* (L.) Moench) landraces assessed by simple sequence repeats. Plant Genetic Resources: Characterization and Utilization. 2015;13:131–141.

[23] Demissew A, Watson G, Shimelis H, Derera J, Twumasi-Afriyie S. Comparison of two PCR-based DNA markers with high resolution melt analysis for the detection of genetic variability in selected quality protein maize inbred lines. African Journal of Agricultural Research. 2012;742:5692–5700.

[24] Demissew A, Shimelis H, Derera J, Kassa S. Genetic purity and patterns of relationships among tropical highland adapted quality protein and normal maize inbred lines using microsatellite markers. Euphytica. 2015;204:49–61.

[25] Ganapathy KN, Gomashe SS, Rakshit S, Prabhakar B, Ambekar SS, Ghorade RB, Biradar BD, Saxena U, Patil JV. Genetic diversity revealed utility of SSR markers in classifying parental lines and elite genotypes of sorghum (*Sorghum bicolor* L. Moench). Australian Journal of Crop science. 2012;6:1486–1493.

[26] Amelework B, Shimelis H, Laing M. Genetic variation in sorghum as revealed by phenotypic and SSR markers: implications for combining ability and heterosis for grain yield. Plant Genetic Resources 2016:1–13. DOI:10.1017/S1479262115000696

[27] Senior ML, Murphy JP, Goodman MM, Stuber CW. Utility of SSRs for determining genetic similarities and relationships in maize using an agarose gel system. Crop Science. 1998;38:1088–1098.

[28] Dagne W, Vivek B, Abuschagne ML. Association of parental genetic distance with heterosis and specific combining ability in quality protein maize. Euphytica. 2013;191:205–216.

[29] Van-Inghelandt D, Melchinger AE, Lebreton C, Stich B. Population structure and genetic diversity in a commercial maize breeding program assessed with SSR and SNP markers. Theoretical and Applied Genetics. 2010;120:1289–1299.

[30] Hallauer AR, Russell WA, Lamkey KR. Corn breeding. In: Sprague GF and Dudley JW, editors. Corn and Corn Improvement. ASA, Madison, WI, USA; 1988. pp. 469–564.

[31] Gilbert ML. Identification and search for heterotic patterns in sorghum. In: Wilkinson D, editor. Proceedings of 49th Annual Corn and Sorghum Industrial Research Conference, 9–10 December 1994, Chicago, IL. American Seed Trade Associations, Washington, DC; 1994. pp. 117–126.

[32] Melchinger AE. Genetic diversity and heterosis. In: Coors JG, Pandey S, editors. The Genetics and Exploitation of Heterosis in Crops. ASA, CSSA, and SSSA, Madison, WI; 1999. pp. 9–118.

[33] Assar AHA, Uptmoor R, Abdelmula AA, Salih M, Ordon F, Friedt W. Genetic variation in sorghum germplasm from Sudan, ICRISAT, and USA assessed by simple sequence repeats (SSRs). Crop Science. 2005;45:1636–1644.

[34] Mutegi E, Sagnard F, Semagn K, Deu M, Muraya M, Kanyenji B, deVilliers S, Kiambi D, Herselman L, Labuschagne M. Genetic structure and relationships within and between cultivated and wild sorghum (*Sorghum bicolor* (L.) Moench) in Kenya as revealed by microsatellite markers. Theoretical Applied Genetics. 2011;122:989–1004.

[35] Payne RW, Murray DA, Harding SA, Baird DB, Soutar DM. GenStat for Windows (14th Edition) Introduction. VSN International, Hemel Hempstead, UK; 2011.

[36] Perrier X, Jacquemoud-Collet JP. DARwin software. Dissimilarity analysis and representation for windows [Internet]. 2006. Available from: http://www.darwin.cirad.fr/darwin.html [Accessed: 2016-02-15].

[37] Folkertsma RT, Frederick H, Rattunde W, Chandra S, Raju GS, Hash CT. The pattern of genetic diversity of Guinea-race *Sorghum bicolor* (L.) Moench landraces as revealed with SSR markers. Theoretical Applied Genetic. 2005;111:399–409.

[38] Wang ML, Zhu CS, Barkley NA, Chen ZB, Erpelding JE, Murray SC, Tuinstra MR, Tesso T, Pederson GA, Yu JM. Genetic diversity and population structure analysis of accessions in the US historic sweet sorghum collection. Theoretical and Applied Genetics. 2009;120:13–23.

[39] Muraya MM, Mutegi E, Geiger HH, de Villiers SM, Sagnard F, Kanyenji BM, Kiambi D, Parzies HK. Wild sorghum from different eco-geographic regions of Kenya display a mixed mating system. Theoretical and Applied Genetics. 2011, 122:1631–1639.

[40] Barnaud A, Trigueros G, MvKey D, Joly HI. High outcrossing rates in fields with mixed sorghum landraces: how are landraces maintained? Heredity. 2008;101:445–452.

[41] Asif M, Rahman M, Zafar Y. Genotyping analysis of six maize (*Zea mays* L.) hybrids using DNA fingerprinting technology. Pakistan Journal of Botany. 2006;38:1425–1430.

[42] Liu K, Goodman M, Muse S, Smith JS, Buckler E, Doebley J. Genetic structure and diversity among maize inbred lines as inferred from DNA microsatellites. Genetics. 2003;65:2117–2128.

[43] Garcia AFA, Benchimol LL, Barbosa MMA, Geraldi OI, Souza LC, Souza PA. Comparison of RAPD, RFLP, AFLP and SSR markers for diversity studies in tropical maize inbred lines. Genetic and Molecular Biology. 2004;27:579–588.

[44] Makumbi D, Betran JF, Banziger M, Ribaut JM. Combining ability, heterosis and genetic diversity in tropical maize (*Zea mays* L.) under stress and non-stress conditions. Euphytica. 2011;180:143–162.

[45] Beyene Y, Botha AM, Myburg AA. Genetic diversity among traditional Ethiopian highland maize accessions assessed by simple sequence repeat (SSR) markers. Genetic Resource and Crop Evolution. 2006;53:1579–1588.

[46] Wu Y, Zheng Y, Sun R, Wu S, Gu H, Bi Y. Genetic diversity of waxy corn and popcorn landraces in Yunnan by SSR markers. Acta Agronomica Sinica. 2004;30:36–42.

[47] Yao Q, Fang P, Kang K, Pan G. Genetic diversity based on SSR markers in maize (*Zea mays* L.) landraces from WuLing mountain region in China. Journal of Genetics. 2008;87:287–291.

[48] Kassahun B, Prasanna BM. Simple sequence repeat polymorphism in Quality Protein Maize (QPM) lines. Euphytica. 2003;129:337–344.

[49] Babu BK, Agrawal PK, Mahajan V, Gupta HS. Molecular and biochemical characterization of short duration quality protein maize. Journal of Plant Biochemistry and Biotechnology. 2009;18:93–96.

[50] Babu BK, Pooja P, Bhatt JC, Agrawal PK. Characterization of Indian and exotic quality protein maize (QPM) and normal maize (*Zea mays* L.) inbreds using simple sequence repeat (SSR) markers. African Journal of Biotechnology. 2012;11:9691–9700.

[51] Botstein D, White RL, Skolnick M, Davis RW. Construction of a genetic linkage map in man using restriction fragment length polymorphisms. American Journal of Human Genetics. 1980;32:314–331.

[52] Dhliwayo T, Pixley K, Menkir A, Warburton M. Combining ability, genetic distances, and heterosis among elite CIMMYT and IITA tropical maize inbred lines. Crop Science. 2009;49:1201–1210.

[53] Mahar K, Agrawal PK, Babu BK, Gupta HS. Assessment of genetic diversity among the elite maize (*Zea mays* L.) genotypes adapted to North-Western

Himalayan region of India using microsatellite markers. Journal of Plant Biochemistry and Biotechnology. 2009;18:217–220.

[54] Quinby JR. Manifestation of hybrid vigor in sorghum. Crop Science. 1963;3:288–291.

[55] Kambal AE, Webster OJ. Manifestation of hybrid vigor in grain sorghum and relations among the components of yield, weight per bushel and height. Crop Science. 1966;6:513–516.

[56] Kenga R, Alabi SO, Gupta SC. Combining ability studies in tropical sorghum [*Sorghum bicolor* (L.) Moench]. Field Crops Research. 2004;88:251–260.

[57] Haussmann BIG, Obilana AB, Ayiecho PO, Blum A, Schipprack W, Geiger HH. Quantitative-genetic parameters of sorghum (*Sorghum bicolor* (L.) Moench) grown in semi-arid areas of Kenya. Euphytica. 1999;105:109–118.

[58] Reddy BVS, Sharma HC, Thakur RP, Ramesh S, Kumar AA. Characterization of ICRISAT-bred sorghum hybrid parents. International Sorghum and Millets Newsletter. 2007;48:1–123.

[59] Blum A. Heterosis, stress, and the environment: a possible road map towards the general improvement of crop yield. Journal of Experimental Botany. 2013;64:4829–4837.

[60] Zhang Q, Gao YJ, Yang S, Ragab R, Saghai Maroof MA, Li ZB. A diallele analysis of heterosis in elite hybrid rice based on RFLPs and microsatellites. Theoretical and Applied Genetics. 1994;89:185–192.

[61] Rao M, Reddy GL, Kulkarni RS, Ramesh S, Lalitha RSS. Prediction of heterosis based on genetic divergence of parents through regression analysis in sunflower (*Helianthus annuus* L.). Helia. 2004;27:51–58.

[62] Bertan I, Carvalho FIF, Oliveira AC. Parental selection strategies in plant breeding programs. Journal of Crop Science and Biotechnology. 2007;10:211–222.

[63] Hua JP, Xing YZ, Xu CG, Sun XL, Yu SB, Zhang QF. Genetic dissection of an elite rice hybrid revealed that heterozygotes are not always advantageous for performance. Genetics. 2002;162:1885–1895.

[64] Corbellini M, Perenzin M, Accerbi M, Vaccino P, Borghi B. Genetic diversity in breed wheat as revealed by coefficient of parentage and molecular markers, and its relationship to hybrid performance. Euphytica. 2002;123:273–285.

[65] Jordan D, Tao Y, Godwin I, Henzell R, Cooper M, McIntyre QF. Prediction of hybrid performance in grain sorghum using RFLP markers. Theoretical and Applied Genetics. 2003;106:559–567.

[66] Boppenmaier J, Melchinger AE, Brunklaus-Jung E, Geiger HH, Herrmann RG. Genetic diversity for RLFP in European maize inbreds. III. Performance of crosses with versus between heterotic groups for grain traits. Plant Breeding. 1992;111:217–226.

[67] Mosar H, Lee M. RFLP variation of genealogical distance, multivariate distance, heterosis and genetic variation in oats. Theoretical and Applied Genetics. 1994;87:947–956.

[68] Yu CY, Hu SW, Zhao HX, Guo AG, Sun GL. Genetic distance revealed by morphological characters, isozymes, proteins and RAPD markers and their relationships with hybrid performance in oilseed rape (*Brassica napus* L.). Theoretical and Applied Genetics. 2005;110:511–518.

[69] Hamblin MT, Warburton ML, Buckler ES. Empirical comparison of simple sequence repeats and single nucleotide polymorphisms in assessment of maize diversity and relatedness. PLoS One. 2007;2:e1367.

[70] Bantte K, Prasanna BM. Simple sequence repeat polymorphism in Quality Protein Maize (QPM) lines. Euphytica. 2003;129:337–344.

[71] Rajab C, Abdolahadi H, Ghannadha MR, Warburton ML, Talei AR, Mohammadi SA. Use of SSR data to determine relationships and potential heterotic groupings within medium to late maturing Iranian maize inbred lines. Field Crops Research. 2006;95:212–222.

[72] Semagn K, Magorokosho C, Vivek BS, Makumbi D, Beyene Y, Mugo S, Prasanna BM, Warburton ML. Molecular characterization of diverse CIMMYT maize inbred lines from eastern and southern Africa using single nucleotide polymorphic markers. BMC Genomics. 2012;13:113. DOI:10.1186/1471-2164-13-113.

[73] Warburton ML, Ribaut JM, Franco J, Crossa J, Dubreuil P, Betran FJ. Genetic characterization of 218 elite CIMMYT maize inbred lines using RFLP markers. Euphytica. 2005;142:97–106.

[74] Xia XC, Reif JC, Melchinger AE, Frisch M, Hoisington DA, Beck D, Pixley K, Warburton ML. Genetic diversity among CIMMYT maize inbred lines investigated with SSR markers: II. Subtropical, tropical mid-altitude, and highland maize inbred lines and their relationships with elite U.S. and European maize. Crop Science. 2005;45:2573–2582.

[75] Shehata AI, Al-Ghethar HA, Al-Homaidan AA. Application of simple sequence repeat (SSR) markers for molecular diversity and heterozygosity analysis in maize inbred lines. Sudan's Journal of Biological Sciences. 2009;16:57–62.

[76] Hallauer AR, Carena MJ, Filho JBM. Quantitative genetics in maize breeding. Springer, New York; 2010.

[77] Semagn K, Beyene Y, Makumbi D, Mugo S, Prasanna BM, Magorokosho C, Atlin G. Quality control genotyping for assessment of genetic identity and purity in diverse tropical maize inbred lines. Theoretical and Applied Genetics. 2012;125:1487–1501.

Section 3

Microsatellite Markers in Animal Genetics and Breeding

Chapter 7

Practical Applications of Microsatellite Markers in Goat Breeding

Yuta Seki, Kenta Wada and Yoshiaki Kikkawa

Additional information is available at the end of the chapter

http://dx.doi.org/10.5772/64780

Abstract

To date, the genetic loci associated with disease and economic traits have been identified in livestock based on linkage analysis or genome-wide association studies. These analyses require the use of numerous genetic markers, of which microsatellites have been utilized most extensively because they allow for the easy genotyping of allelic variation at each locus using PCR. In the domestic goat (*Capra hircus*), microsatellite markers are powerful tools for various genetic studies, such as the estimation of intra- and interpopulation genetic diversity, linkage analyses of phenotypic traits, and marker-assisted selection of favorable phenotypes; however, the studies on goats are less extensive than those on other major livestock. The aim of this chapter is to summarize the currently available information on goat breeding using microsatellite markers. In particular, we use various studies, including our own recent work, to illustrate how these markers may be used to identify phenotypic traits.

Keywords: animal breeding, domestic goats, linkage analysis, population structure, quantitative trait locus

1. Introduction

Over the past few decades, several genetic markers have been developed and have contributed to the progress of various biological fields. Microsatellites, which are composed of between one and six nucleotide repeats, are some of the most frequently used genetic markers for genomics [1, 2]. In animal breeding, microsatellite markers have become valuable tools for the estimation of population genetic structure [3–5] and for marker-assisted selection based on the genetic mapping of disease and economic traits [6]. Although single nucleotide polymorphism (SNP) markers are widely used for genetic studies of livestock, microsatellite markers are still in great demand worldwide because they can be identified using simple detection protocols. In addition, microsatellites have several advantages, such as a high level of polymorphism, a codominant mode of inheritance, and high reproducibility [2].

The domestic goat (*Capra hircus*) was one of the first animals to be domesticated, with domestication occurring approximately 10,000 years ago [7, 8]. The domestic goat is bred worldwide as an important resource for animal products, such as meat, milk, and coat, particularly in China, India, and other developing countries [9, 10]. Despite this economic importance, considerably fewer genetic studies have been conducted on goat breeding than on the breeding of other livestock. This is largely because the genomic information available for goats is scarce and of low quality. In particular, information regarding the number and chromosomal location of goat genetic markers is limited. Although in a previous study we developed a large number of new microsatellite markers [11], these were insufficient for linkage analyses of phenotypic traits. Recently published studies have reported on whole-genome mapping technologies [12] and on the sequencing data of the goat genome obtained by integrating next-generation sequencing [10]. Therefore, it is now easier to conduct linkage analyses for phenotypic traits using these genome resources.

In the following sections, we will critically discuss the information on and advantages and applications of some of the important aspects of microsatellite markers to genetic studies and the breeding of domestic goats, including (1) the development of markers, (2) the characterization of intrapopulation and interpopulation genetic diversity, (3) linkage analyses of disease and economic traits, and (4) marker-assisted selection using microsatellites.

2. Development of microsatellite markers in goats

Several researchers have developed microsatellite markers for goats. In the initial development, several polymorphic microsatellite loci were screened from the goat genomic library using hybridization with an end-labeled microsatellite probe [13–16]. However, many researchers used the microsatellite markers developed in cattle and sheep genetic studies because several markers were available through sequence conservation among the Artiodactyls. Luikart et al. [17] reported that nine microsatellite markers from cattle and five from sheep were useful for parentage testing in goats. Moreover, a large number of microsatellite markers derived from cattle and sheep were used to construct the first goat linkage map [18]. This linkage map was constructed using 612 microsatellite markers, and most were markers from cattle (approximately 80%) and sheep (approximately 18%).

Although some microsatellite markers from cattle and sheep can be utilized for goats, few goat genetic markers have been identified for use in genetic studies. Therefore, we sought to develop new microsatellite markers that are derived from the goat genome. Many methodologies for obtaining microsatellite loci have been reported. The most common method is the combination of cloning small genomic fragments and hybridization with an end-labeled oligonucleotide probe, as mentioned above [13–16]. We also used this approach but found it ineffective, probably because microsatellite repeats are less abundant within the goat genomic sequence. This lack of repeats indicates that the enrichment of genomic sequences, including microsatellites, is indispensable to the efficient isolation of the sequences. Although enrichment strategies have been developed for microsatellite screening, we used the protocol described by Glenn and Schable [19]. This protocol is based on linker ligation-mediated PCR using a unique SuperSNX linker. The amplification of DNA using the SuperSNX linker primer is biased against producing small PCR products, and PCR products obtained after enrichment can be cloned directly without contaminating a large proportion of the small DNA fragments [19]. We succeeded in developing 260 novel microsatellite loci using hybridization with biotinylated microsatellite oligonucleotide $(TG)_{12}$ or $(AG)_{12}$ probes [11]. These developed markers were composed of two types of repeat motifs containing interrupted DNA sequences: 15 markers contained compound repeats such as $(CA)_n$ and $(AT)_n$, and 243 were composed of simple repeats such as dinucleotide motifs (239 markers), trinucleotide motifs (two markers), tetranucleotide motifs (one marker), and heptanucleotide motifs (one marker). These results were the most efficient of the protocols we used. We recommend this protocol for the isolation of DNA fragments, including microsatellites, if the genome sequence is not available.

In 2013, the ~2.66-Gb genome sequence of a female Yunnan black goat was reported [10]. The genome project is ongoing. The sequence can be downloaded from the Goat Genome database [20]. Moreover, the potential microsatellite sequences can be easily identified using web-based software such as MIcroSAtellite [21], and design primers can then be used to amplify the genomic region including microsatellites.

3. Characterization of intrapopulation and interpopulation genetic diversity in goats

Intrapopulation and interpopulation genetic diversity in livestock is required to produce food in diverse environments, allow sustained genetic improvement, and rapidly respond to changing breeding objectives [22]. In addition, intrapopulation and interpopulation genetic information is occasionally required to establish a novel strain that exhibits a similar phenotype. Microsatellite markers are often used to estimate genetic diversity because they have higher polymorphism and reproducibility than other genetic markers.

Several studies have analyzed genetic diversity in Asian goat populations. Goats are an important livestock in Asia. There are large numbers of individuals, populations, and breeds of goats in Asia [23]. Moreover, archeological analysis has revealed that the ancestor of domestic goats was initially domesticated in the Iranian Zagros Mountains [7], in the high Euphrates valley, and in Southeastern Anatolia [24], which is located in Western Asia. Wei et al. [25] investigated the genetic diversity of 40 goat populations in China using 30 microsatellite markers and revealed that the average number of alleles ranged from 4.33 to 8.23 and the expected and observed heterozygosity (H_E and H_O) ranged from 0.5070 to 0.7378 and from 0.4336 to 0.6730, respectively. Wei et al. [25] also reported that the Chinese goat population could be divided into at least four genetic clusters using phylogenetic analysis. In India, Rout et al. [26] investigated microsatellite-based genetic diversity in seven Indian goat breeds using 17 markers and detected that the average number of alleles ranged from 0.739 to 0.783 and that the H_E of the goats they assessed ranged from 0.739 to 0.783. In addition, the authors also suggested that the seven populations of Indian goats could be classified into distinct genetic groups or breeds using microsatellite markers [26]. Nomura et al. [27] investigated genetic diversity in East Asian indigenous goat breeds derived from Korea, Taiwan, the Philippines, Indonesia, Bangladesh, and Mongolia using 26 microsatellite markers and found that the Mongolian indigenous goat population had higher genetic diversity than the other populations. Moreover, Nomura et al. [27] also revealed that Shiba goats, which were established as a small experimental breed in Japan, exhibited lower genetic diversity, indicating that this breed is composed of genetically homogeneous individuals.

In this study, we demonstrate the structural analysis of intrapopulation genetic diversity in goats. We analyzed native Korean and Japanese Saanen breed populations using microsatellite markers. The native Korean population used in this study is a closed herd due to more than 20 years of assortative mating [9]. By contrast, the Japanese Saanen population, which was established by mating native Japanese goats and European Saanen breeds, constitutes a large proportion of the dairy goats in Japan. **Table 1** shows general information on the genetic diversity and differentiation of the native Korean and Japanese Saanen breeds. The average number of alleles (N_A) was 3.09 and 4.82 in the native Korean and Japanese Saanen breeds, respectively. The average expected heterozygosity (H_E) and observed heterozygosity (H_O) in the native Korean breeds were 0.48 and 0.45, respectively. In the Japanese Saanen breed, the H_E and H_O were 0.64 and 0.57, respectively. Although within-population inbreeding (F_{IS}) of the native Korean breed was lower than in the Japanese Saanen breed, both the N_A and H_E/H_O in the native Korean breed indicate that the native Korean breed has lower genetic diversity than the Japanese Saanen breed. Therefore, the loss of genetic diversity in the native Korean breed through assortative mating was confirmed using this microsatellite-based analysis. In contrast, genetic differentiation between the native Korean and Japanese Saanen breeds was indicated by the among-population genetic differentiation (F_{ST}), which was highly significant ($P < 0.001$). In the STRUCTURE analysis [28], $K = 2$ was the most appropriate number of partitions [mean Ln P (D) = −480.2], indicating that the native Korean and Japanese Saanen breeds are clearly distinguished by large genetic differentiation (**Figure 1**).

Strain	**N_A (SD)**	**H_E (SD)**	**H_O (SD)**	**F_{IS}**	**F_{ST}**
Native Korean ($n = 9$)	3.09 (1.30)	0.48 (0.25)	0.45 (0.30)	0.035	0.34**
Saanen ($n = 9$)	4.82 (1.33)	0.64 (0.17)	0.57 (0.31)	0.107	

N_A, average number of alleles; H_E, expected heterozygosity; H_O, observed heterozygosity; F_{IS}, population inbreeding coefficient; and F_{ST}, population genetic differentiation.
**$P < 0.01$.

Table 1. Intra- and interstrain genetic diversity in native Korean and Japanese Saanen goat breeds calculated using polymorphisms of 11 microsatellite markers.

http://dx.doi.org/10.5772/64780

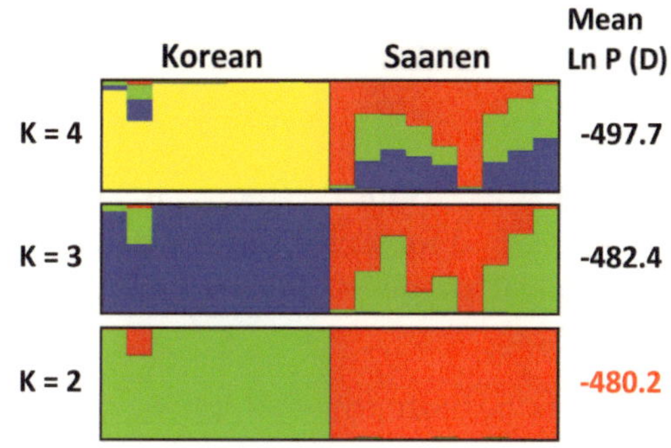

Figure 1. Clustering assignments based on the genotypes of 11 microsatellite markers in native Korean and Japanese Saanen goat breeds using STRUCTURE software ver. 2.3.4.

Figure 2 shows the results of the structural analysis of the interpopulation genetic diversity of the native Korean and Japanese Saanen populations, including four native goats [Indonesian, Mongolian, Bangladeshi, and Japanese (Shiba)] and a wild goat (Bezoar). A neighbor-joining tree, which was constructed based on the genetic distance among the individuals, was calculated using GenAlEx ver. 6.5 [29]. Similar to the results obtained using F_{ST} and STRUCTURE, the native Korean and Japanese Saanen populations were distinctly clustered into different clades in the neighbor-joining tree (**Figure 2**). Therefore, our simple analysis using closed goat populations as a model demonstrates that microsatellite markers are a useful tool for estimating intrapopulation and interpopulation genetic diversity.

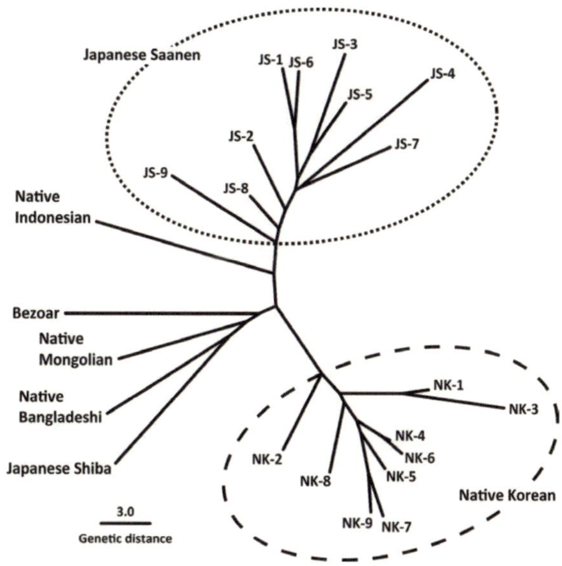

Figure 2. Neighbor-joining tree constructed based on genetic distance calculated using the genotypes of 10 microsatellite loci in domestic and wild goats. The genetic distance among 23 individuals was calculated using GenAlEx ver. 6.502, and the phylogenetic tree was constructed using the neighbor-joining method with the PHYLIP package. NK, native Korean and JS, Japanese Saanen breeds.

4. Linkage analysis of disease and economic traits using microsatellite markers in goats

In animal breeding, it is important to exclude deleterious traits and to select desirable traits. Linkage analysis is a powerful method for identifying the traits associated with disease and the productivity/quality of animal products. Microsatellite markers have provided the genotyping for linkage analysis.

Polled intersex syndrome (PIS) is the most profound genetic disorder in goats and results in the absence of horns in males and females and sex reversal that exclusively affects XX individuals [30]. The sex reversal of XX individuals leads to a reduction of milk production and reproductive efficiency in farmed goats. Based on the development of genomic tools such as microsatellite markers, the identification of the causative genetic locus for PIS has become possible. The PIS locus was mapped to the ~1 centimorgan (cM) region of CHI1q43 on goat chromosome 1 by linkage analysis using microsatellite markers and comparative genomic analysis [31, 32]. An 11.7-kb deletion of this genomic interval was detected in PIS individuals and was shown to be the causative mutation for PIS in goats [33]. Recently, Boulanger et al. [34] demonstrated that the loss of *FOXL2*, which is encoded in this genomic interval, causes an XX female to male sex reversal in the goat.

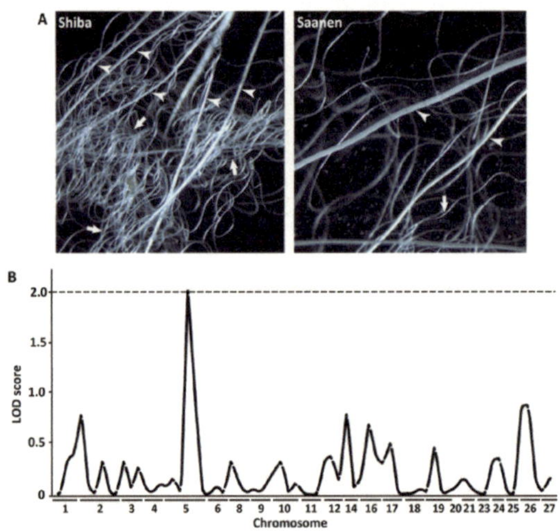

Figure 3. Identification of the genetic locus associated with cashmere productivity using linkage analysis of polymorphic microsatellite markers. (A) Strain differences in cashmere productivity between the Shiba (left panel) and Japanese Saanen breeds (right panel). The Shiba breed produces a higher amount of cashmere than the Japanese Saanen breed. The thin curly hairs and thick straight hairs represent the cashmere (arrows) and the guard hairs (arrowheads), respectively. (B) Genome-wide linkage analysis using 70 microsatellite markers and 35 backcrossed progenies between the Shiba and Japanese Saanen breeds. A suggestive linkage associated with cashmere productivity in the backcrossed progenies was detected on chromosome 5.

In contrast, several economic traits are quantitative traits. Generally, quantitative traits are influenced by polygenes, namely, quantitative trait loci (QTLs). In goat, traits for fecal worm egg count [35] and for resistance to gastrointestinal nematode infections [36] were detected by QTL linkage analysis using microsatellite markers. Of the goat economic traits, cashmere productivity is one of the most important traits because of the high market value of cashmere. We attempted to detect QTLs for cashmere productivity using linkage analysis based on microsatellite markers in an experimental family generated by backcrossing Shiba and Japanese Saanen populations, which have high and low cashmere productivity, respectively. **Figure 3A** shows the amount of cashmere hair in the Shiba (*left panel*) and Japanese Saanen (*right panel*) populations. Measurement of cashmere production in the 10 F_1 hybrid individuals and 35 backcrossed progeny suggested that a major gene associated with cashmere production had the dominant effect (data not shown). We performed genome-wide genotyping of the backcrossed progeny and detected a suggestive linkage (LOD score = 2.0) on chromosome 5 associated with cashmere productivity. Although our mapping data are preliminary because the sample size and markers are small, a previous study also mapped a QTL associated with cashmere yield in Rayini goats to an overlap region of chromosome 5 [37].

5. Marker-assisted selection using microsatellite markers in goats

Detection of single locus and QTLs associated with disease and economic traits has led to enhanced genetic improvement of livestock through marker-assisted selection [37, 38]. Marker-assisted selection is the indirect selection of animals by linking a marker with a trait but is not based on the trait itself. All genetic markers, such as morphological and biochemical markers, are available for marker-assisted selection. However, detection is difficult for some traits because environmental effects influence these markers. Moreover, these markers cannot genotype all traits, particularly if the traits are controlled by QTLs on multiple chromosomal regions. Molecular markers usually do not have any biological effect and can be used for genome-wide genotyping. Microsatellites are suitable genetic markers for marker-assisted selection because they have a high degree of polymorphism, are abundantly distributed throughout the genome, and can be used as the basis of accurate and simple detection protocols. To date, several economically important QTLs have been reported in goats using QTL linkage analysis [39]. The microsatellite markers linked with QTLs have also been reported. We predict that several phenotypes are commonly found in various goat populations and that the microsatellite markers linked with traits are suitable for marker-assisted selection to establish highly productive goats in several countries.

6. Concluding remarks

Although we described the advantages of microsatellite markers for breeding goats, the applications of microsatellite markers have been discussed in a wide range of genetic studies. Moreover, microsatellite markers are commonly used in other livestock to estimate population structures and detect QTLs. Recently, SNPs have become a popular genetic marker for genetic analyses in humans, mice, and livestock, and several SNP genotyping technologies have been developed [40–42]. In the future, SNPs may become the main tool for genetic analysis because large-scale genomic sequences will be published for several breeds and populations. However, we predict that microsatellite markers will also be used for genetic studies because the procedure is simple. Above all, we suggest that microsatellite markers are accessible markers for use at a small scale, such as in a laboratory, because of economic concerns such as cost, time, and labor.

Acknowledgements

This work was supported by the Advanced Research Project Type A, Tokyo University of Agriculture, No. 02, 2006-2008. We thank Mr. M. Fujita and Miss M. Kotani of the National Livestock Breeding Center, Nagano Station, for their assistance in animal keeping and data collection.

Author details

Yuta Seki[1], Kenta Wada[1,2] and Yoshiaki Kikkawa[1*]

*Address all correspondence to: kikkawa-ys@igakuken.or.jp

1 Mammalian Genetics Project, Tokyo Metropolitan Institute of Medical Science, Tokyo, Japan

2 Department of Bioproduction, Tokyo University of Agriculture, Abashiri, Japan

References

[1] Zane L, Bargelloni L, Patarnello T. Strategies for microsatellite isolation: a review. Mol Ecol. 2002;11:1-16. DOI: 10.1046/j.0962-1083.2001.01418.x

[2] Miah G, Rafii MY, Ismail MR, Puteh AB, Rahim HA, Islam KhN, Latif MA. A review of microsatellite markers and their applications in rice breeding programs to improve blast disease resistance. Int J Mol Sci. 2013;14:22499-22528. DOI: 10.3390/ijms141122499

[3] Revidatti MA, Delgado Bermejo JV, Gama LT, Landi Periati V, Ginja C, Alvarez LA, Vega-Pla JL, Martínez AM; BioPig Consortium. Genetic characterization of local Criollo pig breeds from the Americas using microsatellite markers. J Anim Sci. 2014;92:4823-4832. DOI: 10.2527/jas.2014-7848

[4] Sharma R, Kishore A, Mukesh M, Ahlawat S, Maitra A, Pandey AK, Tantia MS. Genetic diversity and relationship of Indian cattle inferred from microsatellite and mitochondrial DNA markers. BMC Genet. 2015;16:73. DOI: 10.1186/s12863-015-0221-0

[5] Brenig B, Schütz E. Recent development of allele frequencies and exclusion probabilities of microsatellites used for parentage control in the German Holstein Friesian cattle population. BMC Genet. 2016;17:18. DOI: 10.1186/s12863-016-0327-z

[6] Setoguchi K, Furuta M, Hirano T, Nagao T, Watanabe T, Sugimoto Y, Takasuga A. Crossbreed comparisons identified a critical 591-kb region for bovine carcass weight QTL (*CW-2*) on chromosome 6 and the Ile-442-Met substitution in *NCAPG* as a positional candidate. BMC Genet. 2009;10:43. DOI: 10.1186/1471-2156-10-43

[7] Zeder MA. Hesse B. The initial domestication of goats (*Capra hircus*) in the Zagros mountains 10,000 years ago. Science. 2000;287:2254-2257. DOI: 10.1126/science.287.5461.2254

[8] Groeneveld LF, Lenstra JA, Eding H, Toro MA, Scherf B, Pilling D, Negrini R, Finlay EK, Jianlin H, Groeneveld E, Weigend S; GLOBALDIV Consortium. Genetic diversity in farm animals - A review. Anim Genet. 2010;41 (Suppl 1):6-31. DOI: 10.1111/j.1365-2052.2010.02038.x

[9] Seki Y, Yokohama M, Wada K, Fujita M, Kotani M, Nagura Y, Kanno M, Nomura K, Amano T, Kikkawa Y. Expression analysis of the type I keratin protein keratin 33A in goat coat hair. Anim Sci J. 2011;82:773-781. DOI: 10.1111/j.1740-0929.2011.00912.x

[10] Dong Y, Xie M, Jiang Y, Xiao N, Du X, Zhang W, Tosser-Klopp G, Wang J, Yang S, Liang J, Chen W, Chen J, Zeng P, Hou Y, Bian C, Pan S, Li Y, Liu X, Wang W, Servin B, Sayre B, Zhu B, Sweeney D, Moore R, Nie W, Shen Y, Zhao R, Zhang G, Li J, Faraut T, Womack J, Zhang Y, Kijas J, Cockett N, Xu X, Zhao S, Wang J, Wang W. Sequencing and automated whole-genome optical mapping of the genome of a domestic goat (*Capra hircus*). Nat Biotechnol. 2013;31:135-141. DOI: 10.1038/nbt.2478

[11] Seki Y, Yokohama M, Ishikawa D, Ikehara N, Wada K, Nomura K, Amano T, Kikkawa Y. Development and characterization of 260 microsatellite loci in the domestic goat, *Capra hircus*. Anim Genet. 2012;43:365-366. DOI: 10.1111/j.1365-2052.2011.02262.x

[12] Du X, Servin B, Womack JE, Cao J, Yu M, Dong Y, Wang W, Zhao S. An update of the goat genome assembly using dense radiation hybrid maps allows detailed analysis of evolutionary rearrangements in *Bovidae*. BMC Genomics. 2014;15:625. DOI: 10.1186/1471-2164-15-625

[13] Arevalo E, Holder DA, Derr JN, Bhebhe E, Linn RA, Ruvuna F, Davis SK, Taylor JF. Caprine microsatellite dinucleotide repeat polymorphisms at the SR-CRSP-1, SR-CRSP-2, SR-CRSP-3, SR-CRSP-4 and SR-CRSP-5 loci. Anim Genet. 1994;25:202. DOI: 10.1111/j.1365-2052.1994.tb00124.x

[14] Bhebhe E, Kogi J, Holder DA, Arevalo E, Derr JN, Linn RA, Ruvuna F, Davis SK, Taylor JF. Caprine microsatellite dinucleotide repeat polymorphisms at the SR-CRSP-6, SR-CRSP-7, SR-CRSP-8, SR-CRSP-9 and SR-CRSP-10 loci. Anim Genet. 1994;25:203. DOI: 10.1111/j.1365-2052.1994.tb00125.x

[15] Kogi J, Yeh CC, Bhebhe E, Burns BM, Ruvuna F, Davis SK, Taylor JF. Caprine microsatellite dinucleotide repeat polymorphisms at the SR-CRSP-11, SR-CRSP-12, SR-CRSP-13, SR-CRSP-14 and SR-CRSP-15 loci. Anim Genet. 1995;26:449. DOI: 10.1111/j.1365-2052.1995.tb02705.x

[16] Yeh CC, Kogi JK, Holder MT, Guerra TM, Davis SK, Taylor JF. Caprine microsatellite dinucleotide repeat polymorphisms at the SR-CRSP21, SR-CRSP22, SR-CRSP23, SR-CRSP24, SR-CRSP25, SR-CRSP26 and SR-CRSP27 loci. Anim Genet. 1997;28:380-381. DOI: 10.1111/j.1365-2052.1997.tb03284.x

[17] Luikart G, Biju-Duval MP, Ertugrul O, Zagdsuren Y, Maudet C, Taberlet P. Power of 22 microsatellite markers in fluorescent multiplexes for parentage testing in goats (*Capra hircus*). Anim Genet. 1999;30:431-438. DOI: 10.1046/j.1365-2052.1999.00545.x

[18] Vaiman D, Schibler L, Bourgeois F, Oustry A, Amigues Y, Cribiu EP. A genetic linkage map of the male goat genome. Genetics. 1996;144:279-305.

[19] Glenn TC, Schable NA. Isolating microsatellite DNA loci. Methods Enzymol. 2005;395:202-222. DOI: 10.1016/S0076-6879(05)95013-1

[20] International Goat Genome Consortium. Goat Genome [Internet]. 2016 Available from: http://www.goatgenome.org/home.html [Accessed: 2016-06-29]

[21] Thomas Thiel. MISA - MIcroSAtellite identification tool [Internet]. 2016. Available from: http://pgrc.ipk-gatersleben.de/misa/ [Accessed: 2016-06-29]

[22] Notter DR. The importance of genetic diversity in livestock populations of the future. J Anim Sci. 1999;77:61-69. DOI: /1999.77161x

[23] Food and Agriculture Organization of the United Nations Statistics Division. FAOSTAT [Internet]. 2016. Available from: http://www.fao.org/statistics/en/ [Accessed: 2016-06-29]

[24] Peters J, von den Driesch A, Helmer D. The upper Euphrates-Tigris basin: cradle of agro-pastoralism? In: Vigne JD, Peters J, Helmer D, editors. First Steps of Animal Domestication, New Archaeozoological Approaches. Oxford: Oxbow Books; 2005. p. 96–124.

[25] Wei C, Lu J, Xu L, Liu G, Wang Z, Zhao F, Zhang L, Han X, Du L, Liu C. Genetic structure of Chinese indigenous goats and the special geographical structure in the Southwest China as a geographic barrier driving the fragmentation of a large population. PLoS One. 2014;9:e94435. DOI: 10.1371/journal.pone.0094435

[26] Rout PK, Joshi MB, Mandal A, Laloe D, Singh L, Thangaraj K. Microsatellite-based phylogeny of Indian domestic goats. BMC Genet. 2008;9:11. DOI: 10.1186/1471-2156-9-11

[27] Nomura K, Ishii K, Dadi H, Takahashi Y, Minezawa M, Cho CY, Sutopo, Faruque MO, Nyamsamba D, Amano T. Microsatellite DNA markers indicate three genetic lineages

in East Asian indigenous goat populations. Anim Genet. 2012;43:760-767. DOI: 10.1111/j.1365-2052.2012.02334.x

[28] Hubisz MJ, Falush D, Stephens M, Pritchard JK. Inferring weak population structure with the assistance of sample group information. Mol Ecol Resour. 2009;9:1322-1332. DOI: 10.1111/j.1755-0998.2009.02591.x

[29] Peakall R, Smouse PE. GenAlEx 6.5: genetic analysis in Excel. Population genetic software for teaching and research--an update. Bioinformatics. 2012;28:2537-2539. DOI: 10.1093/bioinformatics/bts460

[30] Pailhoux E, Vigier B, Schibler L, Cribiu EP, Cotinot C, Vaiman D. Positional cloning of the PIS mutation in goats and its impact on understanding mammalian sex-differentiation. Genet Sel Evol. 2005;37 (Suppl 1):S55-S64. DOI: 10.1186/1297-9686-37-S1-S55

[31] Vaiman D, Koutita O, Oustry A, Elsen JM, Manfredi E, Fellous M, Cribiu EP. Genetic mapping of the autosomal region involved in XX sex-reversal and horn development in goats. Mamm Genome. 1996;7:133-137. DOI: 10.1007/s003359900033

[32] Vaiman D, Schibler L, Oustry-Vaiman A, Pailhoux E, Goldammer T, Stevanovic M, Furet JP, Schwerin M, Cotinot C, Fellous M, Cribiu EP. High-resolution human/goat comparative map of the goat polled/intersex syndrome (PIS): the human homologue is contained in a human YAC from HSA3q23. Genomics. 1999;56:31-39. DOI: 10.1006/geno.1998.5691

[33] Pailhoux E, Vigier B, Chaffaux S, Servel N, Taourit S, Furet JP, Fellous M, Grosclaude F, Cribiu EP, Cotinot C, Vaiman D. A 11.7-kb deletion triggers intersexuality and polledness in goats. Nat Genet. 2001;29:453-458. DOI: 10.1038/ng769

[34] Boulanger L, Pannetier M, Gall L, Allais-Bonnet A, Elzaiat M, Le Bourhis D, Daniel N, Richard C, Cotinot C, Ghyselinck NB, Pailhoux E. *FOXL2* is a female sex-determining gene in the goat. Curr Biol. 2014;24:404-408. DOI: 10.1016/j.cub.2013.12.039

[35] Bolormaa S, van der Werf JH, Walkden-Brown SW, Marshall K, Ruvinsky A. A quantitative trait locus for faecal worm egg and blood eosinophil counts on chromosome 23 in Australian goats. J Anim Breed Genet. 2010;127:207-214. DOI: 10.1111/j.1439-0388.2009.00824.x

[36] de la Chevrotière C, Bishop SC, Arquet R, Bambou JC, Schibler L, Amigues Y, Moreno C, Mandonnet N. Detection of quantitative trait loci for resistance to gastrointestinal nematode infections in Creole goats. Anim Genet. 2012;43:768-775. DOI: 10.1111/j.1365-2052.2012.02341.x

[37] Mohammad Abadia MR, Askarib N, Baghizadehb A, Esmailizadeha AK. A directed search around caprine candidate loci provided evidence for microsatellites linkage to growth and cashmere yield in Rayini goats. Small Rumin Res. 2009;81:146–151. DOI: 10.1016/j.smallrumres.2008.12.012

[38] Dekkers JC. Commercial application of marker- and gene-assisted selection in livestock: strategies and lessons. J Anim Sci. 2004;82 (E-Suppl):E313-E328.

[39] Wakchaure R, Ganguly S, Praveen KP, Kumar A, Sharma S, Mahajan T. Marker assisted selection (MAS) in animal breeding: a review. J Drug Metab Toxicol. 2015;6:e127. DOI: 10.4172/2157-7609.1000e127

[40] Amills M. The application of genomic technologies to investigate the inheritance of economically important traits in goats. Adv Biol. 2014;2014:904281. DOI: 10.1155/2014/904281

[41] Ragoussis J. Genotyping technologies for genetic research. Annu Rev Genomics Hum Genet. 2009;10:117-133. DOI: 10.1146/annurev-genom-082908-150116

[42] Jiang Z, Wang H, Michal JJ, Zhou X, Liu B, Woods LC, Fuchs RA. Genome wide sampling sequencing for SNP genotyping: methods, challenges and future development. Int J Biol Sci. 2016;12:100-108. DOI: 10.7150/ijbs.13498

Chapter 8

Microsatellites for the Amazonian Fish *Hypophthalmus marginatus*

Emil J. Hernández-Ruz, Evonnildo C. Gonçalves,
Artur Silva, Rodolfo A. Salm,
Isadora F. de França and Maria P.C. Schneider

Additional information is available at the end of the chapter

http://dx.doi.org/DOI: 10.5772/65655

Abstract

We isolated 41 and characterized 17 microsatellite loci for evaluating the genetic structure of the Amazonian fish *Hypophthalmus marginatus*, from the Tocantins and Araguaia River in the Eastern Amazonia. Of the 17 selected microsatellite sequences, 15 were dinucleotide repeats, 9 of which were perfect (5–31 repetitions) and 6 were composite motifs. Among these 17 microsatellites, only two were polymorphic. The average number of alleles (Na) observed in the five examined populations ranged from 3.5 to 4.5, while the average observed heterozygosity (Ho) ranged from 0.3 to 0.6. The allelic frequency was less homogeneous at the locus Hm 5 than that for the Hm 13. Genetic diversity was measured in three upstream and two downstream populations under the influence of the Tucuruí Hydroelectric Dam. Our findings provide evidence for low levels of genetic diversity in *H. marginatus* of the Tocantis basin possibility related to the Dam construction. The F_{st} and R_{st} analysis fits well with migratory characteristics of *H. marginatus*, suggesting the existence of a gene flow mainly in the upstream or downstream directions. To test the hypothesis that the Dam was responsible for the detected reduction on this species genetic diversity, a large number of genetic markers are recommended, covering geographic distribution range of the fish species.

Keywords: hydroelectric dam influence, migratory fishes, population genetic structure

1. Introduction

Migratory freshwater fishes are vulnerable to a variety of anthropogenic impacts, including harvesting, pollution, and other types of habitat disturbance. The impact of dams is not only limited to the transformation of habitats from lentic to lotic but they also isolate the population from their places of spawning to feeding grounds [1–3]. Therefore, a survival and reproduction of migratory fish can be directly affected by changing thermal and hydrodynamic conditions in their habitat [4]. In the Brazilian Amazonia, over 10 million hectares (ha) of forests are expected to become permanently flooded after the construction of new-planned dams [5]. Long-term monitoring of fish populations is available only for Tucuruí Dam in the Tocantins River [6–10], where alterations following impoundment reduced the fish diversity on the reservoir resulting in the increase of predators such as *Cichla* spp. Schneider 1801, and *Serrasalmus* spp. Lacepède 1803 [11]. Furthermore, a drastic reduction in fish production has been observed downstream of the dam, probably due to the low oxygen content of water that runs through the turbines and the blocking of fish migration [6, 12]. Harvesting of freshwater shrimp downstream the dam has dropped from 179 tons in 1981, before the dam construction, to only 62 tons in 1988 three years after dam construction, while fish landings declined from 4726 to 831 tons (the dam was built between 1984 and 1985) [13]. Catches in the reservoir increased to pre-flooding levels by the early 1990s [8], although nowadays migratory species such as *Hypophthalmus marginatus* are still not such abundant as before. Therefore, due to the great economic importance to local fisheries, the current genetic structure and species/biodiversity conservation of *H. marginatus* stocks in the low to medium Tocantins River is a matter of concern and was investigated here. Besides, helping to understand the impact of the construction of the Tucuruí Dam on the genetic variability, our results should contribute to the eventual development of population management strategies for the studied species and will hopefully arise concerns about the building of future dams in the Amazon.

2. Materials and methods

The Tocantins is largely a plateau river, flowing for most of its length within an enclosed valley, draining an area of 343,000 km^2. Over the past three decades, its basin has suffered from huge anthropogenic pressures, including widespread deforestation, mining, and the construction of the Tucuruí between 1984 and 1985. This dam is one of the world's largest hydroelectric dams, which has a reservoir of 2840 km^2, most of which was originally covered with primary *terra firme* forest [9, 10].

2.1. Samples

Eighty-two samples (14–19 per site) obtained from muscle or liver tissue of *H. marginatus* were stored in absolute ethanol and frozen at -20°C for future genomic DNA extraction, which was performed using Sambrook standard protocol [14]. The specimens were preserved in 4% formaldehyde and deposited in the ichthyological collection of the Museu Paraense Emílio Goeldí (MPEG 13375, MPEG 17486, MPEG 17499 and MPEG 17578). Microsatellite loci were characterized in *H. marginatus* individuals from four different points of the Tocantins River: Itupiranga (05°06'51.5"S, 49°21'34.9"W), Tucuruí (04°18'43.06"S, 49°19'58.1"W), Cametá (02° 03'27.5"S, 49°20'31.9"W), and Abaetetuba (01°40'42.6"S, 49°00'16.6"W). Additionally, samples from one point of Araguaia River (Conceição do Araguaia, 07°58'10.8" S, 49°11'0.6" W) were included in the analysis (**Figure 1**).

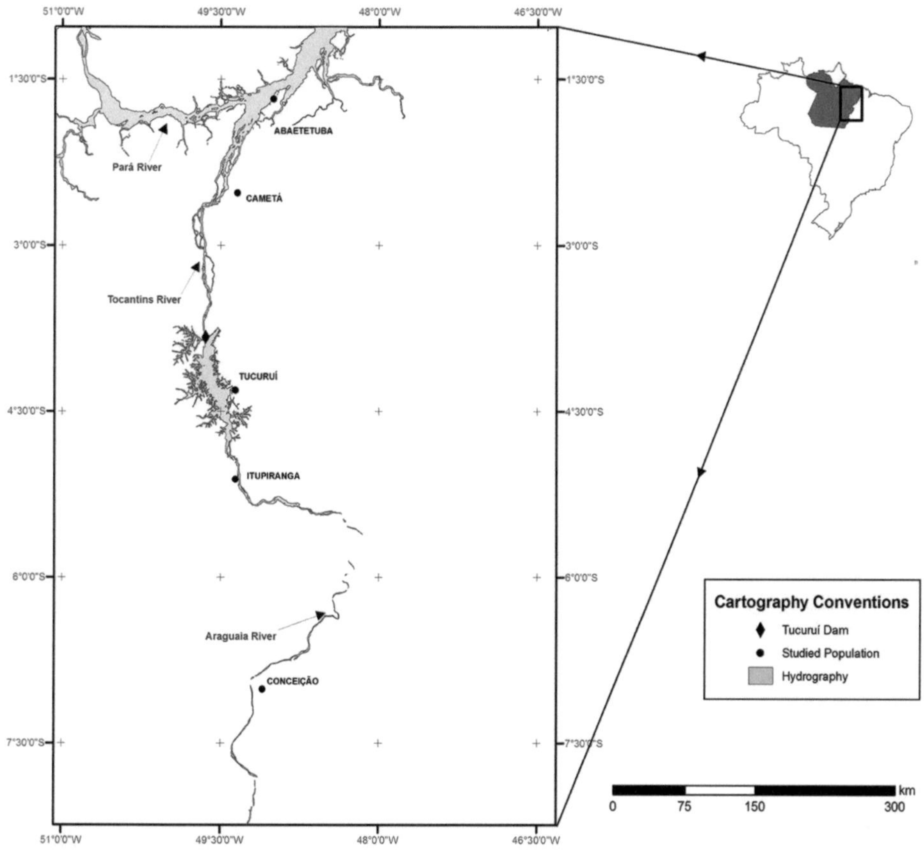

Figure 1. Distribution of the five stocks of *Hypophthalmus marginatus* sampled on the Tocantins and Araguaia Rivers in eastern Amazonia.

2.2. Microsatellite development

Molecular tools such as microsatellites markers can give us a picture of the distribution of the genetic variability of the natural populations of Amazonian fish [15, 16]. To assess the genetic parameters of the *Hypophthalmus* in the Amazon basin, we developed a partial genomic library of these fishes enriched for microsatellites following the method of selective hybridization with biotinylated probe types $(CT)_8$, conjugated to streptavidin-coated magnetic beads [17]. After hybridization, the microsatellite-enriched sequences were amplified by polymerase chain reaction (PCR), ligated into the pGEM-T Easy Vector (Promega Corp., Madison, USA) and transformed into *Escherichia coli* TOP 10 electroporated-competent bacteria. The transformed bacteria were plated on solid medium containing LB-ampicillin (100 mg/ml) + X-gal (2%), and after growth, the white colonies containing inserts were transferred and grown in 96-well plates in a liquid Tartoff-Hobbs Broth/ampicillin medium. A total of 96 positive clones were sequenced in both directions using the BigDye® Terminator v3.1 Cycle Sequencing Kit, according to the manufacturer's instructions (Applied Biosystems, Carlsbad, USA). The sequences were edited and aligned in the software BioEdit [18].

A total of 96 clones were sequenced, and 17 of these were selected for primer design using the software Primer3 [19]. In all primer pairs, the forward primers had an M13(-21) tail added to its 5' end [20]. An optimal annealing temperature was inferred using a gradient PCR with temperatures set between 52.3 and 70.5°C (**Table 1**).

Genotyping reactions were carried out in the Biocycler Thermal Cycler MJ96+/MJ96G (Applied Biosystems), in a final volume of 10 μL. Each reaction contained 3.8 μL of MilliQ water, 1.2 μL of 50 mM $MgCl_2$, 1.0 μL of 10 mM dNTPs, 1.0 μL of PCR buffer (100 mM Tris-HCl, pH 8.5, 500 mM KCl), 0.4 μL of 2 μM tailed forward primer, 0.4 μL of 2 μM fluorescently labeled primer, 0.8 μL of 2 μM reverse primer, 0.3 μL of 2.5 U Taq DNA polymerase, and 1 μL of DNA (50–100 ng/μL). Reactions were submitted to the following cycling profile: hot start at 94°C for 60 s followed by 25 cycles of denaturing at 94°C for 30 s, annealing for 30 s at locus specific temperatures (**Table 1**), and extension at 68°C for 30 s; labeling step consisted of 20 cycles of denaturing at 94°C for 20 s, annealing at 52°C for 30 s, and extension at 72°C for 60 s; final extension was performed at 72°C for 30 min. The fragments present in 1 μL of PCR product were separated in 8% polyacrylamide denaturing gel in an ALFexpressTM II (Amersham Biosciences, Freiburg, Germany) automatic DNA sequencer. Amplicon size was estimated by the Allele Locator 1.03 software (Amersham Biosciences, India), based on the internal and external standards provided by the manufacturer.

Using the program Micro-Checker v2.2.3 [21], we verified that null alleles were not present in the data set. Genetic parameters were obtained with the program Arlequin 3.5 [22].

2.3. Data analysis

To measure the genetic variability within each population, the number of alleles per locus (A), effective number of alleles per locus (Ae), the observed heterozygosity (Ho), and expected (He) under Hardy-Weinberg equilibrium (HWE) for each locus and their averages were calculated using Popgene 32 software [23].

The Genepop 3.1b program [24] was used to test whether the data obtained are significant deviations from Hardy-Weinberg equilibrium and the occurrence of connection imbalance between the loci analyzed. This program uses a method of Markov chain to get an unbiased estimate of Fisher's exact test to detect a significant deficiency or excess of heterozygotes [25].

The differentiation between the populations was evaluated by comparing peer-to-peer two ways: 1. Estimates F_{ST} [26], using the Arlequin 3.5 program [22] and 2. Estimates R_{ST} [27], by program RSTCalc [28].

R_{ST} is an analog of Wright F_{ST}, which is based on the stepwise mutation model (SMM) for microsatellite loci and has the particularity of not displaying associated bias to differences in the size of the alleles in the samples of populations and / or differences the variance between

Locus	Primer sequences (5'–3')	Repeat motif (5'–3')	T (°C)	Size range
Hm 2	GTTACTCGGGCTCATGGGTA	(GT)8A(TG)21	66.5	171
	TAGGGCTGAAGGTGAGTGCT			
Hm 4	CGTGCATCACTGGAGTCTTC	(TAAAAA)3	64.5	204
	ATGAAGGATGTCTGCGCTTT			
Hm 5*	GCAGCTACAGGGCATACTCC	$(AC)_9TG(CA)_5$	66	183
	CTCCCTGTCTCTGCACTTCC			
Hm 6	ACCACCATGCTTTAGCCAAG	(TG)5	64.5	178
	CTCTTGAGCCAGGAAACAGG			
Hm 7	GCCCCACGGCTATACATACA	(CA)23	56.4	222
	CTCTTGCTTACGCGTGGACT			
Hm 9	CCCCTTCTCATCGGAGAGTT	(TG)5	64.5	298
	CACAGACTGCATGCCACAC			
Hm 10	CCCGAGGCACTGTAGGTTAG	(GA)9	66	239
	ATGTGGGAATCCTGGTTCAG			
Hm 11	ATCAGTGCACCAGCATCAAG	(TG)5CA(TG)7	64.5	285
	CATCCTTGTGGGGATTTTTG			
Hm 12	CACCAGCACAGCTGATGATTA	(GA)12GC(GA)11	63.5	127
	GAGGCCCCTACAGTCACATT			
Hm 13*	GGACAAGGTTGTGTGGGTAAG	$(TG)_8$	66	162
	GGAGTAGTGACCCGTCTTCG			
Hm 14	TGGTGAAACATACCCTGTCG	(TG)31	68.1	125
	GAGGACACGAGAGAGTCACTGATA			
Hm 15	GAGTCTCCACACCACCTGCT	(CA)13CG(CA)5	58.8	125
	GAGCCTTTGTTATCTGGCTCA			
Hm 16	GTGAATTGGTGTTTCTAAAGTGG	(TG)15	60.8	100
	CCCTAGACAGGGTGCTACTCC			
Hm 17	GTTTCTAAAGTGCCCCTTAGTGTG	(TG)19A(GT)5	70.5	113
	GGCGCCACTCCATCGTAG			
Hm EH1	GTCTCCTCCCACAGTCCAAA	(TG)18	53.2	152
	GGGCAGGAACAACCCTAGAC			
Hm EH2	CTGCCCTGCTCTCGTGTTAT	(TG)21	53.2	257
	AATTCATTAAAAATCCTCAGCGTA			
Hm EH3	GTTTCCTCCCACAGTCCAAA	(TGGA)13	53.2	300
	AAAAATCGAAGGACAGGTAAAA			

*Polymorphic.

Table 1. Characteristics of microsatellite loci isolated from *Hypophthalmus marginatus*.

loci. Some authors argue that the estimates of FST show lower when compared to RST estimates in same analysis [29].

The existence of linkage disequilibrium between the loci was evaluated by Genepop 3.4 program [24].

3. Results

Among a total of 98 sequenced recombinant clones, 61 clones presented microsatellites. After sequence analysis, it was found that 41 clones showed more than four repeats of microsatellites and we have designed and purchased primers for 17 of SSRs.

Among the 17 selected microsatellite sequences were a hexanucleotide, a tetranucleotide, and 15 dinucleotide repeats. Of 15 dinucleotide repeats, nine were perfect (5–31 repetitions) and six were composite dinucleotide repeat type (**Table 1**). Of the 17 loci, only two (Hm 5 and Hm 13) were polymorphic among studied samples.

The average number of alleles (A) observed in five populations examined ranged from 3.5 to 4.5, while the average observed heterozygosity (Ho) ranged from 0.3 to 0.6 (**Table 2**). The allelic frequency was less homogeneous to the Hm 5 locus than for the Hm 13; its most frequent allele was the same for all populations (**Table 3**).

Significant values of F_{st} were observed in all comparisons including Abaetetuba and the comparison of Tucuruí × Conceição (**Table 4**) gave negative R_{st} values representing interactions where the variance within a population exceeds the variance between populations.

4. Discussions

Although tested just by two polymorphic SSRs, genetic variability of *H. marginatus* population is under the influence of the Tucuruí Dam on the Tocantis River and as measured by heterozygosity test it is relatively low, regarding the number of alleles (absolute and effective). Few studies use less than six microsatellite markers in population studies [30]. Although we would like to stress that the results presented here are preliminary, they are consistent with results obtained with other molecular markers. The importance of our work is that it described a library that can be used to test for the polymorphism kind of economic importance to the Amazon.

Some populations of *H. marginatus*, such as those of Abaetetuba and Conceição, had remarkable low values. We could indicate that the heterozygosity was similar to that shown by other Siluriformes [31].

A comparison made elsewhere of *H. marginatus* cytochrome b gene with the same genes in other freshwater fishes [32, 33] indicates very low genetic diversity levels in *H. marginatus*, possibly reflecting a low mutation rate in this species [34] or a characteristic of Pimelodidae, as found in other studies [35].

The heterozygosity values provided by two microsatellite loci in *H. marginatus* in five populations analyzed did not differ between populations upstream and downstream of

Locus											
Hm 5						Hm 13					
	Relative frequencies						Relative frequencies				
Size (bps)	Conceição	Abaetetuba	Itupiranga	Cametá	Tucuruí	Size (bps)	Conceição	Abaetetuba	Itupiranga	Cametá	Tucuruí
175			0.1786	0.026		146	0.0667	0.0714			
177		0.786				148	0.1000	0.0714		0.132	0.079
181	0.1000	0.107	0.3571	0.421	0.526	150	0.6333	0.4286	0.6429	0.684	0.632
183					0.053	152	0.200	0.4286	0.3571	0.184	0.289
185	0.133		0.1071	0.132	0.158						
187	0.233		0.1429	0.079	0.158						
189	0.500	0.0714	0.2143	0.316	0.105						
191		0.0357		0.026							
195	0.033										

Table 2. Average allelic frequencies for two microsatellite loci in five populations of *Hypophthalmus marginatus*.

Population (N)	*Locus*	A	Ae	Ho	He	P – EHW
Abaetetuba (14)	Hm 5	4.0	4.0	0.3	0.4	0.3
	Hm 13	4.0	4.0	0.4	0.6	0.1
	Mean (SD)	**4.0 (0.0)**	**4.0 (0.0)**	**0.3 (0.1)**	**0.5 (0.2)**	**0.2 (0.1)**
Cametá (19)	Hm 5	6.0	5.5	0.6	0.7	0.2
	Hm 13	3.0	3.0	0.4	0.5	0.2
	Mean (SD)	**4.5 (2.1)**	**4.2 (1.8)**	**0.5 (0.1)**	**0.6 (0.1)**	**0.2 (0.0)**
Itupiranga (15)	Hm 5	5.0	5.0	0.7	0.8	0.1
	Hm 13	2.0	2.9	0.4	0.5	1.0
	Mean (SD)	**3.5 (2.1)**	**4.0 (1.5)**	**0.6 (0.2)**	**0.6 (0.2)**	**0.5 (0.6)**
Tucuruí (19)	Hm 5	5.0	4.9	0.6	0.7	0.4
	Hm 13	3.0	3.0	0.4	0.5	0.3
	Mean (SD)	**4.0 (1.4)**	**3.9 (1.3)**	**0.5 (0.1)**	**0.6 (0.1)**	**0.3 (0.1)**
Conceição (15)	Hm 5	5.0	4.9	0.5	0.7	0.4
	Hm 13	4.0	4.0	0.5	0.6	0.9
	Mean (SD)	**4.5 (0.7)**	**4.4 (0.6)**	**0.5 (0.0)**	**0.6 (0.1)**	**0.6 (0.3)**

N = sample size; A = number of alleles; Ae = allelic richness; Ho = observed heterozygosity; He = expected heterozygosity second Nei (1973); SD = Standard deviation.

Table 3. Variability intrapopulation in five populations of *Hypophthalmus marginatus*.

Population	*Conceição*	*Abaetetuba*	*Itupiranga*	*Cametá*	*Tucuruí*
Conceição	****	0.28 (0.000)	0.05 (0.05)	0.04 (0.09)	0.10 (0.001)
Abaetetuba	0.71 (0.0000)	****	0.24 (0.00)	0.28 (0.00)	0.27 (0.000)
Itupiranga	0.35 (0.0006)	0.26 (0.0061)	****	0.005 (0.41)	0.006 (0.350)
Cametá	0.20 (0.0100)	0.47 (0.0002)	0.04 (0.19)	****	0.008 (0.350)
Tucuruí	0.41 (0.0000)	0.42 (0.0000)	-0.02 (0.63)	0.02 (0.223)	****

Table 4. Comparisons of peer to peer between the populations of *H. marginatus* analyzed, with F_{ST} values (above the diagonal) calculated [21]according to Weir and Cockerham (1984), with their respective *P*-values (in quotes) and values of R_{st} (below the diagonal) calculated according to Michalakis and Excoffier (1996) with their respective *P*-values (in quotes).

Tucuruí Dam. In these populations, the observed heterozygosity was lower than expected heterozygosity for all populations, thus indicating that there is no evidence of population bottleneck. On the other hand, the distribution of heterozygosity did not vary much in comparison with other species of commercial fish such as arowana (*Osteoglossum bicirrhosum* (Vandelli 1829)) [15] or pirarucu (*Arapaima gigas*) [16].

There is no much information on populations of *H. marginatus*, or other *Hypophthalmus*, as this knowledge would have been instrumental in understanding the effects of the Tucuruí Dam on the populations of *H. marginatus* Tocantins and Araguaia. The values of F_{st} and R_{st} showed little differentiation among populations of the same side of the current course of the Tocantins River, for example, populations of Conceição and Itupiranga upstream of Tucuruí Dam or

http://dx.doi.org/DOI: 10.5772/65655

Abaetetuba and Cametá downstream of the same dam gave values of F_{st} low, as between populations separated by the dam as Abaetetuba and Conceição, accented F_{st} values indicating greater differentiation among populations, probably generated by low levels of gene flow.

Laroche and Durand [36] studied the genetic structure of the Percidae *Zinger asper* populations, an endangered endemic species, affected by the construction of a dam built on the River Rhone in France, and found significant genetic differences between upstream and downstream populations.

5. Preliminary conclusions

If low differentiation is prevalent, the geographic distribution range of large samples would be recommended for genetic analyses. It would also be useful to assess the levels of genetic variability within and among populations from different basins for a better understanding of population dynamics of these species. Although our conclusions were made by using only two microsatellite loci analyses, results are consistent with data from mitochondrial markers.

Acknowledgments

This study was supported by CAPES, and CNPq. We are also grateful to IBAMA, for providing the authorization 013-2007 to capture, collect, and transport the biological material to the Centrais Elétricas do Norte do Brasil S.A. (ELETRONORTE S.A.) as well as for logistic support at Tucuruí. We thank Cassio Andrade (EMATER/PA) and Comunidade Jaraqüera Grande for providing logistic support at Cametá; Aparecida, Jhonis, and Leo for providing logistic support at Conceição de Araguaia. Special thanks to Soraya Andrade, Silvanira Ribeiro Barbosa for helping in laboratory. EJHR thanks Mauricio Papa de Arruda for collaboration with ALFexpress management.

Author details

Emil J. Hernández-Ruz[1]*, Evonnildo C. Gonçalves[2], Artur Silva[3], Rodolfo A. Salm[1], Isadora F. de França[1] and Maria P.C. Schneider[3]

*Address all correspondence to: emilhjh@yahoo.com

1 Laboratory of Zoology, School of Biological Sciences, Federal University of Para/UFPA, Altamira, PA, Brazil

2 Biomolecular Technology Laboratory, Institute of Biological Sciences, Federal University of Para/UFPA, Belém, Pará, Brazil

3 Laboratory of Genomics and Bioinformatics, Federal University of Para/UFPA, Belém, Pará, Brazil

References

[1] Barthem R, Lambert M, Petrere M. Life strategies of some long-distance migratory catfish in relation to hydroelectric/dams in the Amazon Basin. Biological Conservation. 1991;**55**:339–345. DOI:10.1016/0006-3207(91)90037-A.

[2] Wei Q, Ke F, Zhang J, Zhuang P, Luo J, Zhou R, Yang W. Biology, fisheries, and conservation of sturgeons and paddlefish in China. Environmental Biology of Fishes. 1997;**48**:241–255. DOI: 10.1007/0-306-46854-9_14.

[3] Ruban GI. Species structure, contemporary distribution and status of the Siberian sturgeon, *Acipenser baerii*. Environmental Biology of Fishes. 1997;**48**:221–230. DOI: 10.1007/0-306-46854-9_12.

[4] Agostinho AA, Júlio HF Jr, Borghetti JR. Considerations on the impacts of dams on fish populations and measures for mitigation - a case study: Itaipu reservoir. Revista UNIMAR. 1992; **14**:89-107

[5] Fearnside PM. Dams in the Amazon: Belo Monte and Brazil's hydroelectric development of the Xingu River Basin. Environment Management. 2006;**38(1)**:16–27. DOI:10.1007/s00267-005-0113-6.

[6] Carvalho JL, Mérona B. Studies on two migratory fish from lower Tocantins River, before closure of Tucuruí dam. Amazoniana. 1986;**9**:595-607.

[7] Mérona B, Carvalho JL, Bittencourt MM. The immediate effects of the closure dam Tucuruí (Brazil) on the downstream ichthyofauna. Revue d'Hydrobiologie Tropicale. 1987;**20**:73–84.

[8] Ribeiro MCLB, Petrere M, Juras AA. Ecological integrity and fisheries ecology of the Araguaia-Tocatins River Basin, Brazil. Rivers Research and Applications. 1995;**11**:325–350. DOI: 10.1002/rrr.3450110308.

[9] Cetra M, Petrere M. Small-scale fisheries in the middle River Tocantins, Imperatriz (MA), Brazil. Fisheries Management and Ecology. 2001;**8**:153-162. doi.org/10.1046/j.1365-2400.2001.00233.x.

[10] Santos GM, Mérona B, Juras AA, Jégu M. Fish and fishing in the Lower Tocantins River twenty years after Tucuruí Hydroelectric Plant . ELECTRONORTE. Brasília. 2004. 216 p.

[11] Leite RAN, Bittencourt MM. Hydropower impact on the Amazon fish fauna: The sample Tucuruí. In: Val AL, Figiuolo R and Feldberg E, editors. Scientific Basis for Preservation Strategies and Development of the Amazon: Facts and Perspectives Vol 1. Instituto Nacional de Pesquisas da Amazônia (INPA). Manaus; 1991. p. 85-100.

[12] Odinetz-Collart O. The shrimps *Macrobrachium amazonicum* (Palaemonidae) in the Lower Tocantins, after closing the dam of Tucuruí (Brazil).Revue d'Hydrobiologie Tropicale. 1987;**20**(2):131-144.

[13] Odinetz-Collart O. Ecology and fishing potential of shrimp cinnamon, *Macrobrachium amazonicum*, in the Amazon Basin In: Ferreira EJG, GM Santos, Leão ELM, Oliveira LA (eds) Scientific Basis for Preservation and Development of the Amazon Strategies, Vol 2 Instituto Nacional de Pesquisas da Amazônia (INPA), Manaus; 1993. p. 147-166.

[14] Sambrook J, EF Fritsch, Maniatis T. Molecular Cloning: A Laboratory Manual. 2nd edn. Cold Spring Harbor Laboratory Press, Cold Spring Harbor, NY, USA. 1989.

[15] Silva T J, Hrbek T, Farias I P. Microsatellite markers for the silver arowana (Osteoglossidae, Osteoglossiformes). Molecular Ecology Notes 2009;**9**:1019–1022. DOI: 10.1111/j.1755-0998.2009.02556.x.

[16] Farias IP, Hrbek T, Brinkmann H, Sampaio I, Meyer A. Characterization and isolation of DNA microsatellite primers for *Arapaima gigas*, an economically important but severely over-exploited fish species of the Amazon basin. Molecular Ecology Notes. 2003;**3**:128–130. DOI:10.1046/j.1471-8286.2003.00375.x.

[17] Refseth UH, Fangan BM, Jakobsen KS. Hybridization capture of microsatellites directly from genomic DNA. Electrophoresis. 1997;**18**:1519–1523. DOI: 10.1002/elps.1150180905.

[18] Hall TA. Bioedit v709: Biological sequence alignment editor analysis program for Windows 95/98/Nt. Nucleic Acids Symposium Series 2007;**41**:95–98.

[19] Rozen S, Skaletsky HJ. Primer 3 on the www for general users and for biologist programmers. In: Krawetz S and Misener S, editors. Bioinformatics Methods and Protocols: Methods in Molecular Biology. Humana Press, Totowa; NJ. 2000. p. 365–386.

[20] Schuelke M. An economic method for the fluorescent labeling of PCR fragments: A poor man's approach to genotyping for research and high-throughput diagnostics. Nature Biotechnology 2000;**18**:233–234. DOI:10.1038/72708.

[21] Van Oosterhout C, Hutchinson WF, Wills DPM, Shipley P. MICROCHECKER: software for identifying and correcting genotyping errors in microsatellite data. Molecular Ecology Notes. 2004;**4**:535–538. DOI: 10.1111/j.1471-8286.2004.00684.x.

[22] Excoffier L, Lischer HEL. Arlequin suite ver 3.5: a new series of programs to perform population genetics analyses under Linux and Windows. Molecular Ecology Resources. 2010;**10**:564–567. DOI: 10.1111/j.1755-0998.2010.02847.x.

[23] Yeh FC, Rong-cai Y, T Boyle. POPGENE VERSION 1.31: Microsoft Window-based Freeware for Population Genetic Analysis. University of Albert, Centre for International Forestry Research. 1999.

[24] Raymond M, Rousset F. Genepop Version 1.2.: Population genetics software for exact tests and ecumenicism. Journal of Heredity. 1995;**86**:248–249.

[25] Eggert LS, Mundy NI, Woodruff DS. Population structure of loggerhead shrikes in the California Channel Islands. Molecular Ecology. 2004:**13**:2121–2133. DOI: 10.1111/j.1365-294X.2004.02218.x.

[26] Wright S. Evolution & genetics for populations, vol.4. Variability Within & Among Natural Populations. University of Chicago Press, Chicago. 1978.

[27] Slatkin MA. Measure of population subdivision based on microsatellite allele frequencies. Genetics. 1995;**139**:457–462.

[28] Goodman SJ. R-ST Calc: a collection of computer programs for calculating estimates of genetic differentiation from microsatellite data & determining their significance. Molecular Ecology. 1997;**6**:881–885. DOI: 10.1111/j.1365-294X.1997.tb00143.x.

[29] Jarne P, Lagoda PJL. Microsatellites, from molecules to populations & back. Trends in Ecology & Evolution. 1996;**11**:424–429.

[30] Ji YJ, Zhang DX, Hewitt GM, Kang L, Li DM. Polymorphic microsatellite loci for the cotton bollworm *Helicoverpa armigera* (Lepidoptera: Noctuidae) and some remarks on their isolation. Molecular Ecology Notes. 2003;**3**:102–104. DOI: 10.1046/j.1471-8286.2003.00366.x.

[31] Revaldaves E, Pereira LHG, Foresti F, Oliveira C. Isolation and characterization of microsatellite loci in *Pseudoplatystoma corruscans* (Siluriformes: Pimelodidae) and cross-species amplification. Molecular Ecology Notes. 2005;**5**:463–465. DOI: 10.1111/j.1471-8286.2005.00883.x.

[32] Sivasundar A, Bermingham E, Ortí G. Population structure and biogeography of migratory freshwater fishes (*Prochilodus*: Characiformes) in major South American rivers. Molecular Ecology. 2001;**10**:407–418.

[33] Turner TF, Mcphee MV, Campbell P, Winemiller KO. Phylogeography and intraspecific genetic variation of prochilodontid fishes endemic to rivers of northern South America. Journal of Fish Biology. 2004;**64**:186–201. DOI: 10.1111/j.1095-8649.2004.00299.x.

[34] Hernández-Ruz EJ, Goncalves EC, Silva A LC, Schneider MPC. Low genetic diversity of *Hypophthalmus marginatus* from the Tocantins River based on cytochrome b sequence data. International Journal of Genetic and Molecular Biology. 2013;**5**(6):71–77. DOI: 10.5897/IJGMB2013.0071.

[35] Du M, Liu YH, Niu BZ. Isolation and characterization of polymorphic microsatellite markers in *Bagarius yarrelli* using RNA-Seq. Genetics and Molecular Research. 2015;**14**(4):16308–16311. DOI: 10.4238/2015.

[36] Laroche J, Durand JD. Genetic structure of fragmented populations of a threatened endemic percid of the Rhône River: *Zingel asper*. Heredity. 2004;**92**:329–334. DOI: 10.1038/sj.hdy.6800424.

Chapter 9

Microsatellite Markers in the Mud Crab (*Scylla paramamosain*) and their Application in Population Genetics and Marker-Assisted Selection

Hongyu Ma, Chunyan Ma, Lingbo Ma,
Xincang Li and Yuanyou Li

Additional information is available at the end of the chapter

http://dx.doi.org/10.5772/65041

Abstract

The mud crab (*Scylla paramamosain*) is a commercially important species for aquaculture and fisheries in China. In this study, a total of 302 polymorphic microsatellite markers have been isolated and characterized. The observed and expected heterozygosity ranged from 0.04 to 1.00 and from 0.04 to 0.96 per locus. The wild populations distributed along South-eastern China coasts showed high genetic diversity (H_O ranged from 0.62 to 0.77) and low genetic differentiation (F_{ST} = 0.018). Meanwhile, a significant association (r^2 = 0.11) was identified between genetic and geographic distance of 11 locations. Furthermore, a PCR-based parentage assignment method was successfully developed using seven polymorphic microsatellite loci that could correctly assign 95% of the progeny to their parents. Moreover, three polymorphic microsatellite loci were identified to be significantly associated with 12 growth traits of *S. paramamosain*, and four genotypes were considered to be great potential for marker-assisted selection. Finally, a first preliminary genetic linkage map with 65 linkage groups and 212 molecular markers was constructed using microsatellite and AFLP markers for *S. paramamosain*. This map was 2746 cM in length, and covered approximately 50% of the estimated genome. This study provides novel insights into genome biology and molecular marker-assisted selection for *S. paramamosain*.

Keywords: genetic linkage map, growth traits linked loci, microsatellite marker, parentage assignment, population genetic diversity

1. Introduction

The mud crab (*Scylla paramamosain*), a big size crustacean, is one of the most important aquaculture species and marine fisheries in China. It is naturally distributed along the coasts of South-eastern China, as well as other East and Southeast Asian countries. Due to the good flavor, high nutrition value, and fast growth speed, *S. paramamosain* is now becoming more and more popular in the above countries. In China, the artificial culture of this crab can date back more than 100 years [1], and in recent years, the culture production is usually above 100,000 tons per year [2]. However, the current culture capacity cannot meet the demands of market. Under the natural conditions, mature *S. paramamosain* mates inshore, then the gravid females migrate offshore for spawning eggs, and finally the offspring return to inshore. Nowadays, the wild resource of this crab including adults and larvae has been decreasing quickly due to seawater pollution and overexploitation. Therefore, for conservation and sustainable utilization of this valuable marine resource, we first need to better understand its population genetic diversity and improve economic traits. Molecular marker-assisted selection (MAS) is thought to be a good method for genetic improvement, because it can shorten the selection period, and increase the accuracy of improvement. Of the many known molecular markers, microsatellite marker is an ideal genetic tool for helping to fulfill this purpose.

Microsatellites, normally known as simple sequence repeats (SSR), are widely used for population structure analysis [3, 4], parentage assignment [5], genetic map construction [6, 7], and marker-assisted selection [8, 9] because they are abundantly distributed throughout genome, codominant, and hyper-variable in most eukaryotic organism genomes. Before this study, there were only 15 polymorphic microsatellite loci available for *S. paramamosain* [10, 11]. The lack of efficient microsatellite markers has severely blocked the genetic studies in *S. paramamosain*.

The purpose of this study is to massively develop polymorphic microsatellite markers, uncover the population genetic diversity, create molecular parentage assignment technique, identify growth performance-associated markers, and construct a genetic linkage map, so as to provide novel insights into population genetic diversity and genetic improvement of economic traits for *S. paramamosain*.

2. Microsatellites and their application in population genetics and MAS

2.1. Material and methods

For microsatellite loci isolation, a total of six different strategies based on PIMA [12], FIASCO [13], GenBank-derived genes [14], 5′ anchored PCR [15], cDNA library [16], and 454 sequencing transcriptome [17, 18] have been employed to isolate microsatellite markers. The polymorphisms of microsatellite loci were evaluated by using a wild population with approximately 30 individuals.

For population genetics analysis, a total of 397 wild individuals were sampled from 11 locations (Sanmen, Ningde, Zhangzhou, Shantou, Shenzhen, Zhanjiang, Haikou, Wenchang, Wanning, Dongfang, and Danzhou) of South-eastern coasts of China. Nine polymorphic microsatellite markers were genotyped in these specimens [19].

For development of parentage assignment technique, four G_1 families were collected, with 46 progenies in each family. Family 1 lost both parents information, and families 2, 3, and 4 only had maternal information. Ten polymorphic microsatellite loci were selected for genotyping the above crabs [20].

For trait-marker association analysis, a total of 96 three-month-old full-sib specimens were randomly sampled from a G_1 family. Sixteen growth traits including carapace length (CL), internal carapace width (ICW), carapace width (CW), body height (BH), carapace frontal width (CFW), carapace width at spine 8 (CWS8), abdomen width (AW), fixed finger length of the claw (FFLC), fixed finger width of the claw (FFWC), fixed finger height of the claw (FFHC), distance between lateral spine 1 (DLS1), distance between lateral spine 2 (DLS2), meropodite length of pereiopod 1 (MLP1), meropodite length of pereiopod 2 (MLP2), meropodite length of pereiopod 3 (MLP3), and body weight (BW) were measured. Moreover, 129 transcriptome-derived polymorphic microsatellite loci were genotyped in these animals [17].

For genetic linkage map construction, a G_1 family with 95 individuals was selected as mapping population. Microsatellite and AFLP markers were employed for linkage analysis. A total of 337 polymorphic microsatellite markers and 64 AFLP selective primer combinations were used in this study [21].

For data analysis, the observed (N_a) and effective (N_e) number of alleles, the observed (H_O) and expected (H_E) heterozygosity, Hardy-Weinberg equilibrium (HWE), and linkage disequilibrium (LD) were calculated by softwares POPGENE 1.31 [22] and ARLEQUIN 3.01 [23]. Significance values for multiple tests were corrected by sequential Bonferroni procedure [24]. The null allele frequency was predicted by MICRO-CHECKER 2.2.3 [25]. Genetic differentiation was tested by AMOVA analysis using software GENA1EX 6.41 [26]. The UPGMA tree among 11 locations was constructed by software MEGA 4.0 [27]. The links between genetic distance and geographic distance were evaluated by Mantel test [28]. The exclusion probability of microsatellite loci and parentage assignment were carried out using software CERVUS 3.0 [29]. Double-blind test was performed using seven most informative microsatellites and 40 specimens. The UPGMA tree of these 40 individuals was created by software MEGA 4.0. The general linear model (GLM) was used to identify the association between microsatellite loci and growth performance. A linear animal model with the fixed effects was used as follows: $Y_{ijk} = \mu + G_i + S_j + e_{ijk}$, where Y_{ijk} is the observed value of the ijkth trait; μ is the mean value of the trait; G_i is the effect of the ith genotype; S_j is the effect of the jth sex; and e_{ijk} is the random error effect. Significant differences in growth traits among the different genotypes were calculated through multiple comparison analysis using the S-N-K method. The software JoinMap 3.0 [30] was used for linkage analysis of microsatellite and AFLP genotypes. The population type was defined as cross-pollination (CP). A critical logarithm of odds (LOD) score threshold ≥2.5 was referenced for markers assignment. Linkage groups were drawn by MapChart 2.1 software [31]. The expected genome size (G_e) was estimated using the formula: $G_e = (G_{e1} + G_{e2})/2$ [32]. The expected genome size is the sum of the revised lengths of all linkage groups [33]. The observed map length (G_{oa}) was the total length of groups, triplets, and doublets. The estimated coverage of the genome (C_{oa}) was calculated as: G_{oa}/G_e accordingly.

2.2. Results and discussion

2.2.1. Isolation and characterization of microsatellite loci

In this study, a total of 302 polymorphic microsatellite markers were successfully developed by using six different strategies. For methods based on PIMA, FIASCO, GenBank-derived genes, 5′ anchored PCR, cDNA library, and 454 sequencing transcriptome, a total of 12, 54, 18, 18, 36, and 164 polymorphic microsatellite loci were identified, respectively. A total of 1858 alleles were detected with an average of 6.15 alleles per locus from these microsatellite markers. The observed and expected heterozygosity ranged from 0.04 to 1.00, and from 0.04 to 0.96 per locus, respectively. The genotype proportions at 45 microsatellite loci significantly deviated from Hardy-Weinberg equilibrium expectations after Bonferroni correction; this could be due to the small sample size or the presence of null alleles, but cannot be attributed to technical or statistical artifacts. No significant linkage disequilibrium was detected between these loci pairs. According to the utilities for comparative mapping, molecular markers are classified into two types: type I markers are linked with genes of known functions, while type II markers are linked with anonymous genomic fragments. Among these 302 microsatellite loci, 218 may be associated with functional genes, which were classified as type I markers that are usually considered to have lower polymorphic level than type II markers. In this study, the genetic diversity level of type I loci was slightly lower than that of genome-derived loci too. Moreover, the polymorphisms of type II loci isolated in this study were lower than those described in previous references [10, 11].

2.2.2. Population genetic diversity and differentiation

The population genetic diversity of *S. paramamosain* distributed along South-eastern coasts of China was found to be high by nine microsatellite markers. A total of 104 alleles were observed at these nine microsatellite loci, with an average of 11.6 alleles per locus. The H_O values ranged from 0.32 to 1.00 per locus-location combination, and from 0.62 to 0.77 per location. This result was in accordance with the previous study by mtDNA marker [34]. Three factors are usually thought to be associated with high genetic variation of marine animals: environmental heterogeneity, the life history characteristics, and large population size [35, 36]. Further, we determined that the genetic diversity level of *S. paramamosain* population was gradually increased from the Northern location to the South. This interesting trend was also found in previous study by mtDNA marker [34].

Approximately 98.2% of variance was within locations and 1.8% of that was among locations, which indicated that the population genetic variation mainly existed within locations, and the genetic differentiation level was very low among locations (**Table 1**).

Source of variation	*df*	Sum of squares	Variance components	Percentage of variation	F_{ST}
Among locations	10	83.706	0.064	1.83	0.0183
Among individuals within locations	386	1465.290	0.388	11.18	
Within individuals	397	1199.000	3.020	86.99	
Total	793	2747.996	3.472	100	

Table 1. AMOVA design and results in 11 locations of *Scylla paramamosain*.

The mtDNA data also indicated that the population genetic structure of this crab was genetically homogeneous [37]. Therefore, we concluded that *S. paramamosain* population distributed along South-eastern coasts of China is a single genetically homogeneous population with low differentiation. Moreover, from the UPGMA tree (**Figure 1**), we observed that there were totally

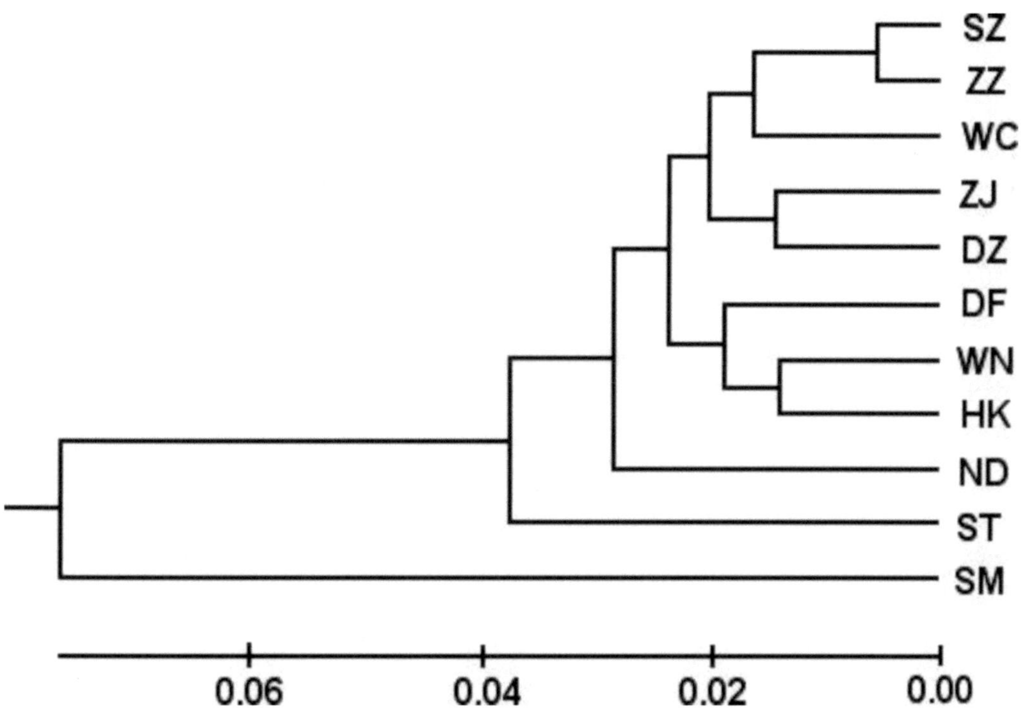

Figure 1. The UPGMA tree constructed among 11 locations of *Scylla paramamosain*. SM, Sanmen; ND, Ningde; ZZ, Zhangzhou; ST, Shantou; SZ, Shenzhen; ZJ, Zhanjiang; HK, Haikou; WC, Wenchang; WN, Wanning; DF, Dongfang; DZ, Danzhou.

two groups: one consisted of 10 locations and the other one contained only one location (Sanmen). Mantel tests showed a significantly positive link between pairwise $F_{ST}/(1 - F_{ST})$ and natural logarithm of geographic distance (km) (**Figure 2**).

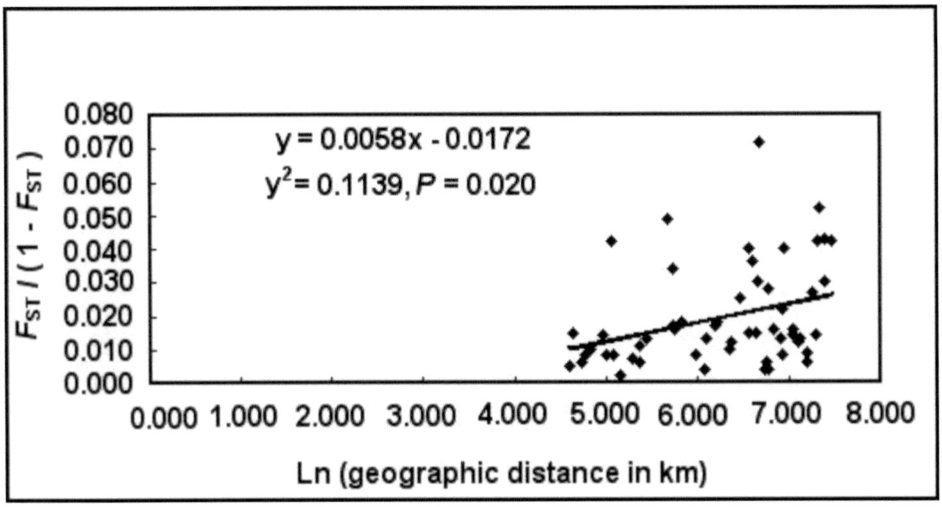

Figure 2. Relationship estimated between genetic differentiation and geographic distance (km) among 11 locations of *Scylla paramamosain*.

2.2.3. Parentage assignment technique based on PCR

In this study, 10 polymorphic microsatellite loci produced 1870 genotypes in 184 offspring and three parents. The genetic diversity indexes showed a relative high variation of these individuals, with H_O and PIC values ranging from 0.38 to 0.99 and from 0.44 to 0.75, respectively. Two loci deviated from HWE in family 1 and 4, four loci in family 2, and six loci in family 3. According to Mendelian inheritance principle, the genotypes of all parents were successfully deduced based on genotypes of offspring, suggesting microsatellites are ideal molecular markers for evaluating genetic relationship among different individuals. In panda and tiger, microsatellite loci were also successfully used to identify the relationship among different specimens [38, 39].

Furthermore, the exclusion probability was used to distinguish the pedigree relationship of *S. paramamosain* individuals. The PIC value was found to be associated with the exclusion probability: when the PIC value went up, the exclusion probability increased accordingly. Moreover, the combined exclusion probability was observed higher than single locus in this study (**Figure 3**). Ten microsatellite loci had 97% exclusion probability under without parent information conditions. The assignment success rate reached to 100% when seven microsatellite markers were combined together under the condition of no any parent information. Practical application showed that seven microsatellite loci combination could accurately assign 95% of the offspring to right parents (**Figure 4**).

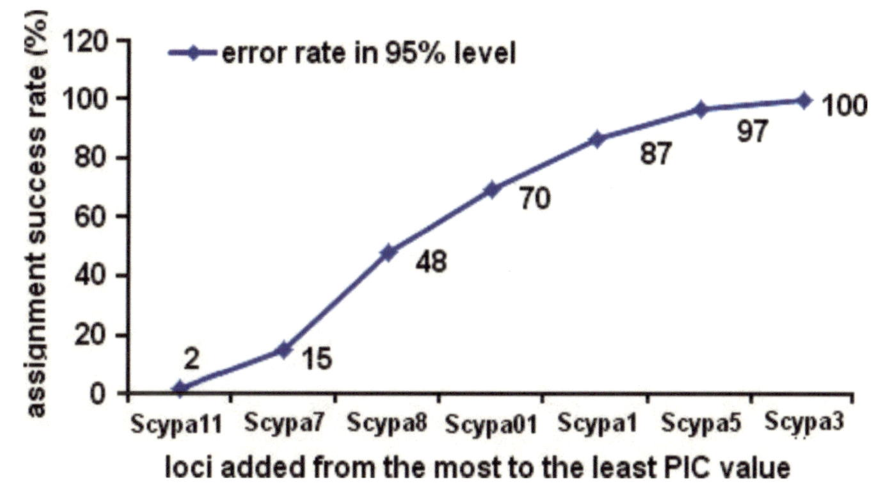

Figure 3. Cumulative assignment success rates of seven most informative microsatellite loci of *Scylla paramamosain*.

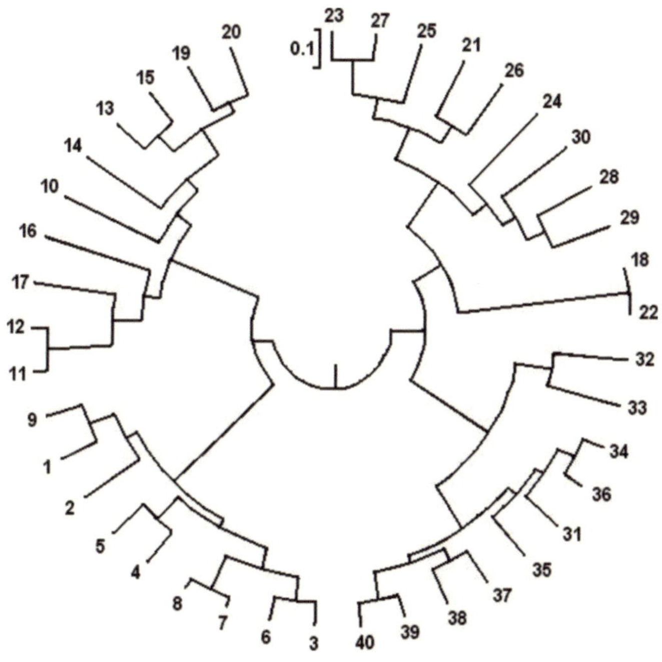

Figure 4. The UPGMA dendrogram of 40 progeny of *Scylla paramamosain* constructed using double-blind test.

2.2.4. Identification of growth performance related microsatellite markers

In aquatic animals, a set of microsatellite markers were identified to link to growth traits [40, 41]. In this study, of 129 polymorphic microsatellite loci, 30 showed polymorphisms in the experimental G_1 family. Statistical analysis indicated that three markers (Scpa36, Scpa75, and Spm30) were significantly linked to 12 growth traits (CL, BH, ICW, AW, FFWC, FFLC, FFHC, CWS8, MLP2, MLP3, DLS2, and BW) in *S. paramamosain*. Microsatellite marker Scpa36 was significantly associated with growth traits CL, FFLC, FFWC, AW, MLP2, BH, FFHC, and MLP3. Out of four genotypes AB, BB, BC, and AC at this locus, the genotype BC had the highest potential for artificial selection (**Table 2**). Microsatellite marker Scpa75 was significantly linked to growth traits ICW, DLS2, MLP3, AW, and CWS8. Among four genotypes AD, AC, BC, and BD at this locus, the genotypes BC and BD showed the highest correlation rate with growth traits in *S. paramamosain* (**Table 3**). Locus Spm30 was significantly associated with three traits BH, BW, and DLS2. Multiple comparison analysis indicated that genotypes AC and BD at this locus had the highest association degree with growth traits (**Table 4**). Moreover, growth traits CW, CFW, DLS1, and MLP1 were not found to link to any microsatellite marker in this study.

Locus	Genotype	Number	Growth trait (Means ± SD, mm)							
			CL	AW	BH	FFLC	FFWC	FFHC	MLP2	MLP3
Scpa36	AB	19	47.87 ± 7.88^{a}	23.85 ± 3.62^{a}	28.37 ± 3.96^{a}	43.98 ± 7.34^{a}	11.80 ± 2.25^{a}	17.10 ± 3.37^{a}	26.58 ± 3.72^{a}	21.88 ± 2.88^{a}
	BB	21	49.80 ± 7.85^{ab}	24.48 ± 4.08^{ab}	28.97 ± 4.68^{a}	46.90 ± 9.20^{ab}	13.01 ± 3.14^{ab}	18.65 ± 4.39^{ab}	27.29 ± 4.71^{ab}	22.98 ± 4.33^{ab}
	AC	23	52.50 ± 8.83^{ab}	26.20 ± 4.86^{ab}	30.73 ± 5.36^{ab}	49.79 ± 9.72^{ab}	14.07 ± 3.25^{b}	19.99 ± 4.86^{ab}	28.70 ± 5.30^{ab}	24.73 ± 3.98^{bc}
	BC	21	54.46 ± 5.01^{b}	27.08 ± 2.75^{b}	32.21 ± 3.10^{b}	52.37 ± 7.57^{b}	14.39 ± 2.68^{b}	21.01 ± 4.29^{b}	30.45 ± 3.36^{b}	25.75 ± 2.64^{c}

CL, carapace length; AW, abdomen width; BH, body height; FFLC, fixed finger length of the claw; FFWC, fixed finger width of the claw; FFHC, fixed finger height of the claw; MLP2, meropodite length of pereiopod 2; MLP3, meropodite length of pereiopod 3.

$^{a, b, ab, bc}$ and ^{c}, the superscripts in different genotypes without a common one are significant different ($P < 0.05$).

Table 2. Association analysis performed between microsatellite locus Scpa36 and eight growth traits of *Scylla paramamosain*.

Locus	Genotype	Number	Growth trait (Means ± SD, mm)				
			ICW	AW	CWS8	DLS2	MLP3
Scpa75	AD	32	69.79 ± 11.83^{a}	24.10 ± 4.20^{a}	71.90 ± 12.50^{a}	43.45 ± 7.18^{a}	22.45 ± 4.20^{a}
	AC	17	74.70 ± 11.75^{a}	24.98 ± 3.75^{a}	77.03 ± 12.06^{a}	46.65 ± 6.50^{ab}	24.63 ± 3.83^{a}
	BD	24	76.82 ± 9.99^{a}	26.85 ± 4.32^{a}	79.15 ± 10.16^{a}	47.21 ± 5.28^{ab}	24.54 ± 3.52^{a}
	BC	14	77.59 ± 7.34^{a}	26.45 ± 2.65^{a}	80.00 ± 7.74^{a}	48.69 ± 4.30^{b}	25.51 ± 2.83^{a}

ICW, internal carapace width; AW, abdomen width; CWS8, carapace width at spine 8; DLS2, distance between lateral spine 2; MLP3, meropodite length of pereiopod 3.

$^{a, b}$ and ^{ab}, the superscripts in different genotypes without a common one are significant different ($P < 0.05$).

Table 3. Association analysis performed between microsatellite locus Scpa75 and five growth traits of *Scylla paramamosain*.

Among 16 growth traits tested in this study, traits AW and MLP3 were associated with two loci Scpa36 and Scpa75, and traits BH and DLS2 were associated with two loci Scpa75 and Spm30. Meanwhile, traits CL, FFWC, FFLC, ICW, MLP2, BW, and CWS8 were associated with only one microsatellite locus. It is considered to be a common event that one locus contributes to several quantitative traits and/or several different loci influence a same quantitative trait [41, 42]. In the next artificial breeding program, these three microsatellite markers should be first considered for marker-assisted selection of *S. paramamosain*.

Locus	Genotype	Number	Growth trait (Means ± SD, mm)		
			BH	DLS2	BW
Spm30	CD	18	27.34 ± 4.47^{a}	42.13 ± 7.28^{a}	57.72 ± 31.66^{a}
	AB	24	29.52 ± 5.24^{ab}	44.78 ± 7.07^{ab}	79.68 ± 38.73^{b}
	BD	33	30.88 ± 4.22^{b}	47.28 ± 5.30^{b}	89.53 ± 32.98^{b}
	AC	21	31.08 ± 3.58^{b}	47.54 ± 4.25^{b}	92.99 ± 31.06^{b}

BH, body height; DLS2, distance between lateral spine 2; BW, body weight.
$^{a, b}$ and ^{ab}, the superscripts in different genotypes without a common one are significant different ($P < 0.05$).

Table 4. Association analysis performed between microsatellite locus Spm30 and three growth traits of *Scylla paramamosain*.

2.2.5. Construction of genetic linkage map

Of 337 microsatellite markers, 118 segregated from parents to offspring of *S. paramamosain* with a rate of 35%. Meanwhile, 64 AFLP selective primer combinations produced 574 segregated bands. After chi-square test according to Mendelian ratio, a total of 470 molecular markers were suitable for genetic map construction. The phenomenon that markers deviated from Mendelian ratio could be caused by small population size, scoring errors, selection pressure, nonrandom segregation, and gametes competition [43].

A first preliminary genetic linkage map was developed for *S. paramamosain* (**Figure 5**). This map contained 65 linkage groups and 212 molecular markers (60 microsatellites and 152 AFLPs). In theory, the number of linkage group is equal to the number of haploid chromosome. In this study, the haploid chromosome number ($N = 49$) [44] was much lower than the total group number ($N = 65$), which indicated that this genetic map may still be preliminary with small number and low resolution of markers. The number of markers per genetic group ranged from 2 to 14, with an average of 3.3. All markers were evenly distributed in genetic groups and no clustering was found. This linkage map was 2746 cM in length with an average resolution of 18.7 cM. The expected genome was estimated to be approximately 5540 cM, which covered about 50% by our preliminary genetic map. In the next step, a high density genetic linkage map needs to be constructed in order to facilitate QTL mapping and marker-assisted selection for *S. paramamosain*.

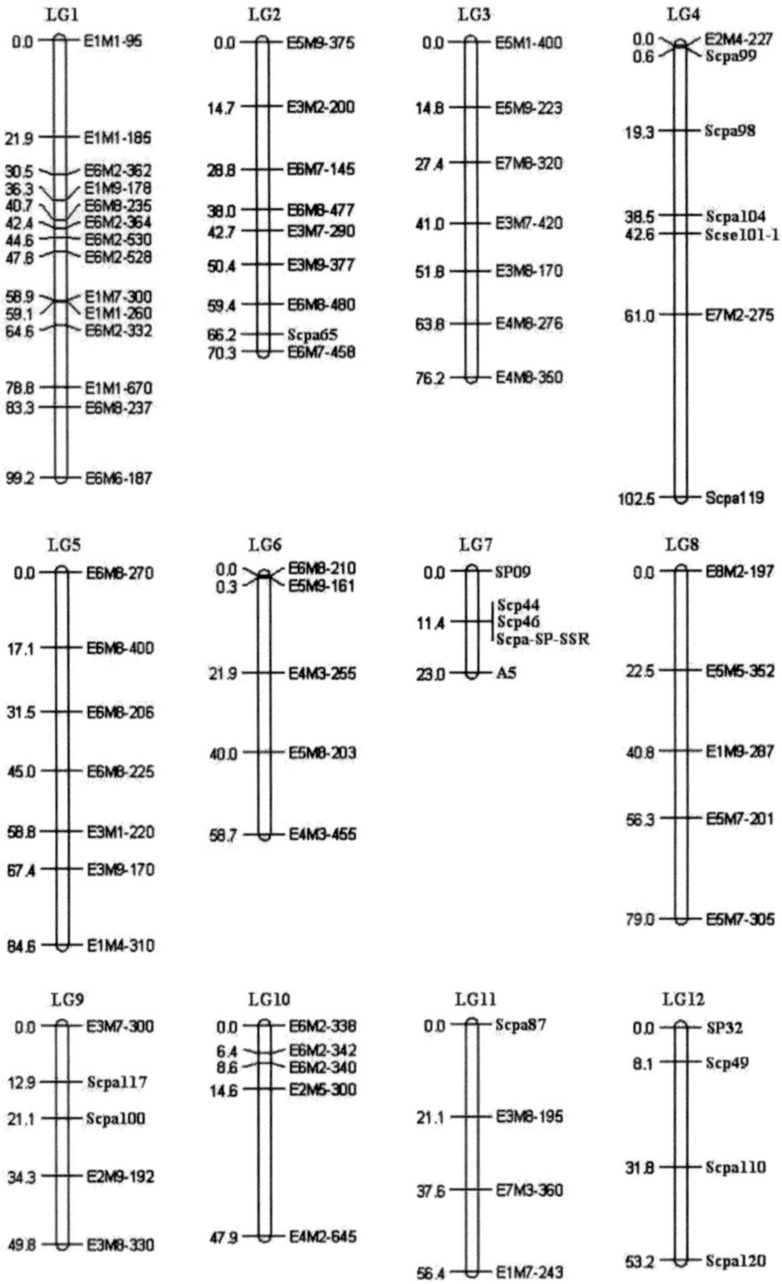

LG1
0.0 E1M1-95
21.9 E1M1-185
30.5 E6M2-362
36.3 E1M9-178
40.7 E6M8-235
42.4 E6M2-364
44.6 E6M2-530
47.8 E6M2-528
58.9 E1M7-300
59.1 E1M1-260
64.6 E6M2-332
78.8 E1M1-670
83.3 E6M8-237
99.2 E6M6-187
LG2
0.0 E5M9-375
14.7 E3M2-200
28.8 E6M7-145
38.0 E6M8-477
42.7 E3M7-290
50.4 E3M9-377
59.4 E6M8-480
66.2 Scpa65
70.3 E6M7-458
LG3
0.0 E5M1-400
14.8 E5M9-223
27.4 E7M8-320
41.0 E3M7-420
51.8 E3M8-170
63.8 E4M8-276
76.2 E4M8-350
LG4
0.0 E2M4-227
0.6 Scpa99
19.3 Scpa98
38.5 Scpa104
42.6 Scse101-1
61.0 E7M2-275
102.5 Scpa119
LG5
0.0 E6M8-270
17.1 E6M8-400
31.5 E6M8-206
45.0 E6M8-225
58.8 E3M1-220
67.4 E3M9-170
84.6 E1M4-310
LG6
0.0 E6M8-210
0.3 E5M9-161
21.9 E4M3-255
40.0 E5M8-203
58.7 E4M3-455
LG7
0.0 SP09
11.4 Scp44
Scp46
Scpa-SP-SSR
23.0 A5
LG8
0.0 E8M2-197
22.5 E5M5-352
40.8 E1M9-287
56.3 E5M7-201
79.0 E5M7-305
LG9
0.0 E3M7-300
12.9 Scpa117
21.1 Scpa100
34.3 E2M9-192
49.8 E3M8-330
LG10
0.0 E6M2-338
6.4 E6M2-342
8.6 E6M2-340
14.6 E2M5-300
47.9 E4M2-645
LG11
0.0 Scpa87
21.1 E3M8-195
37.6 E7M3-360
56.4 E1M7-243
LG12
0.0 SP32
8.1 Scp49
31.8 Scpa110
53.2 Scpa120

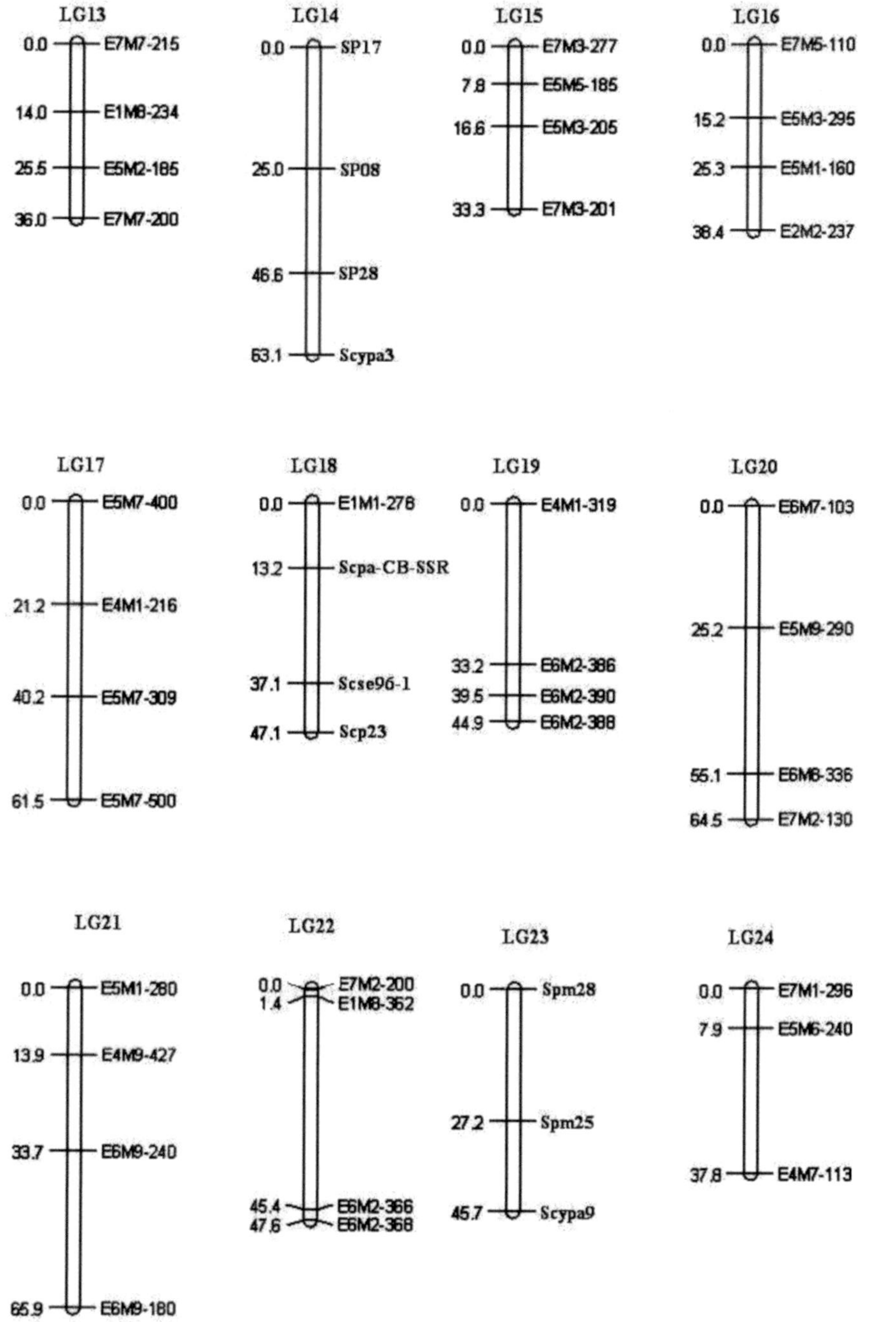
LG13
0.0 E7M7-215
14.0 E1M8-234
25.5 E5M2-185
36.0 E7M7-200
LG14
0.0 SP17
25.0 SP08
46.6 SP28
63.1 Scypa3
LG15
0.0 E7M3-277
7.8 E5M5-185
16.6 E5M3-205
33.3 E7M3-201
LG16
0.0 E7M5-110
15.2 E5M3-295
25.3 E5M1-160
38.4 E2M2-237
LG17
0.0 E5M7-400
21.2 E4M1-216
40.2 E5M7-309
61.5 E5M7-500
LG18
0.0 E1M1-278
13.2 Scpa-CB-SSR
37.1 Scse96-1
47.1 Scp23
LG19
0.0 E4M1-319
33.2 E6M2-386
39.5 E6M2-390
44.9 E6M2-388
LG20
0.0 E6M7-103
25.2 E5M9-290
55.1 E6M8-336
64.5 E7M2-130
LG21
0.0 E5M1-280
13.9 E4M9-427
33.7 E6M9-240
65.9 E6M9-180
LG22
0.0 E7M2-200
1.4 E1M8-362
45.4 E6M2-366
47.6 E6M2-368
LG23
0.0 Spm28
27.2 Spm25
45.7 Scypa9
LG24
0.0 E7M1-296
7.9 E5M6-240
37.8 E4M7-113

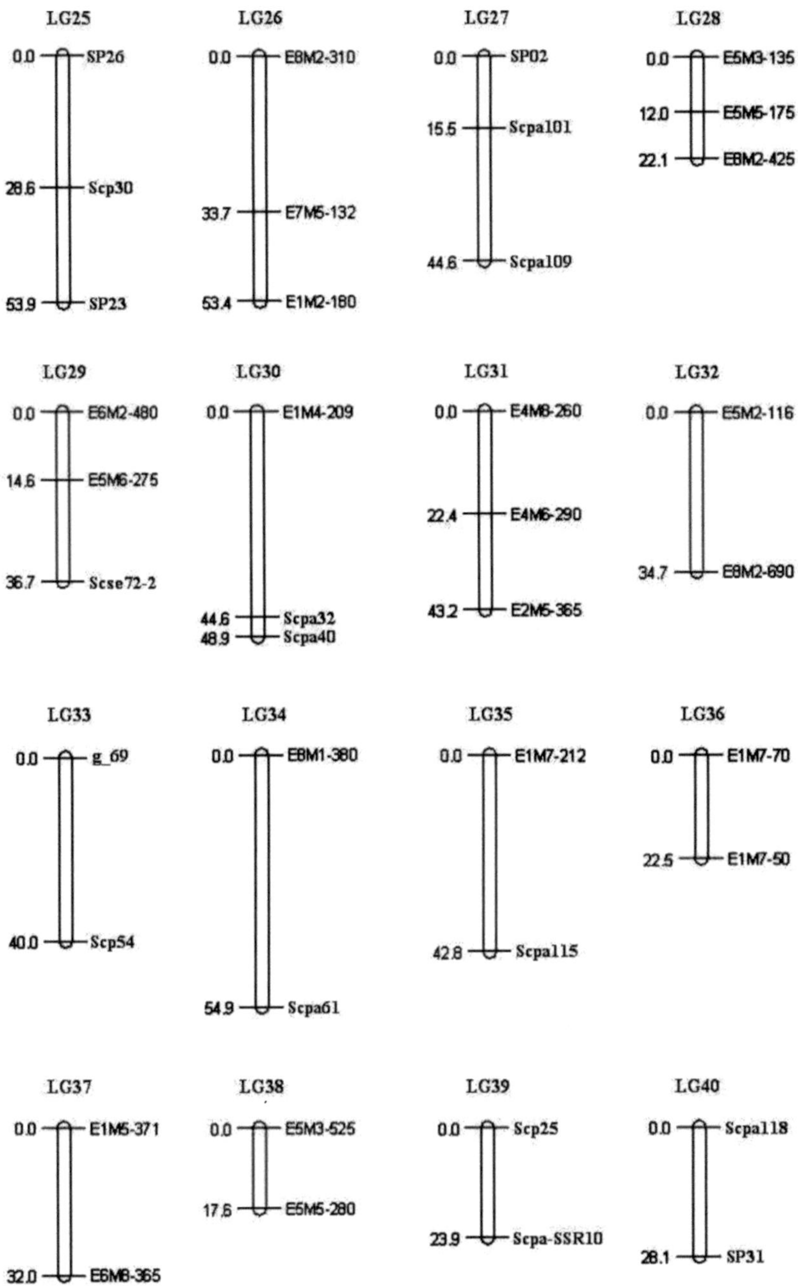

LG25
0.0 SP26
28.6 Scp30
53.9 SP23
LG26
0.0 E8M2-310
33.7 E7M5-132
53.4 E1M2-180
LG27
0.0 SP02
15.5 Scpa101
44.6 Scpa109
LG28
0.0 E5M3-135
12.0 E5M5-175
22.1 E8M2-425
LG29
0.0 E6M2-480
14.6 E5M6-275
36.7 Scse72-2
LG30
0.0 E1M4-209
44.6 Scpa32
48.9 Scpa40
LG31
0.0 E4M8-260
22.4 E4M6-290
43.2 E2M5-365
LG32
0.0 E5M2-116
34.7 E8M2-690
LG33
0.0 g_69
40.0 Scp54
LG34
0.0 E8M1-380
54.9 Scpa61
LG35
0.0 E1M7-212
42.8 Scpa115
LG36
0.0 E1M7-70
22.5 E1M7-50
LG37
0.0 E1M5-371
32.0 E6M8-365
LG38
0.0 E5M3-525
17.6 E5M5-280
LG39
0.0 Scp25
23.9 Scpa-SSR10
LG40
0.0 Scpa118
28.1 SP31

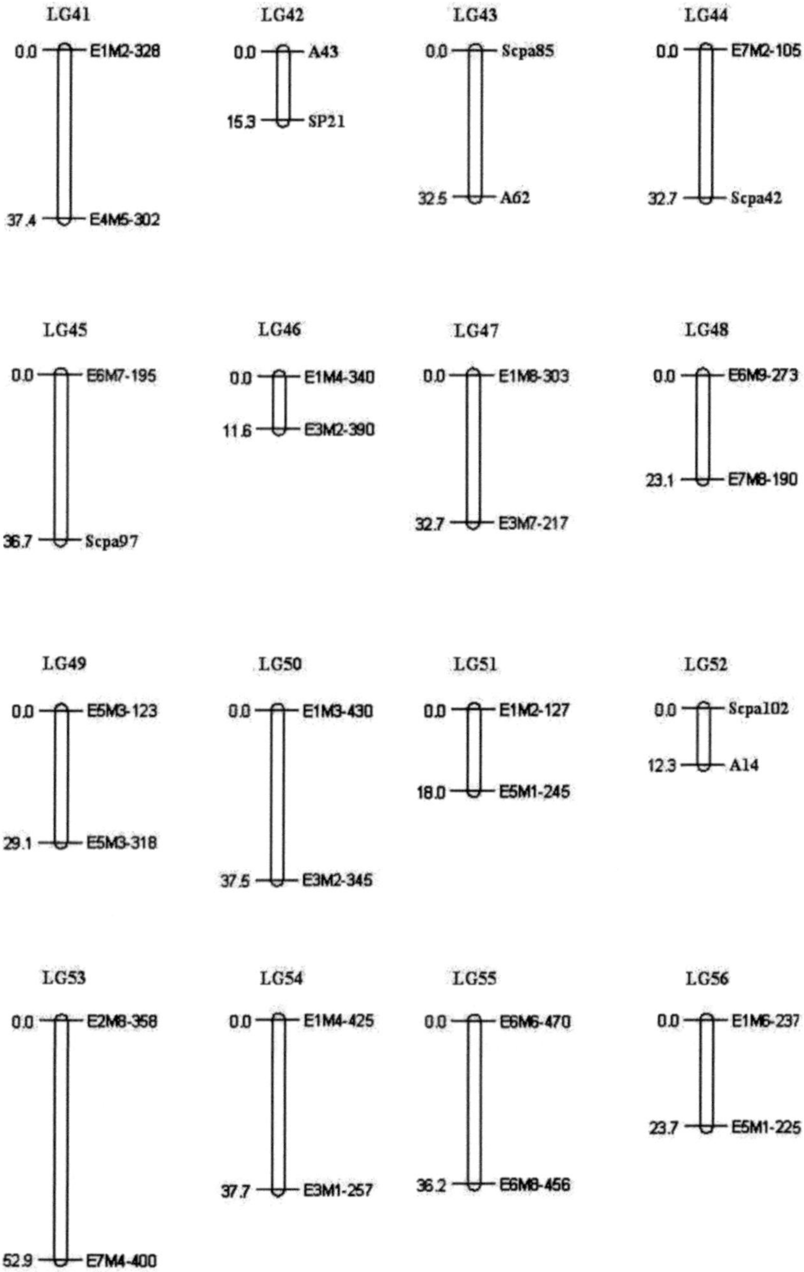
LG41
0.0 E1M2-328
37.4 E4M5-302
LG42
0.0 A43
15.3 SP21
LG43
0.0 Scpa85
32.5 A62
LG44
0.0 E7M2-105
32.7 Scpa42
LG45
0.0 E6M7-195
36.7 Scpa97
LG46
0.0 E1M4-340
11.6 E3M2-390
LG47
0.0 E1M8-303
32.7 E3M7-217
LG48
0.0 E6M9-273
23.1 E7M8-190
LG49
0.0 E5M3-123
29.1 E5M3-318
LG50
0.0 E1M3-430
37.5 E3M2-345
LG51
0.0 E1M2-127
18.0 E5M1-245
LG52
0.0 Scpa102
12.3 A14
LG53
0.0 E2M8-358
52.9 E7M4-400
LG54
0.0 E1M4-425
37.7 E3M1-257
LG55
0.0 E6M6-470
36.2 E6M8-456
LG56
0.0 E1M6-237
23.7 E5M1-225

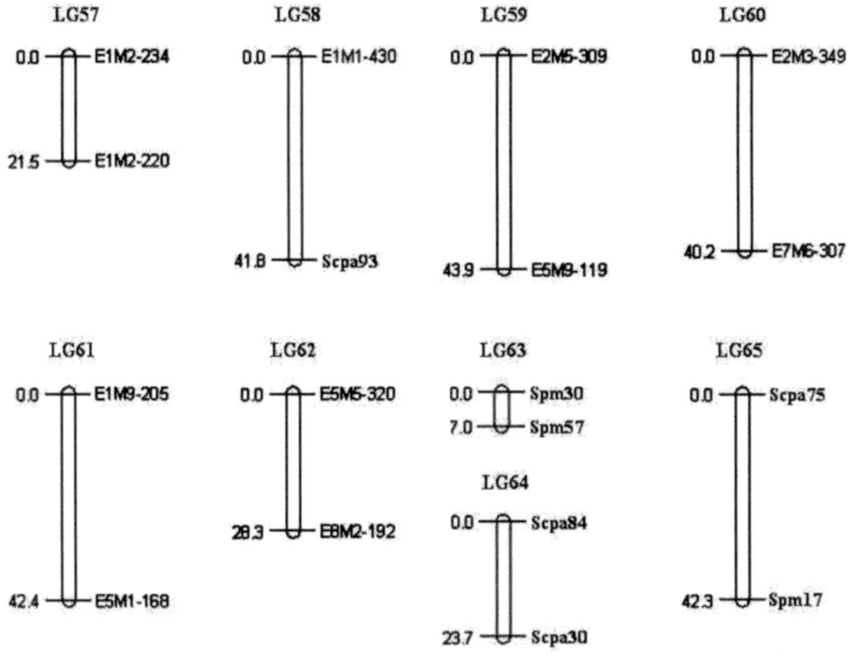

Figure 5. Genetic linkage map constructed for the mud crab (*Scylla paramamosain*). Genetic distances are listed on the left in Kosambi units (cM). Markers are shown on the right of each linkage group. Amplified fragment length polymorphism (AFLP) markers are named by the primer combination and fragment size. Microsatellite markers are in bold.

3. Conclusions

This study isolated and characterized 302 polymorphic microsatellite markers for the mud crab (*S. paramamosain*), and uncovered the high polymorphism and low genetic differentiation of wild populations distributed along South-eastern China coasts. Furthermore, a PCR-based parentage assignment method was well developed which could correctly assign 95% of the offspring to right parents. Moreover, three microsatellite loci were identified to link with growth performance of *S. paramamosain*. Finally, a first preliminary genetic linkage map was created for *S. paramamosain* using microsatellite and AFLP markers. These findings should provide novel insights into genome biology, wild resource background, and molecular marker-assisted selection in *S. paramamosain*.

Acknowledgements

This work was supported by the Top-Notch Young Talents Program of China, the National Natural Science Foundation of China (Grant No. 31001106), and the Fund of Key Laboratory of Sustainable Development of Marine Fisheries, Ministry of Agriculture, China (Grant No. 2013-SDMFMA-KF-5).

Author details

Hongyu Ma[1*], Chunyan Ma[2], Lingbo Ma[2], Xincang Li[2] and Yuanyou Li[1]

*Address all correspondence to: mahongyuhome@163.com

1 Guangdong Provincial Key Laboratory of Marine Biology, Shantou University, Shantou, China

2 East China Sea Fisheries Research Institute, Chinese Academy of Fishery Sciences, Shanghai, China

References

[1] Shen Y, Lai Q. Present status of mangrove crab (*Scylla serrata* (Forskål)) culture in China. The ICLARM Quarterly. 1994; 17: 28–29.

[2] Fishery Bureau of Ministry of Agriculture of China. China Fisheries Yearbook (2014). Beijing: Chinese Agricultural Press. 2015; 219 p.

[3] Ma HY, Bi JZ, Shao CW, Chen Y, Miao GD, Chen SL. Development of 40 microsatellite markers in spotted halibut (*Verasper variegatus*) and the cross-species amplification in barfin flounder (*Verasper moseri*). Animal Genetics. 2009; 40: 576–578. DOI: 10.111/j.1365-2052.2009.01869.x

[4] Hughes JM, Schmidt DJ, Huey JA, Real KM, Espinoza T, McDougall A, Kind PK, Brooks S, Roberts DT. Extremely low microsatellite diversity but distinct population structure in a long-lived threatened species, the Australian lungfish *Neoceratodus forsteri* (Dipnoi). Plos One. 2015; 10: e0121858. DOI: 10.1371/journal.pone.0121858

[5] Bai X, Huang S, Tian X, Cao X, Chen G, Wang W. Genetic diversity and parentage assignment in Dojo loach, *Misgurnus anguillicaudatus* based on microsatellite markers. Biochemical Systematics and Ecology. 2015; 61: 12–18. DOI: 10.1016/j.bse.2015.05.005

[6] Ma HY, Chen SL, Yang JF, Chen SQ, Liu WH. Genetic linkage maps of barfin flounder (*Verasper moseri*) and spotted halibut (*Verasper variegatus*) based on AFLP and microsatellite markers. Molecular Biology Reports. 2011; 38: 4749–4764. DOI: 10.1007/s11033-010-0612-2

[7] Nietlisbach P, Camenisch G, Bucher T, Slate J, Keller LF, Postma E. A microsatellite-based linkage map for song sparrows (*Melospiza melodia*). Molecular Ecology Resources. 2015; 15: 1486–1496. DOI: 10.1111/1755-0998.12414

[8] Ibitoye DO, Akin-Idowu PE. Marker-assisted-selection (MAS): A fast track to increase genetic gain in horticultural crop breeding. African Journal of Biotechnology. 2010; 9: 8889–8895. DOI: 10.5897/AJB2010.000-3318

[9] Chen SL, Ji XS, Shao CW, Li WL, Yang JF, Liang Z, Liao XL, Xu GB, Xu Y, Song WT. Induction of mitogynogenetic diploids and identification of WW super-female using sex-specific SSR markers in half-smooth tongue sole (*Cynoglossus semilaevis*). Marine Biotechnology. 2012; 14: 120–128. DOI: 10.1007/s10126-011-9395-2

[10] Takano M, Barinova A, Sugaya T, Obata Y, Watanabe T, Ikeda M, Taniguchi N. Isolation and characterization of microsatellite DNA markers from mangrove crab, *Scylla paramamosain*. Molecular Ecology Notes. 2005; 5: 794–795. DOI: 10.1111/j. 1471-8286.2005.01065.x

[11] Xu XJ, Wang GZ, Wang KJ, Li SJ. Isolation and characterization of ten new polymorphic microsatellite loci in the mud crab, *Scylla paramamosain*. Conservation Genetics. 2009; 10: 1877–1878. DOI: 10.1007/s10592-009-9843-y

[12] Ma HY, Ma CY, Ma LB, Cui HY. Novel polymorphic microsatellite markers in *Scylla paramamosain*and cross-species amplification in related crab species. Journal of Crustacean Biology. 2010; 30: 441–444. DOI: 10.1651/09-3263.1

[13] Ma HY, Ma CY, Ma LB, Zhang FY, Qiao ZG. Isolation and characterization of 54 polymorphic microsatellite markers in *Scylla paramamosain* by FIASCO approach. Journal of the World Aquaculture Society. 2011; 42: 591–597. DOI: 10.1111/j. 1749-7345.2011.00503.x

[14] Ma HY, Ma CY, Ma LB. Identification of type I microsatellite markers associated with genes and ESTs in *Scylla paramamosain*. Biochemical Systematics and Ecology. 2011; 39: 371–376. DOI: 10.1016/j.bse.2011.05.007

[15] Cui HY, Ma HY, Ma LB. Development of eighteen polymorphic microsatellite markers in *Scylla paramamosain* by 5′ anchored PCR technique. Molecular Biology Reports. 2011; 38: 4999–5002. DOI: 10.1007/s11033-010-0645-6

[16] Ma CY, Ma HY, Ma LB, Jiang KJ, Zhang FY, Song W. Isolation and characterization of polymorphic microsatellite loci from cDNA library of *Scylla paramamosain*. African Journal of Biotechnology. 2011; 10: 11142–11148. DOI: 10.5897/AJB11.973

[17] Ma HY, Jiang W, Liu P, Feng NN, Ma QQ, Ma CY, Li SJ, Liu YX, Qiao ZG, Ma LB. Identification of transcriptome-derived microsatellite markers and their association with the growth performance of the mud crab (*Scylla paramamosain*). Plos One. 2014; 9: e89134. DOI:10.1371/journal.pone.0089134

[18] Ma HY, Ma CY, Li SJ, Jiang W, Li XC, Liu YX, Ma LB. Transcriptome analysis of the mud crab (*Scylla paramamosain*) by 454 deep sequencing: assembly, annotation, and marker discovery. Plos One. 2014; 9: e102668. DOI: 10.1371/journal.pone.0102668

[19] Ma HY, Cui HY, Ma CY, Ma LB. High genetic diversity and low differentiation in mud crab (*Scylla paramamosain*) along the southeastern coast of China revealed by microsatellite markers. The Journal of Experimental Biology. 2012; 215: 3120–3125. DOI: 10.1242/jeb.071654

[20] Ma QQ, Ma HY, Chen JH, Ma CY, Feng NN, Xu Z, Li SJ, Jiang W, Qiao ZG, Ma LB. Parentage assignment of the mud crab (*Scylla paramamosain*) based on microsatellite markers. Biochemical Systematics and Ecology. 2013; 49: 62–68. DOI: 10.1016/j.bse.2013.03.013

[21] Ma HY, Li SJ, Feng NN, Ma CY, Wang W, Chen W, Ma LB. First genetic linkage map for the mud crab (*Scylla paramamosain*) constructed using microsatellite and AFLP markers. Genetics and Molecular Research. 2016; 15: gmr.15026929. DOI: http://dx.doi.org/10.4238/gmr.15026929

[22] Yeh FC, Yang RC, Boyle T. POPGENE version 1.31. Microsoft window-based freeware for population genetic analysis. 1999. Available from: http://www.ualberta.ca/~fyeh/.

[23] Excoffier L, Laval G, Schneider S. ARLEQUIN (version 3.0): an integrated software package for population genetics data analysis. Evolutionary Bioinformatics. 2005; 1: 47–50.

[24] Rice WR. Analyzing tables of statistical tests. Evolution. 1989; 43: 223–225. DOI: 10.2307/2409177

[25] Van OCW, Hutchinson WF, Wills DPM, Shipley P. MICRO-CHECKER: software for identifying and correcting genotyping errors in microsatellite data. Molecular Ecology Notes. 2004; 4: 535–538. DOI: 10.1111/j.1471-8286.2004.00684.x

[26] Peakall R, Smouse PE. GENALEX 6: genetic analysis in excel. Population genetic software for teaching and research. Molecular Ecology Notes. 2006; 6: 288–295. DOI: 10.1111/j.1471-8286.2005.01155.x

[27] Tamura K, Dudley J, Nei M, Kumar S. MEGA 4: molecular evolutionary genetics analysis (MEGA) software version 4.0. Molecular Biology and Evolution. 2007; 24: 1596–1599. DOI: 10.1093/molbev/msm092

[28] Mantel N. The detection of disease clustering and a generalized regression approach. Cancer Research. 1967; 27: 209–220.

[29] Kalinowski ST, Taper ML, Marshall TC. Revising how the computer program CERVUS accommodates genotyping error increases success in paternity assignment. Molecular Ecology. 2007; 16: 1099–1106. DOI: 10.1111/j.1365-294X.2007.03089.x

[30] Van OJW. JoinMap 3.0: software for the calculation of genetic linkage maps. Plant Research International. 2001. Wageningen, the Netherlands.

[31] Voorrips RE. MapChart: software for the graphical presentation of linkage maps and QTLs. Journal of Heredity. 2002; 93: 77–78. DOI: 10.1093/jhered/93.1.77

[32] Fishman L, Kelly AJ, Morgan E, Willis JH. A genetic map in the *Mimulus guttatus* species complex reveals transmission ratio distortion due to heterospecific interactions. Genetics. 2001; 159: 1701–1716.

[33] Chakravarti A, Lasher LK, Reefer JE. A maximum likelihood method for estimating genome length using genetic linkage data. Genetics. 1991; 128: 175–182.

[34] Lu XP, Ma LB, Qiao ZG, Zhang FY, Ma CY. Population genetic structure of *Scylla paramamosain* from the coast of the Southeastern China based on mtDNA COI sequence. Journal of Fisheries of China. 2009; 33: 15–23. DOI: 10.3724/SP.J.00001 (In Chinese with English abstract)

[35] Nei M. Melecular Evolutionary Genetics. New York, Columbia University. 1987.

[36] Avise J. Phylogeography. Cambridge, MA: Harvard University Press. 1998.

[37] He L, Zhang A, Weese D, Zhu C, Jiang C, Qiao Z. Late Pleistocene population expansion of *Scylla paramamosain* along the coast of China: a population dynamic response to the last interglacial sea level highstand. Journal of Experimental Marine Biology and Ecology. 2010; 385: 20–28. DOI: 10.1016/j.jembe.2010.01.019

[38] Zhang YG, Li DQ, Rao LQ, Xiao QM, Liu D. Identification of polymorphic microsatellite DNA loci and paternity testing of Amur tigers. Acta Zoologica Sinica. 2003; 49: 118–123. (In Chinese with English Abstract)

[39] Zhang ZH, Sen FJ, Sun S, David VA, Zhang AJ, O'Brien SJ. Paternity assignment of giant panda by microsatellite genotyping. Hereditas. 2003; 25: 504–510. DOI: 10.3321/j.issn: 0253-9772.2003.05.002 (In Chinese with English Abstract)

[40] Yang J, Zhang XF, Chu ZY, Sun XW. Correlation analysis of microsatellite markers with body weight, length, height and upper jaw length wensize of common carp (*Cyprinus carpio* L.). Journal of Fishery Sciences of China. 2010; 17: 721–730. (In Chinese with English Abstract)

[41] Liu L, Li J, Liu P, Zhao FZ, Gao BQ, Du Y, Ma CY. Correlation analysis of microsatellite DNA markers with growth related traits of swimming crab (*Portunus trituberculatus*). Journal of Fisheries of China. 2012; 36: 1034–1041. DOI: 10.3724/SP.J.1231.2012.27872 (In Chinese with English abstract)

[42] Li XH, Bai JJ, Ye X, Hu YC, Li SJ, Yu LY. Polymorphisms in the 5′ flanking region of the insulin-like growth factor I gene are associated with growth traits in largemouth bass *Micropterus salmoides*. Fisheries Science. 2009; 75: 351–358. DOI: 10.1007/s12562-008-0051-3

[43] Liebhard R, Koller B, Gianfranceschi L, Gessler C. Creating a saturated reference map for the apple (Malus × domesticaBorkh.) genome. Theoretical and Applied Genetics. 2003; 106: 1497–1508. DOI: 10.1007/s00122-003-1209-0

[44] Chen XL, Wang GZ, Chen LH, Li SJ. Methodological improvement and its application effect in chromosome study of mud crab, *Scylla serrata*. Journal of Oceanography in Taiwan Strait. 2004; 23: 347–353. (In Chinese with English Abstract)

Section 4

Microsatellites in Cancer Research

Chapter 10

Microsatellite Instability and its Significance to Hereditary and Sporadic Cancer

Jeffery W. Bacher, Linda Clipson, Leta S. Steffen and
Richard B. Halberg

Additional information is available at the end of the chapter

http://dx.doi.org/10.5772/65065

Abstract

Up to one million people within the United States may have Lynch syndrome (LS), but only 10% have been diagnosed. Early identification of these individuals is critical because they are predisposed to the development of colorectal and several other cancers at a relatively young age. Individuals with LS carry a germline mutation in one of four DNA mismatch repair genes, which leads to hypermutability in simple repetitive DNA sequences. This hallmark molecular phenotype called microsatellite instability (MSI) is now widely used to screen individuals needing germline sequencing to confirm diagnosis of LS. Standardized markers for MSI testing and other improvements in methodology have greatly improved the accuracy and cost-effectiveness of MSI testing. The current trend toward universal MSI screening of all colorectal and endometrial cancers will save lives by identifying LS prior to the development of deadly cancer. New technologies for MSI detection, such as next generation sequencing, open the possibility of a single test for LS that determines both tumor MSI status and germline mutations. Moreover, MSI detection is poised to take on an even greater role in prediction of responses to the new immunotherapies targeted at MSI-positive tumors.

Keywords: colon cancer, DNA mismatch repair, Lynch syndrome, microsatellite instability, MSI

1. Introduction

A form of hereditary colon cancer, we now call Lynch syndrome (LS), was first identified more than 100 years ago, but it was not until 1993 that rapid progress in unraveling the underlying genetic cause of this disease really began with the serendipitous discovery of a "mutator phenotype" in colon cancers. The mutator phenotype observed in colon tumors was manifested as a high level of instability (i.e., insertion and deletion mutations) in simple repetitive sequences called microsatellites [1–3]. This form of genomic instability now referred to as microsatellite instability (MSI) has become the hallmark molecular signature of LS. Shortly after the discovery of MSI, the four DNA mismatch repair (MMR) genes responsible for LS were identified and the genetic basis for the disease was understood. The role of epigenetics in silencing the MMR system was later discovered, first in sporadic MSI cancers, then in LS. With this knowledge and the adoption of standardized guidelines for identifying and testing individuals at risk for LS, large scale screening for LS became possible and has set the stage for universal screening of all colorectal cancer (CRC) patients [4]. This milestone is important as the vast majority of individuals with LS are not diagnosed and an early detection of LS and identification of at-risk relatives is key to save lives. Finally, targeted immunotherapies offer new hope for treating the more challenging cases of hereditary and sporadic of MSI-positive CRC [5, 6].

2. Discovery of microsatellite instability (MSI) and its association with CRC

2.1. Microsatellite repeats

Microsatellite sequences are 1–6 base pair short tandem repeats that are highly mutable and ubiquitous in eukaryotic genomes [7–9]. As a consequence of high mutability, microsatellites tend to be quite variable in populations and therefore are widely used as molecular markers for linkage mapping, lineage mapping, and genotype identification purposes. Approximately 3% of the human genome contains microsatellite sequences, with mononucleotide repeats, predominantly poly (A/T) tracts, being the most abundant [10]. Microsatellite mutation rates vary greatly among loci, ranging from $\sim 10^{-6}$ to $\sim 10^{-2}$ mutations per locus per generation [11, 12]. The tendency of microsatellites to mutate increases with repeat number and can become pronounced beyond a critical number of repeats [10, 11, 13–15]. The vast majority of mutational variation can be attributed to intrinsic features of the locus, including repeat motif size, repeat number, and sequence composition. The major mechanism of mutagenesis in microsatellites is strand slippage during DNA replication, which can result in either insertion or deletion mutations in repetitive sequences, if not repaired effectively [16]. Post-replication, mismatch repair machinery removes any lesions occurring during replication to maintain genome stability.

2.2. Mutator phenotype hypothesis

In the early 1970s, Loeb [17–21] extended the concept of the "mutator phenotype" observed in bacteria to cancer biology. He proposed that high error rates due to alterations in DNA synthesis are causally linked to malignant transformation [18]. Loeb further speculated that high mutation rates caused by deficiencies in DNA repair activity could also contribute to cancer development. While earlier discoveries in bacteria had shown increased mutagenesis

http://dx.doi.org/10.5772/65065

due to defects in DNA polymerases and DNA repair, the contribution of Loeb was to propose a connection between a mutator phenotype and cancer development. The role of a mutator phenotype in cancer development is also integral to Nowell's model [21] on tumor progression that is based on genomic instability providing the variability for clonal outgrowth and tumor evolution. The type of genomic instability that is described in this model is mainly chromosomal instability, in which breaks and rearrangements are increased as a consequence of inherited defects in DNA repair.

By 1991, Loeb [22] had refined his hypothesis arguing that an increased mutation rate or mutator phenotype could explain the high number of mutations believed to be present in many cancers that may be necessary for multistage tumor progression. He speculated that the spontaneous mutation rate in somatic cells is too low to account for the high number of mutations found in cancers and that an early step in tumorigenesis must be one that induces a mutator phenotype. Confirmation that the mutator phenotype contributes to at least some forms of CRC was conclusively demonstrated by the Cancer Genome Atlas Network study by measuring genome-wide mutation frequencies in 276 CRC samples [23]. Some (16%) of CRC samples were found to be hypermutated, with mutation frequencies 100-fold higher than nonhypermutated CRC. Interestingly, the hypermutated CRC tumors were found to have alterations in either DNA MMR genes or DNA polymerases.

2.3. Discovery of MSI in CRC

In 1990, Fearon and Vogelstein [24] published the multistep model of colon tumorigenesis in which they proposed that tumors develop as the result of mutational activation of oncogenes coupled with the mutational inactivation of tumor suppressor genes. Loss of a specific chromosomal region in CRCs was interpreted as evidence that the region contained a tumor suppressor gene and was detected as "loss of heterozygosity" (LOH) in a linked genetic marker. Following the publication of Fearon and Vogelstein, many investigators started looking for LOH events to determine the chromosomal location of potential tumor suppressor genes [24]. In 1993, Perucho and colleagues [1] performed arbitrarily primed polymerase chain reaction (PCR) to identify differences between normal and tumor samples from the colon. They noted that the amplicons actually became shorter in a few (12% of 130) tumors. Sequence analysis revealed that the PCR amplicons were composed of simple repetitive sequences, principally polyadenine tracts associated with Alu sequences in which one or more adenines were lost by somatic deletion in the cancers. These cancers, with an estimated 10^5 ubiquitous somatic mutations in simple repetitive sequences, had unique clinical and pathological characteristics. First, these tumors were more likely to arise in the proximal colon, less likely to be invasive, less likely to harbor mutations in *KRAS* and *TP53*, and more likely to occur in younger patients. Based upon these findings, Perucho and colleagues [1] concluded that these tumors arose from a unique pathway involving the "catastrophic loss of fidelity in the replication machinery from normal cells" that caused them to be hereditary.

At the same time, two other groups were also using microsatellite markers to detect LOH to identify potential tumor suppressor genes [2, 3]. Thibodeau and colleagues [2] found that microsatellite repeats were often mutated in cancers, with alterations occurring in 25 out of 90

CRCs. They called this phenomenon "microsatellite instability" and used the abbreviation of "MIN." The mutations were denoted as "type 1," if the deletion or expansion was large and "type II," if the change was limited to a single 2-basepair repeat change. The significance of this difference has never been fully resolved. CRCs with microsatellite instability were found to be primarily in the proximal colon and were associated with a better prognosis. Based on these findings, Thibodeau and colleagues [2] reasoned that this was a unique pathway to tumorigenesis that involved microsatellite instability and not chromosomal instability.

Another group, led by Vogelstein and de la Chapelle, was looking for LOH in LS families at the microsatellite marker *D2S123*, which they suspected was linked to a tumor suppressor gene causing hereditary CRC [3]. They observed many mutations at *D2S123* and other microsatellites in the LS patients as well as 13% of sporadic CRC and called this phenomenon, replication error phonotype. Thus, three different groups had independently discovered MSI and named it either "ubiquitous somatic mutations in simple repetitive sequences," microsatellite instability, or replication error phenotype. These names persisted until 2004 when the participants of the National Cancer Institute (NCI) workshop on MSI testing decided that the biomarker for identifying LS would be called microsatellite instability or MSI [25].

2.4. DNA mismatch repair systems

In the 1960s, 1970s, and early 1980s, laboratories studying bacteria [17, 26–28] and yeast [16] had discovered DNA mismatch repair and recognized that inactivation of the MMR genes resulted in widespread mutations at microsatellite sequences (i.e., a mutator phenotype). The first *Escherichia coli* mutator strain (*mutS1*) was isolated by Siegel and Byrson in 1967 and key MMR genes including *mutS, mutL, and mutH* were identified through genetic studies in the 1980s [17, 29, 30]. In vitro reconstitution of the *E. coli* MMR system from individual purified components facilitated mechanistic studies of individual *E. coli* MMR proteins [31, 32]. In the *E. coli* MMR system, a mismatched base is recognized by a MutS homodimer (**Table 1**). A MutL homodimer interacts with the MutS DNA complex, and then a MutH restriction endonuclease is activated by MutL. The MMR system recognizes the newly synthesized strand by the lack of methylation at GATC sites. MutH nicks the unmethylated error-containing strand to introduce an entry point for excision by helicases and exonucleases, and subsequent resynthesis by DNA polymerase III.

Shortly after the discovery of MSI in CRC, Strand and colleagues showed that MMR deficient mutants of the yeast strain *Saccharomyces cerevisiae* exhibited 100–700-fold increased instability in dinucleotide repeat tracts, demonstrating a clear link between loss of MMR and MSI [33]. The knowledge that instability in microsatellites was associated with loss of MMR activity, led to the rapid cloning and identification of the human homologs of yeast MMR genes [33–37]. Eukaryotic MMR systems were found to be more complex than in prokaryotes, but many features are conserved (**Table 1**) (recently reviewed by [38–40]). In eukaryotic MMR, MutS and MutL proteins do not function as homodimers, but instead form the heteroduplexes MSH2-MSH6 (MutSα) or MSH2-MSH3 (MutSβ) that bind to specific mismatches to initiate MMR. These heterodimers have different binding specificities, with MutSα being primarily responsible for repairing single base-base and insertion deletion

http://dx.doi.org/10.5772/65065

loop (IDL) mismatches, and MutSβ for repairing IDL mismatches. There are also multiple human homologs of the bacterial gene for *MutL, including MLH1, MLH3, PMS1,* and *PMS2.* Heterodimer MLH1-PMS2 (MutLα), the major MutL complex in humans, is involved in repairing a wide variety of mismatches. Two other MutL heterodimers, MLH1-PMS1 (MutLβ) and MLH1-MLH3 (MutLγ), appear to have a minor role in MMR. Proliferating cell nuclear antigen (PCNA) activates MutLα endonuclease activity to nick the DNA in a strand-specific fashion, which is then removed by EXO1 digestion and the new strand resynthesized by Polymerase δ and subsequently ligated [39, 41]. Mutator phenotypes conferred by defects in *MSH3, PMS1,* and *MLH3* are much milder than those conferred by defects in *MLH1, MSH2, MSH6,* or *PMS2,* which are typically associated with LS.

E. coli	*S. cerevisiae*	*H. sapiens*	Function
MutS	MSH2-MSH6 (MutSα)	MSH2-MSH6 (MutSα)	Mismatch recognition, binds to single base and IDL mismatches
	MSH2-MSH3 (MutSβ)	MSH2-MSH3 (MutSβ)	Mismatch recognition, binds to IDL mismatches
MutL	MLH1-PMS1 (MutLα)	MLH1-PMS2 (MutLα)	Strand incision, endonuclease activity
	MLH1-MLH2 (MutLβ)	MLH1-PMS1 (MutLβ)	Strand incision, endonuclease activity
	MLH1-MLH3 (MutLγ)	MLH1-MLH3 (MutLγ)	Strand incision, endonuclease activity
Dam methylase	Absent	Absent	Methylation of as GATC sites in *E. coli*
MutH	Absent	Absent	Endonuclease nicks daughter strand at GATC sites, serves as strand discrimination signal in *E. coli*
RecJ, ExoI, ExoVII, ExoX	EXO1	EXO1	Strand excision, 5′–3′dsDNA exonuclease
UrvD	None	None	Helicase, promotes strand excision
β-Clamp	PCNA	PCNA	DNA polymerase processivity factor
γ-Clamp	RFC	RFC	Loading of β-clamp/PCNA
SSB	RPA	RPA	ssDNA binding protein, acts in excision & resynthesis
DNA Pol III	Pol delta	Pol delta	DNA polymerase involved in gap filling
DNA ligase	Unknown	Ligase I	Repair synthesis

Table 1. Mismatch repair proteins in *E. coli, S. cerevisiae*, and *H. sapiens.*

The rate of replication errors can vary by more than a million-fold, depending on the DNA polymerase and the local DNA sequence [39]. Correcting replication errors in MMR-deficient and MMR-proficient cells can vary by more than 100,000-fold. The highest error rates in MMR-deficient yeast strains are for single-base insertion or deletion in long mononucleotide repetitive sequences, reflecting increased strand slippage during replication in these sequences. For example, Kunkel and Erie [39] reported the probability that a particular mismatch that will be made by a replicase varies from extremely rare misinsertion of the dCTP opposite template C by Pol α ($\leq 10^{-7}$) to much more frequent single-base deletion mismatches in long mononucleotide runs ($\geq 10^{-3}$). This high intrinsic error rate in replication of mononucleotide runs helps to explain why mononucleotide repeat markers are extremely sensitive to MSI in the absence of a functional MMR system.

2.5. MSI pathway in familial and sporadic CRC tumorigenesis

Many investigators support the view that some type of genomic instability is necessary to generate all the mutations observed in CRC, whereas others reason that mutations required to form cancer are accumulated spontaneously over long periods of time. Recent advances in molecular biology, especially sequencing, have revealed that CRCs are highly heterogeneous arising from several distinct pathways. Four types of genomic or epigenetic instability have been described in CRCs: chromosomal instability (CIN), microsatellite instability (MSI), CpG island methylator phenotype (CIMP), and global DNA hypomethylation.

About 3% of all MSI-positive CRCs are LS and about 15% are sporadic CRC [42, 43]. Tumor development in both LS and sporadic MSI-positive CRC involves the MSI pathway. The difference is that loss of MMR activity in LS tumors is the consequence of germline mutations or epimutations, while sporadic MSI-positive CRCs are caused by somatic methylation of the MLH1 promoter [44]. Sporadic CRCs with MSI are typically diploid, have biallelic methylation of the MLH1 promoter and subsequent loss of MLH1 protein expression, frequently have mutations in the *BRAF* gene, and are associated with better prognosis compared to individuals with non-MSI tumors. LS CRCs are also typically diploid and are associated with better prognosis, but have mutations in *KRAS* instead of *BRAF*, and have germline mutations or epimutations in MMR genes *MLH1, MSH2, MSH6,* and *PMS2*.

Tumorigenesis in MSI-positive CRC involves changes in the same signaling pathways as tumors without MSI, but often alterations occur in different genes and by different mechanisms. For example, initiating mutations in the *APC* gene are common in sporadic CRC. In contrast, a substantial portion of MSI-positive CRCs do not have mutations in the *APC* gene, but rather have mutations with similar consequences in *CTNNB1* or other genes in the WNT signaling pathway. Sporadic non-MSI CRCs typically arise through CIN, whereas MSI-positive CRCs arise through the MSI pathway. The MSI pathway is characterized by a genome-wide increase in mutations, especially in microsatellite sequences. Since most microsatellites are in noncoding regions of the genome, mutations in these loci do not increase cancer risk. In contrast, mutations in short coding microsatellite sequences can lead to frame shift mutations and gene inactivation that are linked to cancer risk. For example, mutations in *TGFβ-R2* occur primarily (>90%) in an A10 microsatellite tract that results in inactivation of the TGFβ-R2 protein [45, 46]. Transforming growth factor-β (TGF-β) signaling inhibits proliferation in the colonic epithelium and MSI-positive tumors often lack inhibitory TGF-β signaling due to mutations in the gene for TGF-β type II receptor (*TGFβ-R2*). Loss of TGFβ signaling is a critical driver in the MSI pathway, but this is just the tip of the iceberg. There are an estimated 17,654 coding mononucleotide repeats in the human genome [47]. Sequencing of MSI-High (MSI-H) CRCs has identified recurring mutations in many other coding microsatellite sequences including tumor suppressor genes and DNA repair genes [48].

Cancer type	MSI-High, % Unselected[1]	Cancer risk, % LS[2]	References unselected; LS
Colon	13%	10–80%	[58]; [49, 51, 59–62]
Endometrium	18–33%	15–71%	[63, 64]; [49–52, 59, 65, 66]
Stomach	22%	1–13%	[67]; [49, 53, 55, 59, 68–70]
Ovary	10%	4–20%	[71]; [49, 53, 54, 58, 59, 69, 72]
Small bowel		<1–12%	[49, 53, 54, 59, 69]
Urinary tract		<1–25%	[49, 53, 54, 69, 72, 73]
Skin (sebaceous tumors)	35–60%	1–9%	[74, 75]; [76–78]
Brain		1–4%	[53, 69, 72, 79]
Prostrate	1%	9–30%	[53, 54, 56, 57]
Breast	0–1%	5–18%	[80–83]; [49, 53–55, 84]
Hepatobiliary tract	16%	<1–4%	[85]; [53, 58, 59, 68, 72]
Pancreas		1–4%	[53, 66, 86]
Thyroid	63%		[87]
Skin (melanoma)	11%		[88]
Cervix	8%		[89]
Esophageal adenocarcinoma	7%		[90]
Sarcoma (soft tissue)	5%		[91]

[1]Percent of MSI-high tumors in unselected population.
[2]Cumulative risks of cancer by 70 years of age in germline MMR mutation carriers (for all MMR genes and both sexes) [49–91].

Table 2. Frequency of MSI cancers in LS and unselected populations.

Lifetime cancer risks for LS individuals vary depending upon which MMR gene is mutated and by gender. The majority (~80%) of LS tumors have mutations in *MLH1* or *MSH2*. Lifetime risk of CRC by 70 years of age for *MLH1* and *MSH2* germline mutation carriers range from 40 to 80%, with higher risk for men (**Table 2**) [49]. The cumulative lifetime risk of CRC in *MSH6* and *PMS2* germline mutation carriers is lower, ranging from 10 to 22% [50–52]. LS individuals also have a significantly increased risk for a variety of extracolonic malignancies (**Table 2**). The highest risk is for endometrial cancer, which occurs in up to 71% of women with *MSH6* mutations, 54% of those with *MLH1* and *MSH2* mutations, and 15% of those with *PMS2* mutations [51, 52]. Significant cumulative risks also exist for cancers of the stomach, ovary, small bowel, urinary tract, skin, pancreas, and brain. Breast and prostate cancers have not generally been considered part of the LS-associated cancer spectrum, but recent studies have found an increased risk for these cancers in germline MMR mutation carriers [53–57]. Dudley and colleagues [6] reviewed reports on the frequency of MSI-H across different tumor types in unselected populations, which includes both sporadic and familial cancers (**Table 2**).

3. Early development of MSI markers

3.1. Standardization of MSI testing

After the discovery of MSI in 1993, many laboratories began developing their own methods for measuring MSI and started to test different types of cancers. Unfortunately, there were no standards for MSI testing. Assays varied as to which and how many microsatellite markers to use. Moreover, investigators differed on the per cent of unstable markers necessary to classify a tumor as MSI-positive. This lack of standardization made it nearly impossible to compare results between laboratories and resulted in considerable variability in the frequency of MSI reported for a given tumor type. A number of studies were conducted to determine which microsatellite markers and what type of repeat motif was most sensitive and specific for the detection of MSI tumors. Two key studies described below provided the basis for markers chosen at the National Cancer Institute (NCI) workshop on MSI [25]. The first was by Dietmaier and colleagues [92] who tested 31 different microsatellites including six mononucleotide, 15 dinucleotide, three trinucleotide, five tetranucleotide, and two pentanucleotide repeats on a series of 58 primary CRCs. They found that sensitivity and specificity of markers were closely related to the type of the repeat (highest for mono and dinucleotide repeats) and that MSI could be subdivided into MSI-H (>20% of markers were unstable), MSI-Low (MSI-L) (<10% unstable markers), and microsatellite stable (0% unstable markers). The vast majority (14/15) of MSI-H tumors failed to express *MSH2* or *MLH1*. In contrast, all of the MSI-L and MSI stable tumors had normal MMR expression. Based on these results, they recommended a diagnostic strategy for MSI assessment that utilizes a uniform panel of 10 microsatellites in which *BAT26, BAT40, MfdlS, D2S123,* and *D5S346* were tested first, followed by *BAT25, D10S197, D18S58, D18S69,* and *MYCLJ* if less than 40% of the initial set were mutated. Tumors were defined as MSI-positive if at least 40% of the tested markers were unstable.

The second study cited by the NCI workshop on MSI testing as a basis for the choice of MSI markers was a multicenter study to test the reliability and quality of MSI analysis [93]. Eight laboratories compared MSI analyses performed on 10 matched pairs of normal and tumor DNA from patients with CRC. They proposed that five microsatellite markers, which were selected from a panel of 30, should be analyzed in the first run and five additional microsatellite loci should be added in cases where less than two markers displayed MSI. A preferred set of five markers was not identified, but they suggested that the microsatellite panel should be comprised of different repeat types including mononucleotide and dinucleotide repeats. Cases with more than 40% unstable markers were classified as MSI-positive and those with less than 10% unstable markers were classified as MSI-negative [93].

In December 1997, the NCI sponsored an international workshop on Microsatellite Instability in Cancer Detection and Familial Predisposition to further review and unify the field [25]. The following recommendations (often referred to as the Bethesda guidelines) were made: (1) the form of genomic instability associated with defective MMR in tumors was to be called microsatellite instability or MSI, (2) a panel of five microsatellites (two mononucleotide repeats, BAT-26 and BAT-25; and three dinucleotide repeats, D5S346, D2S123, and D17S250) was recommended as a reference panel for MSI testing, (3) tumors should be classified as MSI-H if two or more of the five markers show instability, and MSI-L if only one of the five markers show instability, and MSI stable (MSS) if no markers were unstable, and (4) a unique clinical and pathological phenotype is identified for the MSI-H tumors, which comprise about 15% of colorectal cancers, whereas MSI-L and MSS tumors appear to be phenotypically similar. This standard was followed until 2004 when revisions were made at a second workshop.

The sensitivity, reproducibility, and cost effectiveness of MSI testing have improved considerably since the early days thanks to the use of all mononucleotide repeat markers and the introduction of fluorescent multiplex PCR and capillary electrophoresis technologies [94]. Currently, MSI testing involves comparing allelic patterns in microsatellite markers derived from a tumor and a normal (usually blood) samples from the same individual. A change in allele size between the normal and tumor samples indicates MSI. To generate the allelic profiles, DNA is extracted from each sample and amplified by PCR using fluorescently labeled primers flanking each microsatellite repeat locus. This is most efficiently done by multiplexing, allowing for simultaneous amplification and analysis of all markers in the panel. The resulting PCR products are resolved by capillary electrophoresis and the output is analyzed to determine allele sizes in comparison to known size standards [94]. The classification of tumor MSI status is based on the Bethesda guidelines [25].

3.2. Lynch syndrome screening guidelines

A number of different sets of criteria have been developed to identify patients who should be tested for LS (Box 1). The first set was the Amsterdam criteria in 1991, which was later modified to the Amsterdam II criteria in 1999 [95]. The Amsterdam criteria are very stringent and could miss as many as 58% of individuals with LS [96]. To address this limitation, the NCI published the Bethesda guidelines in 1997 and later the revised Bethesda guidelines in 2004 [97, 98]. Still, between 12 and 28% of individuals with LS could be missed using the revised Bethesda guidelines [4, 49]. To further increase sensitivity for the detection of LS, the trend has been

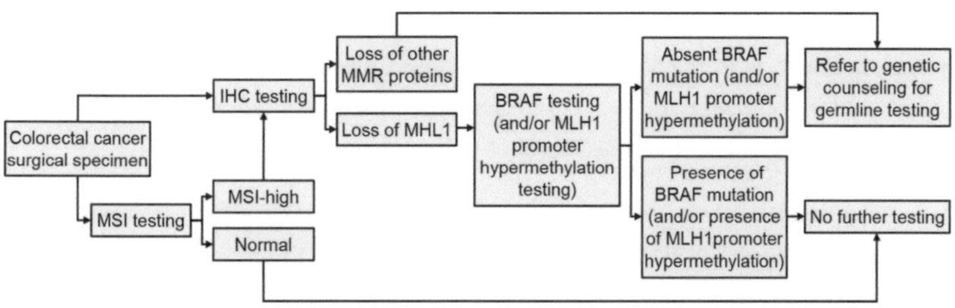

Figure 1. National Comprehensive Cancer Network (NCCN) guidelines for LS testing.

moving toward universal screening of all patients with newly diagnosed CRC. The National Comprehensive Cancer Network (NCCN) recommends either a selective approach using MSI/IHC to screen all patients with CRC diagnosed before 70 years of age and also those older patients who meet the Bethesda guidelines, or universal screening [99] (**Figure 1**). The selective strategy would miss only 4.9% of individuals with LS, whereas, universal screening would theoretically miss none, assuming 100% sensitivity [4].

Box 1. Lynch syndrome screening guidelines

Amsterdam criteria I (1991)

Three or more relatives with colorectal cancer, plus all of the following:

- One affected patient should be a first-degree relative of the other two
- Colorectal cancer should involve at least two generations
- At least one case of colorectal cancer should have been diagnosed before the age of 50 years

Amsterdam II criteria (1999)

Three or more relatives with LS-related cancer (colorectal cancer or cancer of the endometrium, small bowel, ureter, or renal pelvis) plus all of the following:

- One affected patient should be a first-degree relative of the other two
- Two or more successive generations should be affected
- Cancer in one or more affected relatives should be diagnosed before the age of 50 years
- Familial adenomatous polyposis should be excluded in any cases of colorectal cancer
- Tumors should be verified by pathological examination

Bethesda guidelines (1997)

Only one of the following criteria needs to be met:

- Cancer in families that fulfill the Amsterdam criteria
- Two LS-associated cancers in the same individual, including synchronous and metachronous CRC or associated extracolonic cancers (including endometrial, ovarian, gastric, hepatobiliary, or small-bowel cancer, or transitional-cell carcinoma of the renal pelvis or ureter)
- CRC and first-degree relative with CRC and/or LS-associated extracolonic cancers and/or colorectal adenoma; one of the cancers must have been diagnosed before the age of 45 years and the adenoma diagnosed before the age of 40 years
- CRC or endometrial cancer that was diagnosed before the age of 45 years

http://dx.doi.org/10.5772/65065

- Right-sided CRC with an undifferentiated pattern on histology, which is diagnosed before the age of 45 years
- Signet-ring-cell-type CRC that was diagnosed before the age of 45 years
- Adenoma that was diagnosed by the age of 40 years

Revised Bethesda guidelines (2003)

Only one of the following criteria needs to be met:

- CRC before the age of 50 years
- Synchronous or metachronous LS-related tumor
- CRC with 1 or more first-degree relatives with LS-related tumor before the age of 50 years
- CRC with 2 or more first- or second-degree relatives with LS-related tumor
- MSI in CRC in patient before the age of 60 years
- A panel of five quasi-monomorphic mononucleotide repeats may be more sensitive for MSI-High tumors than other microsatellite markers and may obviate the need for normal tissue for comparison

National Comprehensive Cancer Network (NCCN) guidelines (2015)

- Lynch syndrome tumor screening (i.e., MSI or IHC) should be performed for all patients with colorectal cancer diagnosed at or before the age of 70 years and also those after the age of 70 years who meet the Bethesda guidelines
- Or, universal MSI/IHC screening of all CRCs

---

4. Current use of microsatellite markers for detection of MSI

4.1. Mononucleotide repeats

In 2004, the revised Bethesda guidelines recommended the use of a panel of all mononucleotide repeat markers to increase the sensitivity of detection [98]. The recommendation was based on the observation that the original Bethesda MSI panel may underestimate the number of MSI-H tumors because of the use of dinucleotide repeats [100]. The revised guidelines indicate that the use of mononucleotide markers improves the sensitivity; hence, workshop participants suggested that more mononucleotide markers be used to evaluate MSI. The basis for the recommendation for the use of mononucleotide repeat markers is described below.

The *BAT-26* mononucleotide repeat marker in the Bethesda panel is one of the most sensitive markers for MSI testing. Some investigators have suggested that MSI can be identified by analyzing tumor DNA with only *BAT-26* [101, 102]. Zhou and colleagues analyzed 542 tumors from various organs for MSI using a panel of 10 or more microsatellite markers versus *BAT-26* [103]. They found concordance of results in 539 out of 542 (99.5%) cases [103].

An unusual property of *BAT-26* and a few other microsatellite markers is that most individuals in the population have a single allele and are thus quasi-monomorphic, which permits MSI testing using tumor samples only [101, 102]. However, others have shown germline polymorphisms in *BAT-26*, especially in certain racial groups. For example, a study by Samowitz and colleagues found 7.7% of African Americans are polymorphic for *BAT-26* [104]. A more extensive population study performed by Bacher and colleagues, which included individuals of Caucasian, African, and Asian descent, found low-level germline variation in *BAT-26* and other quasi-monomorphic markers (**Table 3**) [94]. Thus, polymorphisms in these microsatellites limit their utility in MSI determinations without the corresponding normal DNA.

	NR-21 (%)	NR-24 (%)	BAT-25 (%)	BAT-26 (%)	MONO-27 (%)
Caucasian-American	1.1	0.0	0.5	0.6	0.0
African-American	0.8	0.9	9.9	9.8	0.8
Asian-American	5.9	0.0	0.0	0.8	0.8

Table 3. Quasi-monomorphic mononucleotide repeat markers (% polymorphic alleles).

Inclusion of dinucleotide repeats in the Bethesda panel might lead to misclassification of some cancers. Incorrect assignments can result from a number of different factors. First, dinucleotide repeats are less sensitive to MSI than mononucleotide repeats [94, 105]. Second, instability involving only dinucleotide markers can occur in MSS tumors [94, 101, 106]. Third, size alterations in dinucleotide repeats can be difficult to interpret. Finally, mutations in *MSH6* often do not lead to alterations in dinucleotide repeats [107]. These limitations lead Suraweera and colleagues [100] to propose using a panel of five quasi-monomorphic mononucleotide repeats (*BAT-25, BAT-26, NR-21, NR-22* and *NR-24*). They determined the MSI status of 124 colon tumors, 50 gastric tumors, 20 endometrial tumors, and 16 colon cancer cell lines that had been previously established. The results were 100% concordant.

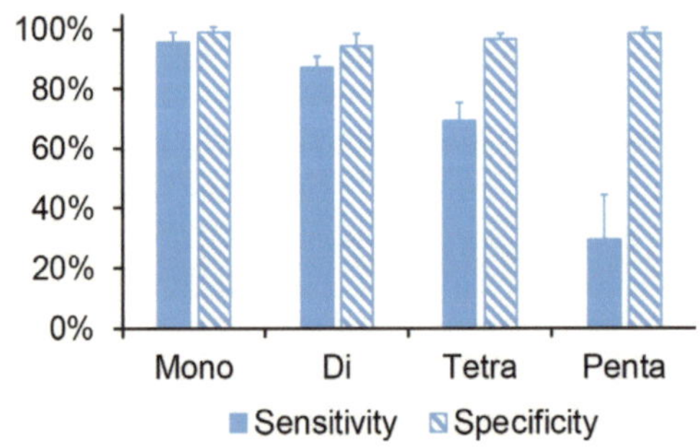

Figure 2. The relative sensitivity and specificity of mono-, di-, tetra- and penta-nucleotide repeats for detection of MSI in mismatch repair deficient CRC.

http://dx.doi.org/10.5772/65065

To determine the best markers for the MSI testing, a study of 266 mono-, di-, tetra-, and pentanucleotide repeat markers was conducted to identify those with the highest sensitivity and specificity for the detection of MSI in MMR deficient tumors [94]. A subset of each marker type was used to screen 225 human colon tumor samples that had been previously characterized for mismatch repair status. Consistent with previous studies, mononucleotide repeats were found to be the most sensitive and specific type of microsatellite marker for the detection of MSI (**Figure 2**). Based on this study, the MSI Analysis System (Promega Corporation, Madison, United States) was developed; it contains five quasi-monomorphic mononucleotide repeats, *BAT-25, BAT-26, NR-21, NR-24,* and *MONO-27*. The MSI Analysis System has several advantages over the Bethesda panel, including: (1) increased sensitivity and specificity, (2) easier interpretation of MSI patterns in mononucleotide repeats compared to dinucleotide repeats, (3) the quasi-monomorphic nature of the markers simplifies analysis and allows MSI classification in cases where only tumor samples are available, and (4) the inclusion of two highly polymorphic pentanucleotide repeats to prevent sample mix-ups (**Figure 3**) [94, 108]. This MSI kit is now a widely used alternative to the Bethesda panel [94, 108, 109].

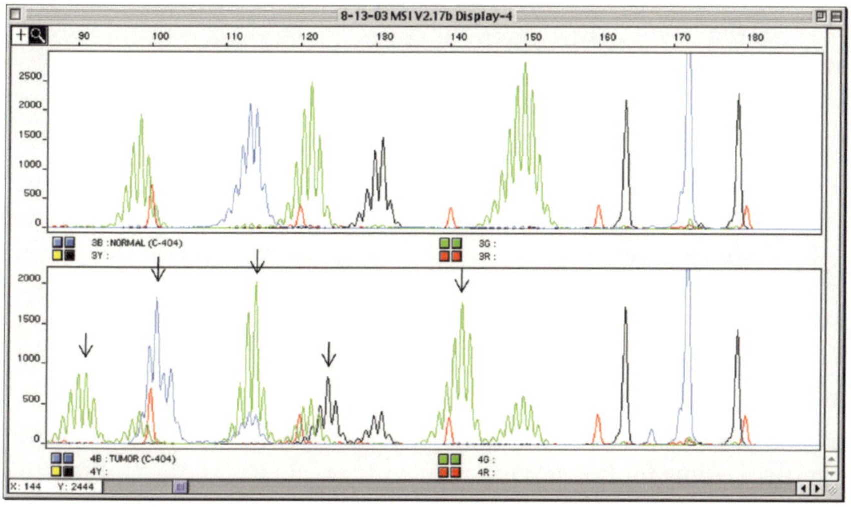

Figure 3. MSI analysis of CRC and the corresponding normal sample using the MSI Analysis System (Promega Corporation, Madison, United States). The electropherogram shows the allelic profile generated from a normal sample (top panel) and a matching MLH1-deficient tumor sample (bottom panel). New alleles in tumor sample that are not found in matching normal are indicated by arrows. The panel contains five quasi-monomorphic mononucleotides for MSI determinations, including: JOE-labeled (green) *NR-21, BAT-25* and *MONO-27*; fluorescein-labeled (blue) *BAT-26* and TMR-labeled (black) *NR-24*. Two highly polymorphic pentanucleotide repeats (Penta-C and Penta-D) are included for sample identification in case of sample mix-ups or contamination problems.

4.2. Relative utility of MSI and IHC for Lynch syndrome screening

Commonly used screening tools for LS include: family history, tumor pathology, MSI, and MMR protein detection by immunohistochemistry (IHC). It has been found that family history and tumor pathology lack sensitivity and specificity for selecting patients for germline mutation analysis [4]. In contrast, both MSI and IHC are highly effective strategies. Which method to use as the primary screening method for the detection of LS is a subject of ongoing debate [110, 111].

As the hallmark molecular signature of LS, MSI is widely accepted as a primary method for identifying individuals at risk for LS. Recent improvements in MSI testing have significantly enhanced accuracy and reduced cost. The *advantages* of MSI as a screening method for LS include: (1) high sensitivity for the detection of MMR loss, (2) use of quasi-monomorphic mononucleotide repeat markers which simplifies data interpretation and allows analysis of tumor samples alone when matching normal is not available, (3) utilization of fluorescent multiplex PCR technology that reduces labor, time, and cost of testing, (4) relatively easy interpretation, and (5) excellent intra- and interlaboratory reproducibility. *Disadvantages* of MSI testing include: (1) lack of specificity for LS as sporadic MSI is common, (2) failure to identify which MMR gene is involved, and (3) 5–10% false negative rate.

Advantages of IHC testing include: (1) high sensitivity and specificity for MMR loss, (2) wide availability in general pathology laboratories, and (3) identification of which MMR gene is mutated. IHC has several *disadvantages* including: (1) requirement for an experienced pathologist to interpret the results, (2) variable staining pattern, resulting in uncertainty in interpretation, (3) dependence of sensitivity on the antibody panel used, (4) possible lack of reliability in small biopsy samples, and (5) potential loss of antigenicity owing to nonpathogenic mutations, which can lead to a 5–10% false negative rate.

The significance, use and implications for MSI and IHC testing are similar, although the tests are slightly complementary. NCCN guidelines state that both MSI and IHC miss about 5–10% of cases [99]. Therefore, many labs have adopted the practice of using both MSI and IHC to maximize sensitivity for the detection of LS.

5. Emerging applications for MSI testing

5.1. Universal screening for Lynch syndrome

Up to one million individuals within the United States may have LS, but less than 5–10% are likely to have been diagnosed [112, 113]. The optimal strategy for identifying individuals with LS is a subject of continued debate. Some advocate targeted screening based on age of onset, family history, and/or histologic criteria to reduce the number of unnecessary tests. Others prefer universal screening of all CRCs to maximize sensitivity and improve outcomes through early monitoring. For example, Moreira and colleagues compared various strategies for identifying patients with LS and found that the revised Bethesda guidelines had a sensitivity of 87.8% compared with 100% sensitivity of the universal screening approach [4].

To help identify the undiagnosed cases of LS, the NCCN recommends that institutions use either a selective approach of testing all patients with CRC diagnosed before 70 years of age plus those diagnosed at older ages who meet the Bethesda Criteria, or universal testing. Universal MSI/IHC testing on all newly diagnosed colorectal and endometrial cancers regardless of family history is practiced by many NCCN member institutions and other comprehensive cancer centers to identify which patients should have genetic testing for LS [114–117]. Universal screening has been shown to be cost effective for colorectal cancers and is endorsed by the Evaluation of Genomic Applications in Practice and Prevention working group at the Centers for Disease Control and Prevention (CDC), the US Multi-society Task Force on Colorectal Cancer, and the European Society of Medical Oncology [118–121]. The Cleveland Clinic has implementing universal MSI/IHC screening since 2004 [122]. Similarly, Ohio State University Comprehensive Cancer Center has screened all CRC patients for LS since 2006 and projects that if universal screening were adopted nationwide it could save thousands of lives every year (**Figure 4**) [112].

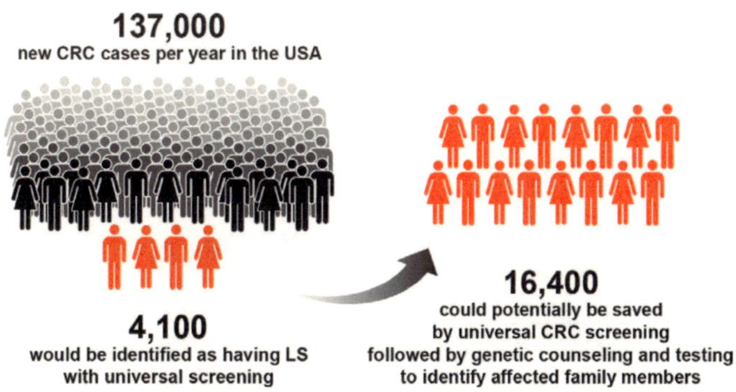

Figure 4. Early identification of Lynch syndrome patients saves lives. In 2014, 4100 or 3% of patients newly diagnosed with CRC carry germline mutations in MMR genes. Each of these individuals will on average have three at-risk relatives. Thus, 16,400 people per year could be potentially saved if all LS patients were identified early by testing CRC for MSI (adapted from Powell [112]).

5.2. Early identification of LS through screening polyps

Early identification of LS is highly desirable as the risk of developing CRC can be significantly reduced with increased cancer surveillance [123]. About 60% of CRC in LS cases are not diagnosed until after the age of 50 [124]. Thus, screening colorectal polyps obtained during colonoscopy that begins at 50 years of age could help identify LS patients and at-risk family members before cancer develops.

Screening for MSI in colon polyps could shift LS diagnosis earlier, allowing for earlier monitoring and improved chances of preventing cancer. However, colorectal polyps exhibit a milder MSI phenotype compared to more advanced neoplasms, limiting adoption of this strategy. Estimates for the incidence of MSI in LS adenomas range from 41 to 86% (average of 70%), which is comparable to IHC sensitivity of 49–82% (average of 72%) [125–131]. A study by Yurgelun and colleagues [130] found that while the overall MSI detection rate in adenomatous polyps from individuals with known pathogenic MMR mutations was 54%, all polyps larger than 10 mm in size exhibited MSI-H and loss of MMR expression by IHC. The higher level of MSI in the larger polyps is likely due to stepwise nature of MSI, in which larger deletions result from multiple smaller sequential replication errors that accumulate throughout many cell divisions [132]. This phenomenon might explain why it is more difficult to detect MSI in small polyps as they would undergo fewer cell divisions after loss of MMR activity. Despite this, MSI can occur at a very early stage of adenoma formation, as it has been found in aberrant crypt foci of microscopic size [133, 134] and has even been observed in normal colonic mucosa of patients with LS [135].

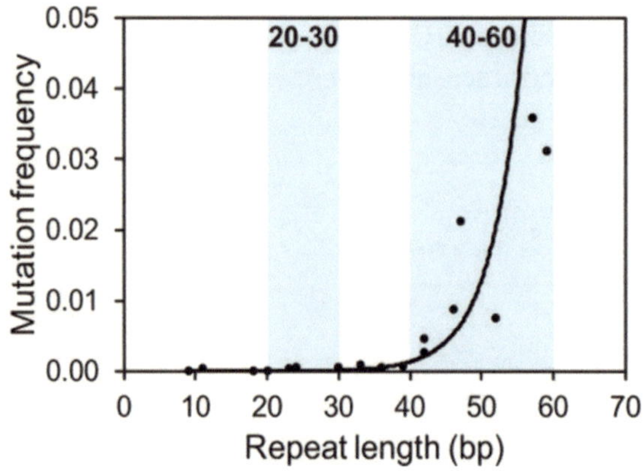

Figure 5. Mutation frequency in mononucleotides increases exponentially with repeat length. Markers with poly-A tracts of 20–30 base pairs are currently used for MSI testing. Markers over 40 base pairs exhibit higher mutability and, therefore, increased MSI sensitivity.

Increasing the sensitivity of MSI testing could facilitate screening adenomas for early identification of LS patients. Bacher and colleagues compared the sensitivity of microsatellite markers with very long poly-A runs of 40–60 base pairs with currently used markers for MSI testing. The long mononucleotide repeat markers were identified from BLAST searches of human genome databases and the frequencies of insertion/deletion mutations were compared to existing markers with shorter poly-A tracks [136, 137]. Mutation frequencies were found to increase exponentially with increasing repeat length (**Figure 5**) in agreement with other studies of microsatellites [13, 15, 138, 139]. This finding is significant as mutation frequencies can serve as a surrogate for MSI sensitivity.

To determine whether the detection of MSI in colorectal polyps could be increased using long mononucleotide repeat markers, 430 polyps from 160 patients were screened using the Bethesda panel, MSI Analysis System (Promega Corporation, Madison, United States), and an experimental panel of long mononucleotide repeats (Promega Corporation, Madison, United States) (**Figure 6**) [140]. Using the long mononucleotide repeat panel, 15 tumors were scored as MSI-H compared to nine for the Bethesda panel and eight for the MSI Analysis System. This difference represented a 1.7–1.9-fold increase in relative sensitivity for the detection of MSI-H polyps over currently used markers. Importantly, a high proportion (80%) of MSI-H polyps was likely from LS patients. The relative MSI sensitivity of the long mononucleotide repeat markers was higher than any markers in the Bethesda panel and the MSI Analysis System (**Figure 7**). The sensitivity and specificity for the detection of MMR-deficient lesions were estimated based on IHC data on MMR protein expression (**Table 4**). The sensitivity and

http://dx.doi.org/10.5772/65065

specificity were 100 and 96% for the long mononucleotide repeat panel compared to 67 and 100% for the MSI Analysis System and 75 and 97% for the Bethesda panel. The difference in sensitivity between the long mononucleotide repeat panel and the other panels was statistically significant.

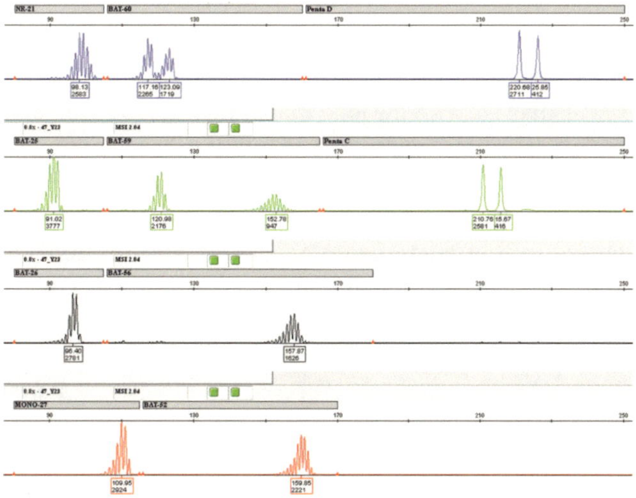

Figure 6. Prototype MSI Analysis System 2.0 (Promega Corporation, Madison, United States). The multiplex contains both short mononucleotide repeat markers, *NR-21, BAT-25, BAT-26,* and *MONO-27,* and new long mononucleotide repeat markers *BAT-52, BAT-56, BAT-59, BAT-60,* and pentanucleotide repeats *Penta-C and Penta-D.* The short mononucleotide repeats have a proven track record for MSI testing of CRC and the longer mononucleotide repeats have increased sensitivity for detection of MSI in colon polyps and extra-colonic tumors that often exhibit attenuated phenotypes. The pentanucleotide repeats are included to confirm sample identity.

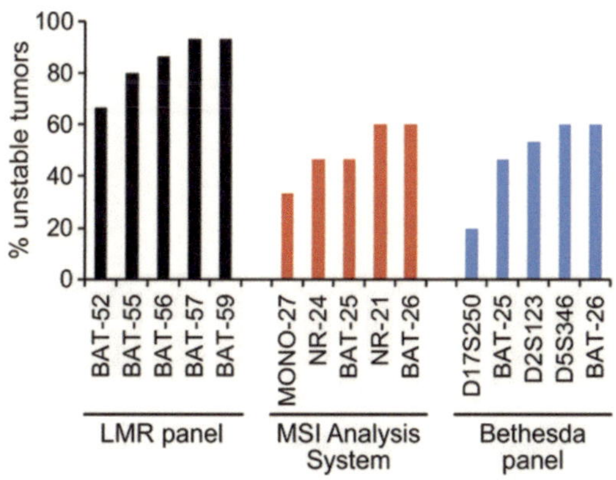

Figure 7. The relative MSI sensitivity of the long mononucleotide repeat (LMR) markers. The percentage of MSI-H tumors that were MSI-positive for each individual marker was determined. The sensitivity of the LMR panel was significantly higher than the Bethesda panel ($p < 0.0038$) and the MSI Analysis System ($p = 0.0012$) using the *t*-test.

Marker	True positive	False negative	True negative	False positive	Sensitivity (%)	Specificity (%)
LMR panel	12	0	67	3	100	96
MSI analysis system	8	4	75	0	67	100
Bethesda panel	9	3	66	2	75	97

Table 4. Sensitivity and specificity of new long mononucleotide repeats (LMR).

The use of the long mononucleotide repeat markers increased confidence in the MSI scoring as a consequence of a higher number of MSI-positive markers and larger allelic size changes for a given sample. MSI analysis with the long mononucleotide repeat panel resulted in MSI-H samples typically (80% of cases) exhibiting instability in four out of five or five out of five markers. With one exception, these cases also exhibited loss of MMR expression by IHC, had a germline MMR mutation, or both. Moreover, the significantly larger size changes in long mononucleotide repeats further simplified MSI classification by reducing the number of ambiguous calls often associated with small changes in the allele size that are observed when assaying shorter mononucleotide repeat sequences (**Figure 8**). The results of this study indicate that these new long mononucleotide repeat markers can increase sensitivity for the detection of MSI in polyps to a level approaching that reported in the literature for CRC with current marker systems. This increased sensitivity opens the possibility of screening polyps for an early detection of LS, while further study will be needed to be fully confident in these results and conclusions.

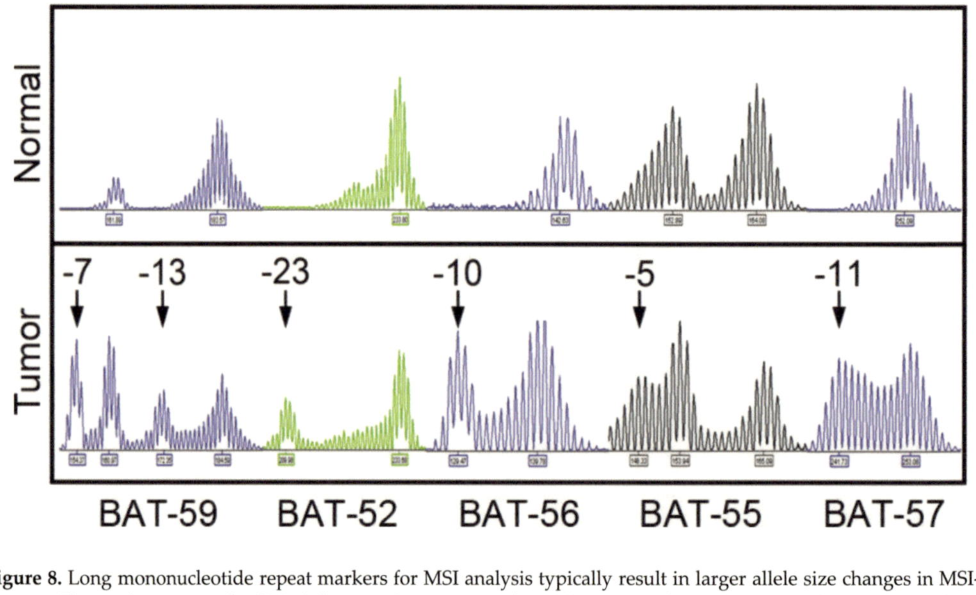

Figure 8. Long mononucleotide repeat markers for MSI analysis typically result in larger allele size changes in MSI-H tumors. Electropherogram of MSH2-deficient colon tumor and matching normal tissue screened for MSI using the experimental long mononucleotide repeat panel which shows all five markers were unstable with size shifts of up to 23 base pairs.

http://dx.doi.org/10.5772/65065

5.3. Alternative methods for LS testing

Current PCR-based MSI testing utilizes a small, standardized panel of highly unstable mononucleotide repeat markers to detect loss of MMR function. An alternative approach for MSI testing is to use highly scalable next generation DNA sequencing (NGS) technologies to infer MSI status. The main advantages of NGS are that multiple targets can be tested simultaneously, more efficiently, more cost effectively, and with higher sensitivity than with traditional Sanger sequencing. The main disadvantages are the greatly increased complexity of results and the return of uncertain or unexpected findings. Because the majority of MSI-positive tumors are due to epigenetic changes rather than genetic changes in MMR genes, even sequencing all MMR genes by NGS will not reliably infer MSI status in a tumor. To address this limitation, Hempelmann and colleagues [141] used NGS to sequence the five standard mononucleotide repeat loci in the MSI Analysis Kit (Promega Corporation, Madison, United States) to determine tumor MSI status. Using NGS they analyzed 81 CRC specimens (44 MSI-H and 37 MSI stable) previously subjected to PCR-based MSI testing. The MSI status of 95% of the specimens was interpretable by NGS and all but four samples were concordant with previous MSI classification. The samples generating ambiguous results were repeated and the result was the same, indicating that the NGS assay may not confidently infer MSI status for a small fraction of samples. While the NGS approach did not substantially improve sensitivity or specificity over existing assays, NGS offers an advantage of automated analysis based on quantitative, descriptive statistics which the authors suggest may improve intra- and interlaboratory variation.

Another approach to diagnose LS is direct sequencing of the MMR genes without previous screening with MSI or IHC. This approach simplifies the traditional multi-step testing procedure, but greatly increases the number of cases receiving costly germline MMR sequencing. Moreover, germline mutations in MMR genes may not be found in up to 30% of suspected LS cases [43]. Heritable, constitutional epimutations in *MLH* and *MSH2* explain many of these cases [142, 143]. Biallelic somatic mutations in MMR genes may account for up to 60–70% of germline MMR-negative cases [144]. Another potential limitation of direct sequencing of MMR genes is the high number of variants of unknown clinical significance, which account for around one third of germline MMR mutations [145]. The International Society of Gastrointestinal Hereditary Tumors currently reports a total of 3104 MMR gene variants (1198 for *MLH1*, 1098 for *MSH2*, 547 for *MSH6*, and 261 for *PMS2*) [146]. Communicating test results showing variants of unknown significance to patients can be challenging due to the potential psychological impact of reporting uncertain test results. Since both LS and MSI are caused by MMR defects, screening with MSI serves as a surrogate marker of LS and is a functional test for loss of MMR. Determining tumor MSI status also provides a prognostic and therapeutic value for individualizing treatment not only for LS patients, but also for those with sporadic MSI-H CRC lacking a germline MMR mutation [5, 6].

5.4. Distinguishing Lynch syndrome from non-Lynch syndrome CRC

There are multiple types of non-Lynch syndrome CRC that can mimic the disease and confound diagnosis [144, 147]. Many of these tumors are MSI-positive or show loss of MMR gene expression by IHC, but lack germline mutations [144, 148]. Distinguishing these mimics from LS is clinically important, as treatment and surveillance for these patients and their at-risk family members differ.

Nonfamilial LS mimics include sporadic MSI-positive CRC and Lynch-like syndrome (LLS) cancers. Hyper-methylation of the *MLH1* gene is responsible for about 80% of cases where MLH1 is missing without *MLH1* germline mutations. These sporadic MSI-positive CRC are fairly easy to distinguish from LS because of older age of onset, lack of family history of cancer, the presence of *BRAF V600E* mutation, and/or methylation of *MLH1*. More challenging are cases where the LLS cancers exhibit MSI and loss of MMR expression, but patients lack germline MMR mutations [149]. Mutations in *EPCAM* explain about 20–25% of LLS cases which show loss of MSH2 expression but no germline *MSH2* mutation. Deletions in the *EPCAM* gene lead to hypermethylation of the MSH2 promoter and subsequent MSH2 silencing. Most (70%) of the remaining unexplained LLS cases have cancers with biallelic somatic MMR mutations [148]. Thus, the distinguishing features of LLS are an MSI-positive phenotype and somatic biallelic MMR gene mutations. LLS has also been shown to occur in some endometrial cancers [148].

Familial CRC mimics include (1) polymerase proofreading associated polyposis (PPAP) caused by mutations in *POLE* or *POLD1*, (2) familial colorectal cancer type X (FCCTX) of unknown etiology, (3) germline *MLH1* methylation, and (4) constitutional mismatch repair-deficiency (CCMRD) caused by biallelic germline MMR mutations. PPAP is a rare inherited form of CRC that is caused by germline mutations in *POLE* (encoding DNA polymerase ε) or *POLD1* (encoding DNA polymerase δ) [150, 151]. Individuals with PPAP can develop CRC as early as 20 years of age and POLD1 mutation carriers are also at increased risk for endometrial and brain cancers. Tumors from PPAP individuals are MSI stable even though they have 100-fold more mutations in nonrepetitive DNA than sporadic MSI-positive tumors [23]. The absence of MSI in these CRCs is a distinguishing feature of PPAP. Another type of familial CRC lacking MSI and germline MMR mutations is familial colorectal cancer type X (FCCTX) [152]. The genetic cause of FCCTX is unknown. FCCTX individuals have about twofold increased risk of CRC compared to the general population, but do not develop other LS-spectrum cancers. Methylation of *MLH1* is usually associated with sporadic MSI-positive CRC and is not heritable. However, in rare cases inherited germline epigenetic silencing of MLH1 has been reported to predispose to cancer development in a pattern typically found in LS families [153]. CRC and other tumors from individuals with *MLH1* germline epimutations exhibit MSI and lack of MLH1 expression. Diagnosis of *MLH1* germline epimutations is accomplished by methylation analysis of tumor and germline samples. Constitutional mismatch repair-deficiency (CMMRD) is another rare disorder that is caused by biallelic germline mutations in MMR genes (most commonly *PMS2* and *MSH6*) that predisposes them to childhood cancers [154]. CMMRD individuals may present with CRC, brain tumors and/or leukemia and lymphoma. These tumors exhibit MSI and loss of MMR protein expression like LS, but can be distinguished by presence of biallelic germline MMR gene mutations. Screening CRC tumors for MSI followed by germline MMR sequencing is an effective strategy to distinguish LS from these non-LS diseases.

5.5. Use of MSI as a predictive biomarker

MSI-positive CRC is associated with a better prognosis and a decreased likelihood of metastasis to lymph nodes and distant organs [155]. A meta-analysis with 7642 cases clearly demonstrated that patients with MSI-H tumors have a significantly better prognosis than those with MSS tumors (hazard ratio for death = 0.65) [156]. There is growing evidence that the improved prognosis of MSI-positive tumors is due to the accumulation of frame shift mutations in genes containing coding microsatellites [157]. Translation of proteins with mutation-induced frame shift peptides renders MSI cancers highly immunogenic, allowing the body's immune system to more effectively target cancer cells.

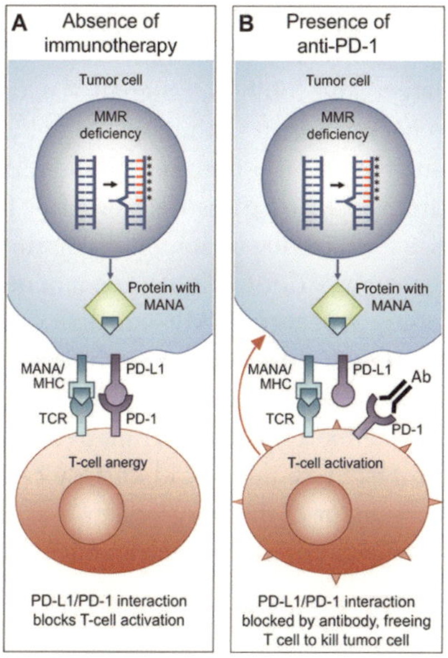

Figure 9. MSI is a biomarker for PD-1 blockage immunotherapy. Increased mutational burden in MMR-deficient tumors creates mutation associated neo-antigens (MANA) responsible for the immune response. Tumors with MSI evade immune surveillance by upregulation of immune checkpoint proteins programmed cell death 1 (PD-1) and its ligand PD-L1. Interaction of the PD-1 co-receptor and its ligand PD-L1 suppresses the immune system, and antibodies to either molecule have shown promise for reinvigorating the immune system, allowing T-cells to target and destroy cancer cells. Ab, antibody; MHC, major histocompatibility complex; TCR, T cell receptor; *, mutation.

While MSI status is a good prognostic factor for CRC, its predictive value for chemosensitivity remains controversial. The initial study on the use of 5-FU-based adjuvant chemotherapy by Ribic and colleagues [158] found that patients with advanced stage MSI-negative CRC benefited, but patients with MSI-H CRC did not. A number of subsequent clinical studies have confirmed these results [159, 160]. The clinical results are supported by *in vitro* evidence showing that MutSα and/or MutSβ binds to 5-FU incorporated DNA resulting in cell death, indicating that a functioning MMR system is required for the cytotoxic effect of 5-FU [161]. In contrast, a number of studies have failed to find any effect of MSI status on 5-FU treatment response [162–164]. A recent meta-analysis involving 9212 patients concluded that there was no clear difference in response to treatment based on MSI status [164]. However, the evidence for a detrimental effect of 5-FU treatment on MSI-positive tumors was sufficiently strong to justify another clinical trial (ClinicalTrials.gov identifier: NCT00217737; this study is ongoing) to assess the role of MSI in predicting response to adjuvant chemotherapy.

One of the most promising new approaches for treating advanced CRC is immune checkpoint therapy, which activates the body's natural antitumor activity (**Figure 9**) [5, 6]. Immune checkpoint therapy is less toxic than chemotherapeutic regimens and has potential for durable responses in advanced cancer patients who may otherwise only live a few months. It is estimated that approximately 50% of CRC in patients will progress to metastatic cancer. Prognosis for advanced CRC remains poor with overall 5-year survival at 70% for patients with localized lymph node metastases and 13% for patients with organ metastases.

Immune surveillance can effectively recognize and eliminate cancerous cells and is regulated by a balance between stimulatory and inhibitory signals (i.e., immune checkpoints). Under normal conditions, immune checkpoints are inhibited to maintain self-tolerance and avoid inappropriate overreaction, such as an auto-immune disease. In the presence of tumor cells, immune surveillance is activated. Selection pressure exerted by the immune system on tumor cells can lead to resistant clones that survive by inhibiting immune surveillance. MSI-positive cancers exhibit active immune response due to high number of neo-antigens that are produced by frameshift mutations in coding repeats in MMR-deficient cells. High expression of checkpoint molecules in MSI CRC creates an immunosuppressive microenvironment that is thought to help MSI tumors evade immune destruction by the infiltrating immune cells. Clinical trials of stage IV CRC with anti-PD-1 antibody pembrolizumab have been shown to be promising for reinvigorating the immune system to target and destroy cancer cells (**Figure 10**) [5]. MSI was found to be a significant predictor of the progression-free survival rate of 78% for MMR deficient CRC, 67% for MMR-deficient non-CRC cancer, and 11% in MMR-proficient CRC.

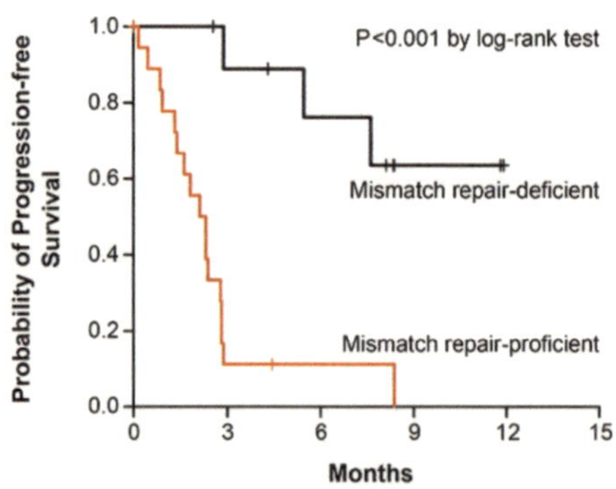

No. at Risk						
Mismatch repair-deficient	11	8	6	2	0	0
Mismatch repair-proficient	21	2	1	0	0	0

Figure 10. Clinical benefit of anti PD-1 antibody pembrolizumab treatment according to MSI status. Kaplan-Meier curves are shown for progression-free survival in the cohorts with CRC (reprinted by permission from Le et al. [5]).

6. Summary and concluding remarks

The vast majority of the estimated one million individuals with LS in the United States are not diagnosed. Early identification of individuals with LS is critical as the risk of developing cancer can be significantly reduced with increased surveillance. It is now recognized that screening strategies which rely on clinical criteria alone for the diagnosis of LS lack the needed sensitivity and that new strategies are required to address the underdiagnoses of the disease. The medical and life costs related with missed diagnosis are substantial due to the high costs and poor prognosis associated with treating advanced cancers. In an effort to increase detection of LS, there has been a growing support for universal screening of all new colorectal and endometrial cancers. Since definitive diagnosis of LS requires expensive germline MMR mutation analysis, cost-effective strategies are needed to prescreen for possible LS patients to triage those who will need germline analysis. In 1993, MSI became the first biomarker to be used for the detection of LS. Subsequent improvements, such as the change to all mononucleotide repeats and the introduction of fluorescent multiplex PCR methodology, have made MSI a highly accurate and cost-effective biomarker for LS (**Figure 11**). New technologies for MSI detection, like next generation sequencing, open the possibility of a single test for LS that determines tumor MSI status and MMR germline mutations. MSI is currently an important prognostic and diagnostic biomarker for LS, but it is poised to take on a much greater role in prediction of responses to the new immunotherapies targeted at MSI-positive tumors.

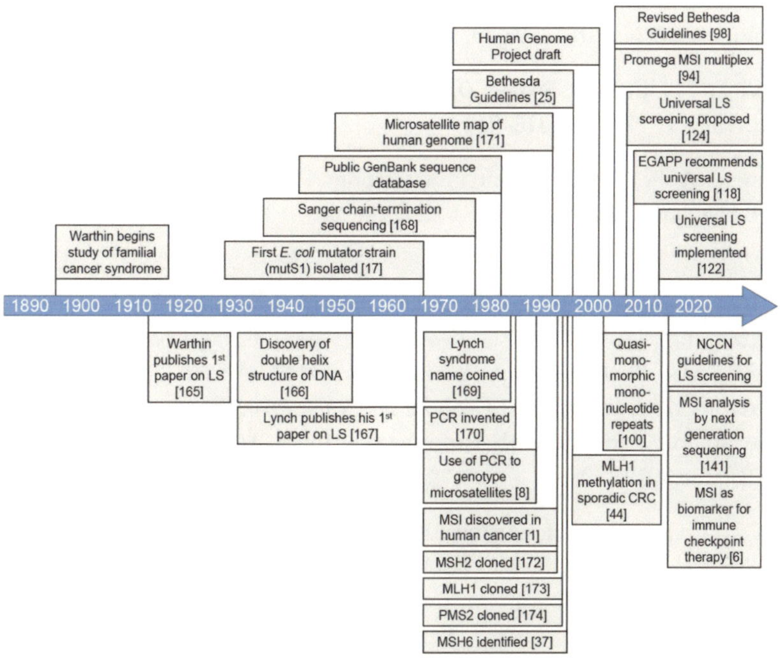

Figure 11. Time line of important events in the development of MSI testing for LS [1, 6, 8, 17, 25, 37, 44, 94, 98, 100, 118, 122, 124, 141, 165–174].

Author details

Jeffery W. Bacher[1,3], Linda Clipson[2], Leta S. Steffen[1] and Richard B. Halberg[2,3,4*]

*Address all correspondence to: rbhalberg@medicine.wisc.edu

1 Research and Development, Promega Corporation, Madison, WI, USA

2 McArdle Laboratory for Cancer Research, Department of Oncology, University of Wisconsin, Madison, WI, USA

3 Division of Gastroenterology & Hepatology, Department of Medicine, University of Wisconsin, WI, USA

4 Carbone Cancer Center, University of Wisconsin, Madison, WI, USA

References

[1] Ionov Y, Peinado MA, Malkhosyan S, Shibata D, Perucho M. Ubiquitous Somatic Mutations in Simple Repeated Sequences Reveal a New Mechanism for Colonic Carcinogenesis. Nature. 1993;363:558–561. DOI: 10.1038/363558a0

[2] Thibodeau SN, Bren G, Schaid D. Microsatellite Instability in Cancer of the Proximal Colon. Science. 1993;260:816–819

[3] Aaltonen LA, Peltomaki P, Leach FS, Sistonen P, Pylkkanen L, Mecklin JP, Jarvinen H, Powell SM, Jen J, Hamilton SR, et al. Clues to the Pathogenesis of Familial Colorectal Cancer. Science. 1993;260:812–816

[4] Moreira L, Balaguer F, Lindor N, de la Chapelle A, Hampel H, Aaltonen LA, Hopper JL, Le Marchand L, Gallinger S, Newcomb PA, Haile R, Thibodeau SN, Gunawardena S, Jenkins MA, Buchanan DD, Potter JD, Baron JA, Ahnen DJ, Moreno V, Andreu M, Ponz de Leon M, Rustgi AK, Castells A, Consortium E. Identification of Lynch Syndrome among Patients with Colorectal Cancer. JAMA. 2012;308:1555–1565. DOI: 10.1001/jama.2012.13088

[5] Le DT, Uram JN, Wang H, Bartlett BR, Kemberling H, Eyring AD, Skora AD, Luber BS, Azad NS, Laheru D, Biedrzycki B, Donehower RC, Zaheer A, Fisher GA, Crocenzi TS, Lee JJ, Duffy SM, Goldberg RM, de la Chapelle A, Koshiji M, Bhaijee F, Huebner T, Hruban RH, Wood LD, Cuka N, Pardoll DM, Papadopoulos N, Kinzler KW, Zhou S, Cornish TC, Taube JM, Anders RA, Eshleman JR, Vogelstein B, Diaz LA, Jr. PD-1 Blockade in Tumors with Mismatch-Repair Deficiency. N Engl J Med. 2015;372:2509–2520. DOI: 10.1056/NEJMoa1500596

[6] Dudley JC, Lin MT, Le DT, Eshleman JR. Microsatellite Instability as a Biomarker for PD-1 Blockade. Clin Cancer Res. 2016;22:813–820. DOI: 10.1158/1078-0432.CCR-15-1678

[7] Tautz D. Hypervariability of Simple Sequences as a General Source for Polymorphic DNA Markers. Nucleic Acids Res. 1989;17:6463–6471

[8] Weber JL, May PE. Abundant Class of Human DNA Polymorphisms Which Can Be Typed Using the Polymerase Chain Reaction. Am J Hum Genet. 1989;44:388–396

[9] Ellegren H. Microsatellites: Simple Sequences with Complex Evolution. Nat Rev Genet. 2004;5:435–445. DOI: 10.1038/nrg1348

[10] Lai Y, Sun F. The Relationship between Microsatellite Slippage Mutation Rate and the Number of Repeat Units. Mol Biol Evol. 2003;20:2123–2131. DOI: 10.1093/molbev/msg228

[11] Sia EA, Kokoska RJ, Dominska M, Greenwell P, Petes TD. Microsatellite Instability in Yeast: Dependence on Repeat Unit Size and DNA Mismatch Repair Genes. Mol Cell Biol. 1997;17:2851–2858

[12] Brinkmann B, Klintschar M, Neuhuber F, Huhne J, Rolf B. Mutation Rate in Human Microsatellites: Influence of the Structure and Length of the Tandem Repeat. Am J Hum Genet. 1998;62:1408–1415. DOI: 10.1086/301869

[13] Bacher JW, Abdel Megid WM, Kent-First MG, Halberg RB. Use of Mononucleotide Repeat Markers for Detection of Microsatellite Instability in Mouse Tumors. Mol Carcinog. 2005;44:285–292. DOI: 10.1002/mc.20146

[14] Kelkar YD, Strubczewski N, Hile SE, Chiaromonte F, Eckert KA, Makova KD. What Is a Microsatellite: A Computational and Experimental Definition Based Upon Repeat Mutational Behavior at A/T and GT/AC Repeats. Genome Biol Evol. 2010;2:620–635. DOI: 10.1093/gbe/evq046

[15] Kelkar YD, Tyekucheva S, Chiaromonte F, Makova KD. The Genome-Wide Determinants of Human and Chimpanzee Microsatellite Evolution. Genome Res. 2008;18:30–38. DOI: 10.1101/gr.7113408

[16] Levinson G, Gutman GA. Slipped-Strand Mispairing: A Major Mechanism for DNA Sequence Evolution. Mol Biol Evol. 1987;4:203–221

[17] Siegel EC, Bryson V. Mutator Gene of *Escherichia coli* B. J Bacteriol. 1967;94:38–47

[18] Loeb LA, Springgate CF, Battula N. Errors in DNA Replication as a Basis of Malignant Changes. Cancer Res. 1974;34:2311–2321

[19] Cox EC, Degnen GE, Scheppe ML. Mutator Gene Studies in *Escherichia coli*: The *mutS* Gene. Genetics. 1972;72:551–567

[20] Speyer JF. Mutagenic DNA Polymerase. Biochem Biophys Res Commun. 1965;21:6–8

[21] Nowell PC. The Clonal Evolution of Tumor Cell Populations. Science. 1976;194:23–28

[22] Loeb LA. Mutator Phenotype May Be Required for Multistage Carcinogenesis. Cancer Res. 1991;51:3075–3079

[23] The Cancer Genome Atlas. Comprehensive Molecular Characterization of Human Colon and Rectal Cancer. Nature. 2012;487:330–337. DOI: 10.1038/nature11252

[24] Fearon ER, Vogelstein B. A Genetic Model for Colorectal Tumorigenesis. Cell. 1990;61:759–767

[25] Boland CR, Thibodeau SN, Hamilton SR, Sidransky D, Eshleman JR, Burt RW, Meltzer SJ, Rodriguez-Bigas MA, Fodde R, Ranzani GN, Srivastava S. A National Cancer Institute Workshop on Microsatellite Instability for Cancer Detection and Familial Predisposition: Development of International Criteria for the Determination of Microsatellite Instability in Colorectal Cancer. Cancer Res. 1998;58:5248–5257

[26] Wildenberg J, Meselson M. Mismatch Repair in Heteroduplex DNA. Proc Natl Acad Sci U S A. 1975;72:2202–2206

[27] Wagner R, Jr., Meselson M. Repair Tracts in Mismatched DNA Heteroduplexes. Proc Natl Acad Sci U S A. 1976;73:4135–4139

[28] Glickman B, van den Elsen P, Radman M. Induced Mutagenesis in Dam-Mutants of *Escherichia coli*: A Role for 6-Methyladenine Residues in Mutation Avoidance. Mol Gen Genet. 1978;163:307–312

[29] Radman M, Wagner R. Mismatch Repair in *Escherichia coli*. Annu Rev Genet. 1986;20:523–538. DOI: 10.1146/annurev.ge.20.120186.002515

[30] Modrich P. DNA Mismatch Correction. Annu Rev Biochem. 1987;56:435–466. DOI: 10.1146/annurev.bi.56.070187.002251

[31] Lu AL, Clark S, Modrich P. Methyl-Directed Repair of DNA Base-Pair Mismatches in Vitro. Proc Natl Acad Sci U S A. 1983;80:4639–4643

[32] Lahue RS, Au KG, Modrich P. DNA Mismatch Correction in a Defined System. Science. 1989;245:160–164

[33] Strand M, Prolla TA, Liskay RM, Petes TD. Destabilization of Tracts of Simple Repetitive DNA in Yeast by Mutations Affecting DNA Mismatch Repair. Nature. 1993;365:274–276. DOI: 10.1038/365274a0

[34] Aebi S, Kurdi-Haidar B, Gordon R, Cenni B, Zheng H, Fink D, Christen RD, Boland CR, Koi M, Fishel R, Howell SB. Loss of DNA Mismatch Repair in Acquired Resistance to Cisplatin. Cancer Res. 1996;56:3087–3090

[35] Baker SM, Bronner CE, Zhang L, Plug AW, Robatzek M, Warren G, Elliott EA, Yu J, Ashley T, Arnheim N, et al. Male Mice Defective in the DNA Mismatch Repair Gene *PMS2* Exhibit Abnormal Chromosome Synapsis in Meiosis. Cell. 1995;82:309–319

[36] Liu B, Nicolaides NC, Markowitz S, Willson JK, Parsons RE, Jen J, Papadopolous N, Peltomaki P, de la Chapelle A, Hamilton SR, et al. Mismatch Repair Gene Defects in Sporadic Colorectal Cancers with Microsatellite Instability. Nat Genet. 1995;9:48–55

[37] Palombo F, Gallinari P, Iaccarino I, Lettieri T, Hughes M, D'Arrigo A, Truong O, Hsuan JJ, Jiricny J. Gtbp, a 160-Kilodalton Protein Essential for Mismatch-Binding Activity in Human Cells. Science. 1995;268:1912–1914

[38] Reyes GX, Schmidt TT, Kolodner RD, Hombauer H. New Insights into the Mechanism of DNA Mismatch Repair. Chromosoma. 2015;124:443–462. DOI: 10.1007/s00412-015-0514-0

[39] Kunkel TA, Erie DA. Eukaryotic Mismatch Repair in Relation to DNA Replication. Annu Rev Genet. 2015;49:291–313. DOI: 10.1146/annurev-genet-112414-054722

[40] Kolodner RD. A Personal Historical View of DNA Mismatch Repair with an Emphasis on Eukaryotic DNA Mismatch Repair. DNA Repair (Amst). 2016;38:3–13. DOI: 10.1016/j.dnarep.2015.11.009

[41] Pluciennika A, Dzantieva L, Iyera RR, Constantina N, Kadyrova FA and Modricha P. PCNA function in the activation and strand direction of MutLα endonuclease in mismatch repair. Proc Natl Acad Sci U S A. 2010;107:16066–16071. DOI: 10.1073/pnas.1010662107

[42] Boland CR, Goel A. Microsatellite Instability in Colorectal Cancer. Gastroenterol. 2010;138:2073–2087 e2073. DOI: 10.1053/j.gastro.2009.12.064

[43] Lynch HT, Snyder CL, Shaw TG, Heinen CD, Hitchins MP. Milestones of Lynch Syndrome: 1895–2015. Nat Rev Cancer. 2015;15:181–194. DOI: 10.1038/nrc3878

[44] Kane MF, Loda M, Gaida GM, Lipman J, Mishra R, Goldman H, Jessup JM, Kolodner R. Methylation of the Hmlh1 Promoter Correlates with Lack of Expression of Hmlh1 in Sporadic Colon Tumors and Mismatch Repair-Defective Human Tumor Cell Lines. Cancer Res. 1997;57:808–811

[45] Parsons R, Myeroff LL, Liu B, Willson JK, Markowitz SD, Kinzler KW, Vogelstein B. Microsatellite Instability and Mutations of the Transforming Growth Factor Beta Type II Receptor Gene in Colorectal Cancer. Cancer Res. 1995;55:5548–5550

[46] Markowitz S, Wang J, Myeroff L, Parsons R, Sun L, Lutterbaugh J, Fan RS, Zborowska E, Kinzler KW, Vogelstein B, et al. Inactivation of the Type II Tgf-Beta Receptor in Colon Cancer Cells with Microsatellite Instability. Science. 1995;268:1336–1338

[47] Woerner SM, Gebert J, Yuan YP, Sutter C, Ridder R, Bork P, von Knebel Doeberitz M. Systematic Identification of Genes with Coding Microsatellites Mutated in DNA Mismatch Repair-Deficient Cancer Cells. Int J Cancer. 2001;93:12–19

[48] The Cancer Genome Atlas. Integrated Genomic Characterization of Endometrial Carcinoma. Nature. 2013;497:67–73. DOI: 10.1038/nature12113

[49] Giardiello FM, Allen JI, Axilbund JE, Boland CR, Burke CA, Burt RW, Church JM, Dominitz JA, Johnson DA, Kaltenbach T, Levin TR, Lieberman DA, Robertson DJ, Syngal S, Rex DK. Guidelines on Genetic Evaluation and Management of Lynch Syndrome: A Consensus Statement by the Us Multi-Society Task Force on Colorectal Cancer. Am J Gastroenterol. 2014;109:1159–1179. DOI: 10.1038/ajg.2014.186

[50] Hendriks YMC, Wagner A, Morreau H, Menko F, Stormorken A, Quehenberger F, Sandkuijl L, Møller P, Genuardi M, van Houwelingen H, Tops C, van Puijenbroek M, Verkuijlen P, Kenter G, van Mil A, Meijers-Heijboer H, Tan GB, Breuning MH, Fodde R, Winjen JT, Bröcker-Vriends AHJT, Vasen H. Cancer Risk in Hereditary Nonpolyposis Colorectal Cancer Due to *MSH6* Mutations: Impact on Counseling and Surveillance. Gastroenterol. 2004;127:17–25. DOI: 10.1053/j.gastro.2004.03.068

[51] Baglietto L, Lindor NM, Dowty JG, White DM, Wagner A, Gomez Garcia EB, Vriends AH, Cartwright NR, Barnetson RA, Farrington SM, Tenesa A, Hampel H, Buchanan D, Arnold S, Young J, Walsh MD, Jass J, Macrae F, Antill Y, Winship IM, Giles GG, Goldblatt J, Parry S, Suthers G, Leggett B, Butz M, Aronson M, Poynter JN, Baron JA, Le Marchand L, Haile R, Gallinger S, Hopper JL, Potter J, de la Chapelle A, Vasen HF, Dunlop MG, Thibodeau SN, Jenkins MA. Risks of Lynch Syndrome Cancers for *MSH6* Mutation Carriers. J Natl Cancer Inst. 2010;102:193–201. DOI: 10.1093/jnci/djp473

[52] ten Broeke SW, Brohet RM, Tops CM, van der Klift HM, Velthuizen ME, Bernstein I, Capella Munar G, Gomez Garcia E, Hoogerbrugge N, Letteboer TG, Menko FH, Lindblom A, Mensenkamp AR, Moller P, van Os TA, Rahner N, Redeker BJ, Sijmons RH, Spruijt L, Suerink M, Vos YJ, Wagner A, Hes FJ, Vasen HF, Nielsen M, Wijnen JT. Lynch Syndrome Caused by Germline *PMS2* Mutations: Delineating the Cancer Risk. J Clin Oncol. 2015;33:319–325. DOI: 10.1200/JCO.2014.57.8088

[53] Barrow E, Robinson L, Alduaij W, Shenton A, Clancy T, Lalloo F, Hill J, Evans DG. Cumulative Lifetime Incidence of Extracolonic Cancers in Lynch Syndrome: A Report of 121 Families with Proven Mutations. Clin Genet. 2009;75:141–149. DOI: 10.1111/j.1399-0004.2008.01125.x

[54] Engel C, Loeffler M, Steinke V, Rahner N, Holinski-Feder E, Dietmaier W, Schackert HK, Goergens H, von Knebel Doeberitz M, Goecke TO, Schmiegel W, Buettner R, Moeslein G, Letteboer TG, Gomez Garcia E, Hes FJ, Hoogerbrugge N, Menko FH, van Os TA, Sijmons RH, Wagner A, Kluijt I, Propping P, Vasen HF. Risks of Less Common Cancers in Proven Mutation Carriers with Lynch Syndrome. J Clin Oncol. 2012;30:4409–4415. DOI: 10.1200/JCO.2012.43.2278

[55] Harkness EF, Barrow E, Newton K, Green K, Clancy T, Lalloo F, Hill J, Evans DG. Lynch Syndrome Caused by *MLH1* Mutations Is Associated with an Increased Risk of Breast Cancer: A Cohort Study. J Med Genet. 2015;52:553–556. DOI: 10.1136/jmedgenet-2015-103216

[56] Grindedal EM, Moller P, Eeles R, Stormorken AT, Bowitz-Lothe IM, Landro SM, Clark N, Kvale R, Shanley S, Maehle L. Germ-Line Mutations in Mismatch Repair Genes

Associated with Prostate Cancer. Cancer Epidemiol Biomarkers Prev. 2009;18:2460–2467. DOI: 10.1158/1055-9965.EPI-09-0058

[57] Raymond VM, Mukherjee B, Wang F, Huang SC, Stoffel EM, Kastrinos F, Syngal S, Cooney KA, Gruber SB. Elevated Risk of Prostate Cancer among Men with Lynch Syndrome. J Clin Oncol. 2013;31:1713–1718. DOI: 10.1200/JCO.2012.44.1238

[58] Hampel H, Stephens JA, Pukkala E, Sankila R, Aaltonen LA, Mecklin JP, de la Chapelle A. Cancer Risk in Hereditary Nonpolyposis Colorectal Cancer Syndrome: Later Age of Onset. Gastroenterol. 2005;129:415–421. DOI: 10.1016/j.gastro.2005.05.011

[59] Bonadona V, Bonaiti B, Olschwang S, Grandjouan S, Huiart L, Longy M, Guimbaud R, Buecher B, Bignon YJ, Caron O, Colas C, Nogues C, Lejeune-Dumoulin S, Olivier-Faivre L, Polycarpe-Osaer F, Nguyen TD, Desseigne F, Saurin JC, Berthet P, Leroux D, Duffour J, Manouvrier S, Frebourg T, Sobol H, Lasset C, Bonaiti-Pellie C, French Cancer Genetics N. Cancer Risks Associated with Germline Mutations in *MLH1, MSH2,* and *MSH6* Genes in Lynch Syndrome. JAMA. 2011;305:2304–2310. DOI: 10.1001/jama.2011.743

[60] Choi YH, Cotterchio M, McKeown-Eyssen G, Neerav M, Bapat B, Boyd K, Gallinger S, McLaughlin J, Aronson M, Briollais L. Penetrance of Colorectal Cancer among *MLH1/MSH2* Carriers Participating in the Colorectal Cancer Familial Registry in Ontario. Hered Cancer Clin Pract. 2009;7:14. DOI: 10.1186/1897-4287-7-14

[61] Senter L, Clendenning M, Sotamaa K, Hampel H, Green J, Potter JD, Lindblom A, Lagerstedt K, Thibodeau SN, Lindor NM, Young J, Winship I, Dowty JG, White DM, Hopper JL, Baglietto L, Jenkins MA, de la Chapelle A. The Clinical Phenotype of Lynch Syndrome Due to Germ-Line *PMS2* Mutations. Gastroenterol. 2008;135:419–428. DOI: 10.1053/j.gastro.2008.04.026

[62] Win AK, Young JP, Lindor NM, Tucker KM, Ahnen DJ, Young GP, Buchanan DD, Clendenning M, Giles GG, Winship I, Macrae FA, Goldblatt J, Southey MC, Arnold J, Thibodeau SN, Gunawardena SR, Bapat B, Baron JA, Casey G, Gallinger S, Le Marchand L, Newcomb PA, Haile RW, Hopper JL, Jenkins MA. Colorectal and Other Cancer Risks for Carriers and Noncarriers from Families with a DNA Mismatch Repair Gene Mutation: A Prospective Cohort Study. J Clin Oncol. 2012;30:958–964. DOI: 10.1200/JCO.2011.39.5590

[63] Hampel H, Frankel W, Panescu J, Lockman J, Sotamaa K, Fix D, Comeras I, La Jeunesse J, Nakagawa H, Westman JA, Prior TW, Clendenning M, Penzone P, Lombardi J, Dunn P, Cohn DE, Copeland L, Eaton L, Fowler J, Lewandowski G, Vaccarello L, Bell J, Reid G, de la Chapelle A. Screening for Lynch Syndrome (Hereditary Nonpolyposis Colorectal Cancer) among Endometrial Cancer Patients. Cancer Res. 2006;66:7810–7817. DOI: 10.1158/0008-5472.CAN-06-1114

[64] Zighelboim I, Goodfellow PJ, Gao F, Gibb RK, Powell MA, Rader JS, Mutch DG. Microsatellite Instability and Epigenetic Inactivation of Mlh1 and Outcome of Patients

with Endometrial Carcinomas of the Endometrioid Type. J Clin Oncol. 2007;25:2042–2048. DOI: 10.1200/JCO.2006.08.2107

[65] Bellcross CA, Bedrosian SR, Daniels E, Duquette D, Hampel H, Jasperson K, Joseph DA, Kaye C, Lubin I, Meyer LJ, Reyes M, Scheuner MT, Schully SD, Senter L, Stewart SL, St Pierre J, Westman J, Wise P, Yang VW, Khoury MJ. Implementing Screening for Lynch Syndrome among Patients with Newly Diagnosed Colorectal Cancer: Summary of a Public Health/Clinical Collaborative Meeting. Genet Med. 2012;14:152–162. DOI: 10.1038/gim.0b013e31823375ea

[66] Win AK, Lindor NM, Young JP, Macrae FA, Young GP, Williamson E, Parry S, Goldblatt J, Lipton L, Winship I, Leggett B, Tucker KM, Giles GG, Buchanan DD, Clendenning M, Rosty C, Arnold J, Levine AJ, Haile RW, Gallinger S, Le Marchand L, Newcomb PA, Hopper JL, Jenkins MA. Risks of Primary Extracolonic Cancers Following Colorectal Cancer in Lynch Syndrome. J Natl Cancer Inst. 2012;104:1363–1372. DOI: 10.1093/jnci/djs351

[67] Cancer Genome Atlas Research Network. Comprehensive Molecular Characterization of Gastric Adenocarcinoma. Nature. 2014;513:202–209. DOI: 10.1038/nature13480

[68] Aarnio M, Salovaara R, Aaltonen LA, Mecklin JP, Jarvinen HJ. Features of Gastric Cancer in Hereditary Non-Polyposis Colorectal Cancer Syndrome. Int J Cancer. 1997;74:551–555

[69] Watson P, Vasen HF, Mecklin JP, Bernstein I, Aarnio M, Jarvinen HJ, Myrhoj T, Sunde L, Wijnen JT, Lynch HT. The Risk of Extra-Colonic, Extra-Endometrial Cancer in the Lynch Syndrome. Int J Cancer. 2008;123:444–449. DOI: 10.1002/ijc.23508

[70] Capelle LG, Van Grieken NC, Lingsma HF, Steyerberg EW, Klokman WJ, Bruno MJ, Vasen HF, Kuipers EJ. Risk and Epidemiological Time Trends of Gastric Cancer in Lynch Syndrome Carriers in the Netherlands. Gastroenterol. 2010;138:487–492. DOI: 10.1053/j.gastro.2009.10.051

[71] Murphy MA, Wentzensen N. Frequency of Mismatch Repair Deficiency in Ovarian Cancer: A Systematic Review This Article Is a Us Government Work and, as Such, Is in the Public Domain of the United States of America. Int J Cancer. 2011;129:1914–1922. DOI: 10.1002/ijc.25835

[72] Aarnio M, Sankila R, Pukkala E, Salovaara R, Aaltonen LA, de la Chapelle A, Peltomaki P, Mecklin JP, Jarvinen HJ. Cancer Risk in Mutation Carriers of DNA-Mismatch-Repair Genes. Int J Cancer. 1999;81:214–218

[73] van der Post RS, Kiemeney LA, Ligtenberg MJ, Witjes JA, Hulsbergen-van de Kaa CA, Bodmer D, Schaap L, Kets CM, van Krieken JH, Hoogerbrugge N. Risk of Urothelial Bladder Cancer in Lynch Syndrome Is Increased, in Particular among *MSH2* Mutation Carriers. J Med Genet. 2010;47:464–470. DOI: 10.1136/jmg.2010.076992

[74] Cesinaro AM, Ubiali A, Sighinolfi P, Trentini GP, Gentili F, Facchetti F. Mismatch Repair Proteins Expression and Microsatellite Instability in Skin Lesions with Sebaceous

Differentiation: A Study in Different Clinical Subgroups with and without Extracutaneous Cancer. Am J Dermatopathol. 2007;29:351–358. DOI: 10.1097/DAD.0b013e318057713c

[75] Kruse R, Rutten A, Schweiger N, Jakob E, Mathiak M, Propping P, Mangold E, Bisceglia M, Ruzicka T. Frequency of Microsatellite Instability in Unselected Sebaceous Gland Neoplasias and Hyperplasias. J Invest Dermatol. 2003;120:858–864. DOI: 10.1046/j.1523-1747.2003.12125.x

[76] Lamba AR, Moore AY, Moore T, Rhees J, Arnold MA, Richard Boland C. Defective DNA Mismatch Repair Activity Is Common in Sebaceous Neoplasms, and May Be an Ineffective Approach to Screen for Lynch Syndrome. Fam Cancer. 2015;14:259–264. DOI: 10.1007/s10689-015-9782-3

[77] Ponti G, Losi L, Di Gregorio C, Roncucci L, Pedroni M, Scarselli A, Benatti P, Seidenari S, Pellacani G, Lembo L, Rossi G, Marino M, Lucci-Cordisco E, Ponz de Leon M. Identification of Muir-Torre Syndrome among Patients with Sebaceous Tumors and Keratoacanthomas: Role of Clinical Features, Microsatellite Instability, and Immunohistochemistry. Cancer. 2005;103:1018–1025. DOI: 10.1002/cncr.20873

[78] South CD, Hampel H, Comeras I, Westman JA, Frankel WL, de la Chapelle A. The Frequency of Muir-Torre Syndrome among Lynch Syndrome Families. J Natl Cancer Inst. 2008;100:277–281. DOI: 10.1093/jnci/djm291

[79] Vasen HF, Stormorken A, Menko FH, Nagengast FM, Kleibeuker JH, Griffioen G, Taal BG, Moller P, Wijnen JT. *MSH2* Mutation Carriers Are at Higher Risk of Cancer Than *MLH1* Mutation Carriers: A Study of Hereditary Nonpolyposis Colorectal Cancer Families. J Clin Oncol. 2001;19:4074–4080

[80] Anbazhagan R, Fujii H, Gabrielson E. Microsatellite Instability Is Uncommon in Breast Cancer. Clin Cancer Res. 1999;5:839–844

[81] Adem C, Soderberg CL, Cunningham JM, Reynolds C, Sebo TJ, Thibodeau SN, Hartmann LC, Jenkins RB. Microsatellite Instability in Hereditary and Sporadic Breast Cancers. Int J Cancer. 2003;107:580–582. DOI: 10.1002/ijc.11442

[82] Kuligina E, Grigoriev MY, Suspitsin EN, Buslov KG, Zaitseva OA, Yatsuk OS, Lazareva YR, Togo AV, Imyanitov EN. Microsatellite Instability Analysis of Bilateral Breast Tumors Suggests Treatment-Related Origin of Some Contralateral Malignancies. J Cancer Res Clin Oncol. 2007;133:57–64. DOI: 10.1007/s00432-006-0146-0

[83] Toyama T, Iwase H, Yamashita H, Iwata H, Yamashita T, Ito K, Hara Y, Suchi M, Kato T, Nakamura T, Kobayashi S. Microsatellite Instability in Sporadic Human Breast Cancers. Int J Cancer. 1996;68:447–451. DOI: 10.1002/(SICI)1097-0215(19961115)68:4<447::AID-IJC8>3.0.CO;2-0

[84] Walsh MD, Buchanan DD, Cummings MC, Pearson SA, Arnold ST, Clendenning M, Walters R, McKeone DM, Spurdle AB, Hopper JL, Jenkins MA, Phillips KD, Suthers GK, George J, Goldblatt J, Muir A, Tucker K, Pelzer E, Gattas MR, Woodall S, Parry S,

Macrae FA, Haile RW, Baron JA, Potter JD, Le Marchand L, Bapat B, Thibodeau SN, Lindor NM, McGuckin MA, Young JP. Lynch Syndrome-Associated Breast Cancers: Clinicopathologic Characteristics of a Case Series from the Colon Cancer Family Registry. Clin Cancer Res. 2010;16:2214–2224. DOI: 10.1158/1078-0432.CCR-09-3058

[85] Chiappini F, Gross-Goupil M, Saffroy R, Azoulay D, Emile JF, Veillhan LA, Delvart V, Chevalier S, Bismuth H, Debuire B, Lemoine A. Microsatellite Instability Mutator Phenotype in Hepatocellular Carcinoma in Non-Alcoholic and Non-Virally Infected Normal Livers. Carcinogenesis. 2004;25:541–547. DOI: 10.1093/carcin/bgh035

[86] Kastrinos F, Mukherjee B, Tayob N, Wang F, Sparr J, Raymond VM, Bandipalliam P, Stoffel EM, Gruber SB, Syngal S. Risk of Pancreatic Cancer in Families with Lynch Syndrome. JAMA. 2009;302:1790–1795. DOI: 10.1001/jama.2009.1529

[87] Mitmaker E, Alvarado C, Begin LR, Trifiro M. Microsatellite Instability in Benign and Malignant Thyroid Neoplasms. J Surg Res. 2008;150:40–48. DOI: 10.1016/j.jss.2007.12.760

[88] Palmieri G, Ascierto PA, Cossu A, Colombino M, Casula M, Botti G, Lissia A, Tanda F, Castello G. Assessment of Genetic Instability in Melanocytic Skin Lesions through Microsatellite Analysis of Benign Naevi, Dysplastic Naevi, and Primary Melanomas and Their Metastases. Melanoma Res. 2003;13:167–170. DOI: 10.1097/01.cmr.0000056222.78713.8c

[89] Lazo PA. The Molecular Genetics of Cervical Carcinoma. Br J Cancer. 1999;80:2008–2018. DOI: 10.1038/sj.bjc.6690635

[90] Farris AB, 3rd, Demicco EG, Le LP, Finberg KE, Miller J, Mandal R, Fukuoka J, Cohen C, Gaissert HA, Zukerberg LR, Lauwers GY, Iafrate AJ, Mino-Kenudson M. Clinicopathologic and Molecular Profiles of Microsatellite Unstable Barrett Esophagus-Associated Adenocarcinoma. Am J Surg Pathol. 2011;35:647–655. DOI: 10.1097/PAS.0b013e31820f18a2

[91] Kawaguchi K, Oda Y, Takahira T, Saito T, Yamamoto H, Kobayashi C, Tamiya S, Oda S, Iwamoto Y, Tsuneyoshi M. Microsatellite Instability and hMLH1 and hMSH2 Expression Analysis in Soft Tissue Sarcomas. Oncol Rep. 2005;13:241–246

[92] Dietmaier W, Wallinger S, Bocker T, Kullmann F, Fishel R, Ruschoff J. Diagnostic Microsatellite Instability: Definition and Correlation with Mismatch Repair Protein Expression. Cancer Res. 1997;57:4749–4756

[93] Bocker T, Diermann J, Friedl W, Gebert J, Holinski-Feder E, Karner-Hanusch J, von Knebel-Doeberitz M, Koelble K, Moeslein G, Schackert HK, Wirtz HC, Fishel R, Ruschoff J. Microsatellite Instability Analysis: A Multicenter Study for Reliability and Quality Control. Cancer Res. 1997;57:4739–4743

[94] Bacher JW, Flanagan LA, Smalley RL, Nassif NA, Burgart LJ, Halberg RB, Megid WM, Thibodeau SN. Development of a Fluorescent Multiplex Assay for Detection of MSI-High Tumors. Dis Markers. 2004;20:237–250

[95] Vasen HF, Watson P, Mecklin JP, Lynch HT. New Clinical Criteria for Hereditary Nonpolyposis Colorectal Cancer (HNPCC, Lynch Syndrome) Proposed by the International Collaborative Group on HNPCC. Gastroenterol. 1999;116:1453–1456

[96] Barnetson RA, Tenesa A, Farrington SM, Nicholl ID, Cetnarskyj R, Porteous ME, Campbell H, Dunlop MG. Identification and Survival of Carriers of Mutations in DNA Mismatch-Repair Genes in Colon Cancer. N Engl J Med. 2006;354:2751–2763. DOI: 10.1056/NEJMoa053493

[97] Rodriguez-Bigas MA, Boland CR, Hamilton SR, Henson DE, Jass JR, Khan PM, Lynch H, Perucho M, Smyrk T, Sobin L, Srivastava S. A National Cancer Institute Workshop on Hereditary Nonpolyposis Colorectal Cancer Syndrome: Meeting Highlights and Bethesda Guidelines. J Natl Cancer Inst. 1997;89:1758–1762

[98] Umar A, Boland CR, Terdiman JP, Syngal S, de la Chapelle A, Ruschoff J, Fishel R, Lindor NM, Burgart LJ, Hamelin R, Hamilton SR, Hiatt RA, Jass J, Lindblom A, Lynch HT, Peltomaki P, Ramsey SD, Rodriguez-Bigas MA, Vasen HF, Hawk ET, Barrett JC, Freedman AN, Srivastava S. Revised Bethesda Guidelines for Hereditary Nonpolyposis Colorectal Cancer (Lynch Syndrome) and Microsatellite Instability. J Natl Cancer Inst. 2004;96:261–268

[99] National Comprehensive Cancer Network. Clinical Practice Guidelines in Oncology: Colon Cancer (Version 2.2016). [Internet] 2016 Available at: wwwnccnorg [Accessed: 2016-07-12].

[100] Suraweera N, Duval A, Reperant M, Vaury C, Furlan D, Leroy K, Seruca R, Iacopetta B, Hamelin R. Evaluation of Tumor Microsatellite Instability Using Five Quasimonomorphic Mononucleotide Repeats and Pentaplex Pcr. Gastroenterol. 2002;123:1804–1811. DOI: 10.1053/gast.2002.37070

[101] Hoang JM, Cottu PH, Thuille B, Salmon RJ, Thomas G, Hamelin R. *BAT-26*, an Indicator of the Replication Error Phenotype in Colorectal Cancers and Cell Lines. Cancer Res. 1997;57:300–303

[102] de la Chapelle A. Testing Tumors for Microsatellite Instability. Eur J Hum Genet. 1999;7:407–408. DOI: 10.1038/sj.ejhg.5200335

[103] Zhou BB. Determination of the Replication Error Phenotype in Human Tumors without the Requirement for Matching Normal DNA by Analysis of Mononucleotide Repeat Microsatellites. Genes Chrom Cancer. 1998;221:101–107

[104] Samowitz WS, Slattery ML, Potter JD, Leppert MF. *BAT-26* and *BAT-40* Instability in Colorectal Adenomas and Carcinomas and Germline Polymorphisms. Am J Pathol. 1999;154:1637–1641. DOI: 10.1016/S0002-9440(10)65418-1

[105] Sutter C, Gebert J, Bischoff P, Herfarth C, von Knebel Doeberitz M. Molecular Screening of Potential HNPCC Patients Using a Multiplex Microsatellite PCR System. Mol Cell Probes. 1999;13:157–165. DOI: 10.1006/mcpr.1999.0231

[106] Loukola A, Eklin K, Laiho P, Salovaara R, Kristo P, Jarvinen H, Mecklin JP, Launonen V, Aaltonen LA. Microsatellite Marker Analysis in Screening for Hereditary Nonpolyposis Colorectal Cancer (Hnpcc). Cancer Res. 2001;61:4545–4549

[107] Akiyama Y, Sato H, Yamada T, Nagasaki H, Tsuchiya A, Abe R, Yuasa Y. Germ-Line Mutation of the *hMSH6/GTBP* Gene in an Atypical Hereditary Nonpolyposis Colorectal Cancer Kindred. Cancer Res. 1997;57:3920–3923

[108] Murphy KM, Zhang S, Geiger T, Hafez MJ, Bacher J, Berg KD, Eshleman JR. Comparison of the Microsatellite Instability Analysis System and the Bethesda Panel for the Determination of Microsatellite Instability in Colorectal Cancers. J Mol Diagn. 2006;8:305–311

[109] Patil DT, Bronner MP, Portier BP, Fraser CR, Plesec TP, Liu X. A Five-Marker Panel in a Multiplex PCR Accurately Detects Microsatellite Instability-High Colorectal Tumors without Control DNA. Diagn Mol Pathol. 2012;21:127–133. DOI: 10.1097/PDM. 0b013e3182461cc3

[110] Shia J. Immunohistochemistry Versus Microsatellite Instability Testing for Screening Colorectal Cancer Patients at Risk for Hereditary Nonpolyposis Colorectal Cancer Syndrome. Part I. The Utility of Immunohistochemistry. J Mol Diagn. 2008;10:293–300. DOI: 10.2353/jmoldx.2008.080031

[111] Zhang L. Immunohistochemistry Versus Microsatellite Instability Testing for Screening Colorectal Cancer Patients at Risk for Hereditary Nonpolyposis Colorectal Cancer Syndrome. Part II. The Utility of Microsatellite Instability Testing. J Mol Diagn. 2008;10:301–307. DOI: 10.2353/jmoldx.2008.080062

[112] Powell K. Going Statewide. Frontiers Ohio State Comprehensive Cancer Center–The James Columbus, Ohio. 2013;Summer 2013:19–23

[113] Scahill E. Statewide Screening Initiative Launched by Ohio State Has Life-Saving Potential. [Internet] 2016 Available at: https://cancerosuedu/news-and-media/news/statewide-screening-initiative-launched-by-ohio-state-has-life-saving-potential [Accessed: 2016-07-12].

[114] Beamer LC, Grant ML, Espenschied CR, Blazer KR, Hampel HL, Weitzel JN, MacDonald DJ. Reflex Immunohistochemistry and Microsatellite Instability Testing of Colorectal Tumors for Lynch Syndrome among Us Cancer Programs and Follow-up of Abnormal Results. J Clin Oncol. 2012;30:1058–1063. DOI: 10.1200/JCO.2011.38.4719

[115] Burt RW. Who Should Have Genetic Testing for the Lynch Syndrome? Ann Intern Med. 2011;155:127–128. DOI: 10.7326/0003-4819-155-2-201107190-00009

[116] Ward RL, Turner J, Williams R, Pekarsky B, Packham D, Velickovic M, Meagher A, O'Connor T, Hawkins NJ. Routine Testing for Mismatch Repair Deficiency in Sporadic Colorectal Cancer Is Justified. J Pathol. 2005;207:377–384. DOI: 10.1002/path.1851

[117] Matloff J, Lucas A, Polydorides AD, Itzkowitz SH. Molecular Tumor Testing for Lynch Syndrome in Patients with Colorectal Cancer. J Natl Compr Canc Netw. 2013;11:1380–1385

[118] Evaluation of Genomic Applications in Practice and Prevention Working Group. Recommendations from the Evaluation of Genomic Applications in Practice and Prevention Working Group: Genetic Testing Strategies in Newly Diagnosed Individuals with Colorectal Cancer Aimed at Reducing Morbidity and Mortality from Lynch Syndrome in Relatives. Genet Med. 2009;11:35–41. DOI: 10.1097/GIM.0b013e31818fa2ff

[119] Ladabaum U, Wang G, Terdiman J, Blanco A, Kuppermann M, Boland CR, Ford J, Elkin E, Phillips KA. Strategies to Identify the Lynch Syndrome among Patients with Colorectal Cancer: A Cost-Effectiveness Analysis. Ann Intern Med. 2011;155:69–79. DOI: 10.7326/0003-4819-155-2-201107190-00002

[120] Palomaki GE, McClain MR, Melillo S, Hampel HL, Thibodeau SN. Egapp Supplementary Evidence Review: DNA Testing Strategies Aimed at Reducing Morbidity and Mortality from Lynch Syndrome. Genet Med. 2009;11:42–65. DOI: 10.1097/GIM.0b013e31818fa2db

[121] Balmana J, Balaguer F, Cervantes A, Arnold D, Group EGW. Familial Risk-Colorectal Cancer: Esmo Clinical Practice Guidelines. Ann Oncol. 2013;24 Suppl 6:vi73–80. DOI: 10.1093/annonc/mdt209

[122] Heald B, Plesec T, Liu X, Pai R, Patil D, Moline J, Sharp RR, Burke CA, Kalady MF, Church J, Eng C. Implementation of Universal Microsatellite Instability and Immunohistochemistry Screening for Diagnosing Lynch Syndrome in a Large Academic Medical Center. J Clin Oncol. 2013;31:1336–1340. DOI: 10.1200/JCO.2012.45.1674

[123] Vasen HF, Abdirahman M, Brohet R, Langers AM, Kleibeuker JH, van Kouwen M, Koornstra JJ, Boot H, Cats A, Dekker E, Sanduleanu S, Poley JW, Hardwick JC, de Vos Tot Nederveen Cappel WH, van der Meulen-de Jong AE, Tan TG, Jacobs MA, Mohamed FL, de Boer SY, van de Meeberg PC, Verhulst ML, Salemans JM, van Bentem N, Westerveld BD, Vecht J, Nagengast FM. One to 2-Year Surveillance Intervals Reduce Risk of Colorectal Cancer in Families with Lynch Syndrome. Gastroenterology. 2010;138:2300–2306. DOI: 10.1053/j.gastro.2010.02.053

[124] Hampel H, Frankel WL, Martin E, Arnold M, Khanduja K, Kuebler P, Clendenning M, Sotamaa K, Prior T, Westman JA, Panescu J, Fix D, Lockman J, LaJeunesse J, Comeras I, de la Chapelle A. Feasibility of Screening for Lynch Syndrome among Patients with Colorectal Cancer. J Clin Oncol. 2008;26:5783–5788. DOI: 10.1200/JCO.2008.17.5950

[125] Iino H, Simms L, Young J, Arnold J, Winship IM, Webb SI, Furlong KL, Leggett B, Jass JR. DNA Microsatellite Instability and Mismatch Repair Protein Loss in Adenomas Presenting in Hereditary Non-Polyposis Colorectal Cancer. Gut. 2000;47:37–42

[126] Giuffre G, Muller A, Brodegger T, Bocker-Edmonston T, Gebert J, Kloor M, Dietmaier W, Kullmann F, Buttner R, Tuccari G, Ruschoff J, German Hnpcc Consortium GCA. Microsatellite Analysis of Hereditary Nonpolyposis Colorectal Cancer-Associated Colorectal Adenomas by Laser-Assisted Microdissection: Correlation with Mismatch Repair Protein Expression Provides New Insights in Early Steps of Tumorigenesis. J Mol Diagn. 2005;7:160–170. DOI: 10.1016/S1525-1578(10)60542-9

[127] Muller A, Beckmann C, Westphal G, Bocker Edmonston T, Friedrichs N, Dietmaier W, Brasch FE, Kloor M, Poremba C, Keller G, Aust DE, Fass J, Buttner R, Becker H, Ruschoff J. Prevalence of the Mismatch-Repair-Deficient Phenotype in Colonic Adenomas Arising in Hnpcc Patients: Results of a 5-Year Follow-up Study. Int J Colorectal Dis. 2006;21:632–641. DOI: 10.1007/s00384-005-0073-6

[128] Ferreira AM, Westers H, Sousa S, Wu Y, Niessen RC, Olderode-Berends M, van der Sluis T, Reuvekamp PT, Seruca R, Kleibeuker JH, Hollema H, Sijmons RH, Hofstra RM. Mononucleotide Precedes Dinucleotide Repeat Instability During Colorectal Tumour Development in Lynch Syndrome Patients. J Pathol. 2009;219:96-102. DOI: 10.1002/path.2573

[129] Walsh MD, Buchanan DD, Pearson SA, Clendenning M, Jenkins MA, Win AK, Walters RJ, Spring KJ, Nagler B, Pavluk E, Arnold ST, Goldblatt J, George J, Suthers GK, Phillips K, Hopper JL, Jass JR, Baron JA, Ahnen DJ, Thibodeau SN, Lindor N, Parry S, Walker NI, Rosty C, Young JP. Immunohistochemical Testing of Conventional Adenomas for Loss of Expression of Mismatch Repair Proteins in Lynch Syndrome Mutation Carriers: A Case Series from the Australasian Site of the Colon Cancer Family Registry. Mod Pathol. 2012;25:722–730. DOI: 10.1038/modpathol.2011.209

[130] Yurgelun MB, Goel A, Hornick JL, Sen A, Turgeon DK, Ruffin MTt, Marcon NE, Baron JA, Bresalier RS, Syngal S, Brenner DE, Boland CR, Stoffel EM. Microsatellite Instability and DNA Mismatch Repair Protein Deficiency in Lynch Syndrome Colorectal Polyps. Cancer Prev Res (Phila). 2012;5:578–582. DOI: 10.1158/1940-6207.CAPR-11-0519

[131] Shia J, Klimstra DS, Nafa K, Offit K, Guillem JG, Markowitz AJ, Gerald WL, Ellis NA. Value of Immunohistochemical Detection of DNA Mismatch Repair Proteins in Predicting Germline Mutation in Hereditary Colorectal Neoplasms. Am J Surg Pathol. 2005;29:96–104

[132] Blake C, Tsao JL, Wu A, Shibata D. Stepwise Deletions of polyA37 Sequences in Mismatch Repair-Deficient Colorectal Cancers. Am J Pathol. 2001;158:1867–1870. DOI: 10.1016/S0002-9440(10)64143-0

[133] Heinen CD, Shivapurkar N, Tang Z, Groden J, Alabaster O. Microsatellite Instability in Aberrant Crypt Foci from Human Colons. Cancer Res. 1996;56:5339–5341

[134] Beggs AD, Domingo E, Abulafi M, Hodgson SV, Tomlinson IP. A Study of Genomic Instability in Early Preneoplastic Colonic Lesions. Oncogene. 2013;32:5333–5337. DOI: 10.1038/onc.2012.584

[135] Kloor M, Huth C, Voigt AY, Benner A, Schirmacher P, von Knebel Doeberitz M, Blaker H. Prevalence of Mismatch Repair-Deficient Crypt Foci in Lynch Syndrome: A Pathological Study. Lancet Oncol. 2012;13:598–606. DOI: 10.1016/S1470-2045(12)70109-2

[136] Megid WA, Ensenberger MG, Halberg RB, Stanhope SA, Kent-First MG, Prolla TA, Bacher JW. A Novel Method for Biodosimetry. Radiat Environ Biophys. 2007;46:147–154. DOI: 10.1007/s00411-006-0072-1

[137] Steffen LS, Bacher JW, Peng Y, Le PN, Ding LH, Genik PC, Ray FA, Bedford JS, Fallgren CM, Bailey SM, Ullrich RL, Weil MM, Story MD. Molecular Characterisation of Murine Acute Myeloid Leukaemia Induced by ^{56}Fe Ion and ^{137}Cs Gamma Ray Irradiation. Mutagenesis. 2013;28:71–79. DOI: 10.1093/mutage/ges055

[138] Lang GI, Parsons L, Gammie AE. Mutation Rates, Spectra, and Genome-Wide Distribution of Spontaneous Mutations in Mismatch Repair Deficient Yeast. G3:Genes, Genomes and Genetics. 2013;3:1453–1465. DOI: 10.1534/g3.113.006429

[139] Koole W, Schafer HS, Agami R, van Haaften G, Tijsterman M. A Versatile Microsatellite Instability Reporter System in Human Cells. Nucleic Acids Res. 2013:1–9. DOI: 10.1093/nar/gkt615

[140] Bacher JW, Sievers CK, Albrecht DM, Grimes IC, Weiss JM, Matkowskyj KA, Agni RM, Vyazunova I, Clipson L, Storts DR, Thliveris AT, Halberg RB. Improved Detection of Microsatellite Instability in Early Colorectal Lesions. PLoS One. 2015;10:e0132727. DOI: 10.1371/journal.pone.0132727

[141] Hempelmann JA, Scroggins SM, Pritchard CC, Salipante SJ. MSIplus for Integrated Colorectal Cancer Molecular Testing by Next-Generation Sequencing. J Mol Diagn. 2015;17:705–714. DOI: 10.1016/j.jmoldx.2015.05.008

[142] Gazzoli I, Loda M, Garber J, Syngal S, Kolodner RD. A Hereditary Nonpolyposis Colorectal Carcinoma Case Associated with Hypermethylation of the *MLH1* Gene in Normal Tissue and Loss of Heterozygosity of the Unmethylated Allele in the Resulting Microsatellite Instability-High Tumor. Cancer Res. 2002;62:3925–3928

[143] Ligtenberg MJ, Kuiper RP, Chan TL, Goossens M, Hebeda KM, Voorendt M, Lee TY, Bodmer D, Hoenselaar E, Hendriks-Cornelissen SJ, Tsui WY, Kong CK, Brunner HG, van Kessel AG, Yuen ST, van Krieken JH, Leung SY, Hoogerbrugge N. Heritable Somatic Methylation and Inactivation of *MSH2* in Families with Lynch Syndrome Due to Deletion of the 3′ Exons of *TACSTD1*. Nat Genet. 2009;41:112–117. DOI: 10.1038/ng.283

[144] Carethers JM, Stoffel EM. Lynch Syndrome and Lynch Syndrome Mimics: The Growing Complex Landscape of Hereditary Colon Cancer. World J Gastroenterol. 2015;21:9253–9261. DOI: 10.3748/wjg.v21.i31.9253

[145] Sijmons RH, Greenblatt MS, Genuardi M. Gene Variants of Unknown Clinical Significance in Lynch Syndrome. An Introduction for Clinicians. Fam Cancer. 2013;12:181–187. DOI: 10.1007/s10689-013-9629-8

[146] International Society for Gastrointestinal Hereditary Tumours. [Internet] 2016 Available at: http://insight-grouporg/ [Accessed: 2016-07-12].

[147] Boland CR. Recent Discoveries in the Molecular Genetics of Lynch Syndrome. Fam Cancer. 2016;15:395–403. DOI: 10.1007/s10689-016-9885-5

[148] Haraldsdottir S, Hampel H, Tomsic J, Frankel WL, Pearlman R, de la Chapelle A, Pritchard CC. Colon and Endometrial Cancers with Mismatch Repair Deficiency Can Arise from Somatic, Rather Than Germline, Mutations. Gastroenterol. 2014;147:1308–1316. DOI: 10.1053/j.gastro.2014.08.041

[149] Rodriguez-Soler M, Perez-Carbonell L, Guarinos C, Zapater P, Castillejo A, Barbera VM, Juarez M, Bessa X, Xicola RM, Clofent J, Bujanda L, Balaguer F, Rene JM, de-Castro L, Marin-Gabriel JC, Lanas A, Cubiella J, Nicolas-Perez D, Brea-Fernandez A, Castellvi-Bel S, Alenda C, Ruiz-Ponte C, Carracedo A, Castells A, Andreu M, Llor X, Soto JL, Paya A, Jover R. Risk of Cancer in Cases of Suspected Lynch Syndrome without Germline Mutation. Gastroenterol. 2013;144:926–932. e921; quiz e913–924. DOI: 10.1053/j.gastro.2013.01.044

[150] Palles C, Cazier JB, Howarth KM, Domingo E, Jones AM, Broderick P, Kemp Z, Spain SL, Almeida EG, Salguero I, Sherborne A, Chubb D, Carvajal-Carmona LG, Ma Y, Kaur K, Dobbins S, Barclay E, Gorman M, Martin L, Kovac MB, Humphray S, The CC, Thomas HJ, Maher E, Evans G, Lucassen A, Cummings C, Stevens M, Walker L, Halliday D, Armstrong R, Paterson J, Hodgson S, Homfray T, Side L, Izatt L, Donaldson A, Tomkins S, Morrison P, Goodman S, Brewer C, Henderson A, Davidson R, Murday V, Cook J, Haites N, Bishop T, Sheridan E, Green A, Marks C, Carpenter S, Broughton M, Greenhalge L, Suri M, The WGSC, Steering C, Donnelly PC, Bell J, Bentley D, McVean G, Ratcliffe P, Taylor J, Wilkie A, Operations C, Donnelly PC, Broxholme J, Buck D, Cazier JB, Cornall R, Gregory L, Knight J, Lunter G, McVean G, Taylor J, Tomlinson I, Wilkie A, Sequencing, Experimental F-u, Buck DL, Gregory L, Humphray S, Kingsbury Z, Data A, McVean GL, Donnelly P, Cazier JB, Broxholme J, Grocock R, Hatton E, Holmes CC, Hughes L, Humburg P, Kanapin A, Lunter G, Murray L, Rimmer A, Lucassen A, Holmes CC, Bentley D, Donnelly P, Taylor J, Petridis C, Roylance R, Sawyer EJ, Kerr DJ, Clark S, Grimes J, Kearsey SE, Thomas HJ, McVean G, Houlston RS, Tomlinson I. Germline Mutations Affecting the Proofreading Domains of *POLE* and *POLD1* Predispose to Colorectal Adenomas and Carcinomas. Nat Genet. 2012;45:136–144. DOI: 10.1038/ng.2503

[151] Spier I, Holzapfel S, Altmuller J, Zhao B, Horpaopan S, Vogt S, Chen S, Morak M, Raeder S, Kayser K, Stienen D, Adam R, Nurnberg P, Plotz G, Holinski-Feder E, Lifton RP, Thiele H, Hoffmann P, Steinke V, Aretz S. Frequency and Phenotypic Spectrum of Germline Mutations in *POLE*

and Seven Other Polymerase Genes in 266 Patients with Colorectal Adenomas and Carcinomas. Int J Cancer. 2014;137:320–331. DOI: 10.1002/ijc.29396

[152] Lindor NM, Rabe K, Petersen GM, Haile R, Casey G, Baron J, Gallinger S, Bapat B, Aronson M, Hopper J, Jass J, LeMarchand L, Grove J, Potter J, Newcomb P, Terdiman JP, Conrad P, Moslein G, Goldberg R, Ziogas A, Anton-Culver H, de Andrade M, Siegmund K, Thibodeau SN, Boardman LA, Seminara D. Lower Cancer Incidence in Amsterdam-I Criteria Families without Mismatch Repair Deficiency: Familial Colorectal Cancer Type X. JAMA. 2005;293:1979–1985. DOI: 10.1001/jama.293.16.1979

[153] Hitchins MP, Wong JJ, Suthers G, Suter CM, Martin DI, Hawkins NJ, Ward RL. Inheritance of a Cancer-Associated *MLH1* Germ-Line Epimutation. N Engl J Med. 2007;356:697–705. DOI: 10.1056/NEJMoa064522

[154] Bakry D, Aronson M, Durno C, Rimawi H, Farah R, Alharbi QK, Alharbi M, Shamvil A, Ben-Shachar S, Mistry M, Constantini S, Dvir R, Qaddoumi I, Gallinger S, Lerner-Ellis J, Pollett A, Stephens D, Kelies S, Chao E, Malkin D, Bouffet E, Hawkins C, Tabori U. Genetic and Clinical Determinants of Constitutional Mismatch Repair Deficiency Syndrome: Report from the Constitutional Mismatch Repair Deficiency Consortium. Eur J Cancer. 2014;50:987–996. DOI: 10.1016/j.ejca.2013.12.005

[155] Gryfe R, Kim H, Hsieh ET, Aronson MD, Holowaty EJ, Bull SB, Redston M, Gallinger S. Tumor Microsatellite Instability and Clinical Outcome in Young Patients with Colorectal Cancer. N Engl J Med. 2000;342:69–77. DOI: 10.1056/NEJM200001133420201

[156] Popat S, Hubner R, Houlston RS. Systematic Review of Microsatellite Instability and Colorectal Cancer Prognosis. J Clin Oncol. 2005;23:609–618. DOI: 10.1200/JCO.2005.01.086

[157] Kloor M, von Knebel Doeberitz M. The Immune Biology of Microsatellite-Unstable Cancer. Trends in Cancer. 2016;2:121–133. DOI: 10.1016/j.trecan.2016.02.004

[158] Ribic CM, Sargent DJ, Moore MJ, Thibodeau SN, French AJ, Goldberg RM, Hamilton SR, Laurent-Puig P, Gryfe R, Shepherd LE, Tu D, Redston M, Gallinger S. Tumor Microsatellite-Instability Status as a Predictor of Benefit from Fluorouracil-Based Adjuvant Chemotherapy for Colon Cancer. N Engl J Med. 2003;349:247–257. DOI: 10.1056/NEJMoa022289

[159] Sargent DJ, Marsoni S, Monges G, Thibodeau SN, Labianca R, Hamilton SR, French AJ, Kabat B, Foster NR, Torri V, Ribic C, Grothey A, Moore M, Zaniboni A, Seitz JF, Sinicrope F, Gallinger S. Defective Mismatch Repair as a Predictive Marker for Lack of Efficacy of Fluorouracil-Based Adjuvant Therapy in Colon Cancer. J Clin Oncol. 2010;28:3219–3226. DOI: 10.1200/JCO.2009.27.1825

[160] Carethers JM, Smith EJ, Behling CA, Nguyen L, Tajima A, Doctolero RT, Cabrera BL, Goel A, Arnold CA, Miyai K, Boland CR. Use of 5-Fluorouracil

and Survival in Patients with Microsatellite-Unstable Colorectal Cancer. Gastroenterol. 2004;126:394–401

[161] Tajima A, Iwaizumi M, Tseng-Rogenski S, Cabrera BL, Carethers JM. Both Hmutsalpha and Hmutsss DNA Mismatch Repair Complexes Participate in 5-Fluorouracil Cytotoxicity. PLoS One. 2011;6:e28117. DOI: 10.1371/journal.pone.0028117

[162] Des Guetz G, Uzzan B, Nicolas P, Schischmanoff O, Perret GY, Morere JF. Microsatellite Instability Does Not Predict the Efficacy of Chemotherapy in Metastatic Colorectal Cancer. A Systematic Review and Meta-Analysis. Anticancer Res. 2009;29:1615–1620

[163] Sinicrope FA, Foster NR, Thibodeau SN, Marsoni S, Monges G, Labianca R, Kim GP, Yothers G, Allegra C, Moore MJ, Gallinger S, Sargent DJ. DNA Mismatch Repair Status and Colon Cancer Recurrence and Survival in Clinical Trials of 5-Fluorouracil-Based Adjuvant Therapy. J Natl Cancer Inst. 2011;103:863–875. DOI: 10.1093/jnci/djr153

[164] Webber EM, Kauffman TL, O'Connor E, Goddard KA. Systematic Review of the Predictive Effect of MSI Status in Colorectal Cancer Patients Undergoing 5fu-Based Chemotherapy. BMC Cancer. 2015;15:156. DOI: 10.1186/s12885-015-1093-4

[165] Warthin A. Heredity with Reference to Carcinoma: As Shown by the Study of the Cases Examined in the Pathological Laboratory of the University of Michigan, 1895–1913. Arch Intern Med. 1913;XII:546–555. DOI: 10.1001/archinte.1913.00070050063006

[166] Watson JD, Crick FH. Molecular Structure of Nucleic Acids: A Structure for Deoxyribose Nucleic Acid. Nature. 1953;171:737–738

[167] Lynch HT, Shaw MW, Magnuson CW, Larsen AL, Krush AJ. Hereditary Factors in Cancer. Study of Two Large Midwestern Kindreds. Arch Intern Med. 1966;117:206–212

[168] Sanger F, Nicklen S, Coulson AR. DNA Sequencing with Chain-Terminating Inhibitors. Proc Natl Acad Sci U S A. 1977;74:5463–5467

[169] Boland CR, Troncale FJ. Familial Colonic Cancer without Antecedent Polyposis. Ann Intern Med. 1984;100:700–701

[170] Saiki RK, Scharf S, Faloona F, Mullis KB, Horn GT, Erlich HA, Arnheim N. Enzymatic Amplification of Beta-Globin Genomic Sequences and Restriction Site Analysis for Diagnosis of Sickle Cell Anemia. Science. 1985;230:1350–1354

[171] Weissenbach J, Gyapay G, Dib C, Vignal A, Morissette J, Millasseau P, Vaysseix G, Lathrop M. A Second-Generation Linkage Map of the Human Genome. Nature. 1992;359:794–801. DOI: 10.1038/359794a0

[172] Fishel R, Lescoe MK, Rao MR, Copeland NG, Jenkins NA, Garber J, Kane M, Kolodner R. The Human Mutator Gene Homolog *MSH2* and Its Association with Hereditary Nonpolyposis Colon Cancer. Cell. 1993;75:1027–1038

[173] Bronner CE, Baker SM, Morrison PT, Warren G, Smith LG, Lescoe MK, Kane M, Earabino C, Lipford J, Lindblom A, et al. Mutation in the DNA Mismatch Repair Gene Homologue *hMLH1* Is Associated with Hereditary Non-Polyposis Colon Cancer. Nature. 1994;368:258–261. DOI: 10.1038/368258a0

[174] Nicolaides NC, Papadopoulos N, Liu B, Wei YF, Carter KC, Ruben SM, Rosen CA, Haseltine WA, Fleischmann RD, Fraser CM, et al. Mutations of Two P/WS Homologues in Hereditary Nonpolyposis Colon Cancer. Nature. 1994;371:75–80. DOI: 10.1038/371075a0

Chapter 11

Microsatellite Instability in Colorectal Cancer

Narasimha Reddy Parine, Reddy Sri Varsha and
Mohammad Saud Alanazi

Additional information is available at the end of the chapter

http://dx.doi.org/10.5772/65429

Abstract

Cancer is a genetic disease. Cancer cells contain various mutations, which includes SNPs to chromosomal aberrations. Together, these changes are referred to as genome instability. Genetic instability is one of the common characteristics of colorectal cancer. In colorectal cancer three major types of genetic instability have been reported. They are chromosomal translocations, microsatellite instability (MSI), and chromosome instability (CIN). Microsatellite instability occurs due to variations in DNA mismatch repair genes, while chromosomal instability is distinguished by major chromosomal alterations occurring at cell division and usually involves β-catenin and Adenomatous polyposis coli protein (APC) mutations. This chapter summarizes the major molecular mechanisms leading to genomic and microsatellite instability and tumorigenesis.

Keywords: cancer, colorectal cancer, genomic instability, microsatellite instability, mismatch repair

1. Introduction

Genomic and microsatellite instability (MSI) play critical roles in both cancer initiation and progression. This instability can manifest itself genetically on several different levels, ranging from simple deoxyribonucleic acid (DNA) sequence changes to structural and numerical abnormalities at the chromosomal level [1]. Since 1990s many researchers reported the presence of microsatellite instability as a common molecular mechanism in colorectal cancers [2]. Since then, several studies using numerous methods have characterized MSI molecular subtype [3]. Around 15% of colorectal cancer tumors with a mismatch repair (MMR) system deficiency is owing to germline, somatic, or epigenetic inactivation [4]. Large number of CRC patients is reported to have deficient MMR system [5]. MSI has only slowly been accepted as a clinically significant aspect of tumor biology even though it is a well-established molecular marker for Lynch syndrome patients [6]. The present chapter provides an overview of genomic instability and molecular basis of the MMR system, the detection of MSI, and the molecular features of these tumors.

2. Genomic instability

Genetic instability is one of the common characteristics of colorectal cancer. Three major types of genetic instability have been reported in colorectal cancer [7–10]. Microsatellite instability occurs due to variations in DNA mismatch repair genes, while chromosomal instability (CIN) is distinguished by major chromosomal alterations occurring at cell division and usually involves β-catenin and Adenomatous polyposis coli protein (APC) mutations [11–13]. Less prevalent are mutations (germline) in DNA stability genes, including the DNA MMR genes, MSH6, MSH2, PMS2, and MLH1, which are connected with frameshift mutations and base pair substitutions in short-tandem repeat sequences causing microsatellite instability in HNPCC [14, 15].

Key changes in chromosomal instability in CRC consist of prevalent alterations in chromosome number and noticeable losses at the molecular level on 5q, 18q, and 17p chromosomes; and KRAS oncogene mutation. Major genes involved in these alterations are TP53 (17p), Adenomatous polyposis coli protein (APC) (5q), and MADH2/MADH4/DCC (18q) [16, 17]. The loss of chromosome is linked with instability at the chromosomal and molecular level. In approximately 13% of colorectal cancer tumors, MMR deficiency leads to MSI [18]. About 40% of colorectal cancer cases are distinguished by epigenetic alterations particularly DNA methylation, a phenomenon called CpG islands methylator phenotype (CIMP) [19, 20]. In the other 47% of colorectal cancers, CIN affects the tumors by insertions and deletions in chromosomes [18]. The chromosomal instability group includes cancers with polypoid or aneuploid karyotypes, and cancers which have numerous insertions or losses of chromosomal arms. Chromosomal instability results from specific molecular alterations, gene silencing, and also result from structural defects occurred during cell cycle [21]. In some of the colorectal adenomas it was observed that the tumor progression starts with chromosome 7 amplification. After this event, the other specific chromosomal alterations, such as losses on 17p, 8p, 18q, 20q, and 15q and gains on 20q, 8q, 13, and 7 will generally occur in the colorectal cancers [21–24].

Tumors with microsatellite instability are well known to possess more mutations than other tumors. Chromosomal instability and microsatellite instability tumors were primarily considered as equally special, as microsatellite instability tumors usually have constant and diploid karyotypes [25, 26]. Recent reports have illustrated that the microsatellite instability and chromosomal instability can arise in the same tumor [27, 28]. Trautmann et al. [29] found have observed that approximately 50% of hereditary microsatellite instability (MSI-H) tumors have similar level of chromosomal aberrations. Although confirmation for similar level of chromosomal instability can be observed in the majority of hereditary microsatellite instability tumors, the specific mutations recognized differed between hereditary microsatellite instability and microsatellite stability tumors [30]. Hereditary microsatellite instability tumors harbor losses of 15q and 18q and gains of chromosomes 8, 12, and 13, whereas microsatellite stability tumors have a high level and variable range of chromosomal aberration [29, 31]. In a recent study by Lassmann et al. [32] in 22 Caucasian colorectal tumors on about 287 sequences found frequent aberrations in specific regions of chromosomes. This study suggested few candidate genes with frequent deletion and amplifications in these chromosome regions. A recent exome analysis of colorectal cancer genomes identified approximately eightfold more nonsynonymous variation in a tumor that displayed microsatellite instability [33].

Genomic instability is a basic feature of tumorigenesis. Three types of genomic instability have been reported in colon cancer: (i) chromosomal translocations, (ii) microsatellite instability, and (iii) chromosome instability [34]. The origin of chromosomal instability has been reported in few subsets of colorectal cancers. Nonetheless, microsatellite instability is renowned to result from inactivating variations or from unusual methylation of genes in the DNA MMR gene family. The MMR genes repair nucleotide mismatches arising during the replication [8]. Variations leading to inactivation of MMR system occur in 1–2% of colorectal cancers due to germline mutations in members of the mismatch repair genes, MSH2, MLH1, MSH6, and PMS2. Mutations in MMR system are one of the major causes of the familial adenomatous polyposis syndrome and hereditary nonpolyposis colon cancer syndrome [35].

In microsatellite instability or chromosomal instability the loss of genomic instability occurs after adenoma formation, but before progression to frank malignancy [36]. However, genomic instability can be a striking target for anticancer therapies as it is almost omnipresent in colorectal cancer and is a distinctive feature of cancerous cells. The possibility of targeting genomic instability for anticolorectal cancer therapy has been proved in *in vitro* systems [37]. Exploring the basis and roles of genetic and epigenetic instability in colorectal carcinogenesis has the potential to result in further development of efficient prevention methods and therapeutics for colorectal cancer [2].

According to the proposed theories, mutations in many pathways have major role in adenoma carcinoma progression series. In colon cancer, mutations in Adenomatous polyposis coli protein (APC) as well as the p53 pathways are seen in approximately 95% of the cases [38]. It has been reported that in approximately 70% of the tumors somatic mutations lead to alteration of the Ras/Raf pathway. The effect and particular roles of somatic mutations in other genes and pathways of colorectal cancer are less examined and less understood [36].

Mutational profiling and comparative studies require both tumor and normal tissue samples. Attaining tumor samples for colorectal cancer studies poses significant technical difficulty. The signal and noise are indistinguishable when the tumor samples render contamination with normal tissue. Very few studies have conducted a systematical analysis to resolve the spectrum of particular mutations in a series of genes in colon cancer tissues and their matching normal tissues, i.e., a systematic analysis of all genes in the Adenomatous polyposis coli protein (APC) pathway (Adenomatous polyposis coli protein, axin, and β-catenin), p53 pathway (BAX, p53, and MDM2), and RAS pathway (B-Raf and K-Ras) in the colorectal cancer tissues [39]. Few such studies have reported specific variations among the mutations observed in chromosomal instability and microsatellite instability tumors. Most of the microsatellite instability tumors have 30% more mutations in β-catenin when compared to Adenomatous polyposis coli protein (APC), while β-catenin mutations are exceptionally rare in nonmicrosatellite instability cancers [40]. This is an indirect confirmation recommending that the microsatellite instability occurs prior to the inactivation of the Adenomatous polyposis coli protein Adenomatous polyposis coli protein (APC) pathway. Moreover, the spectrum of mutations is different in the Adenomatous polyposis coli protein (APC) pathway in many of the microsatellite instability tumors without β-catenin mutations when compared to nonmicrosatellite instability tumors. Specially, in simple repeat sequences of microsatellite instability there is an elevated rate of recurrence of mutations than in the nonmicrosatellite instability cancers [33].

3. Genomic instability in cancer

Genomic instability is a common symptom of most of the tumors and it includes several genomic alterations ranging from SNPs to large-scale chromosomal aberrations [41]. This can be classified into three groups based on the type of genetic changes.

3.1. Nucleotide instability (NIN)

NIN has several genetic variations which includes one or more nucleotide substitutions, deletions, and insertions. These errors may occur during DNA replication or due to faults in DNA repair mechanism, such as nucleotide excision repair (NER) and base excision repair (BER) [42]. These variations in DNA may lead to variations in gene structure and function.

3.2. Chromosomal instability

CIN is one of the common forms of genomic instability, reported in more than 90% of all cancers. CIN is detected in all stages of cancer [43]. For example, chr 10 is frequently lost in glioblastomas, which leads to the inactivation of the tumor-suppressor gene, PTEN. Generally, CIN refers to changes of chromosomal segments, or entire chromosomes, in terms of their structure or number, including translocations, additions, deletions, insertions, inversions and loss of heterozygosity (LOH) [43]. Variation in chromosome numbers is a condition known as aneuploidy. Chromosome translocation involves the merging of various chromosomes, or of two distant parts on the same chromosome, which results in the formation of a chimeric chromosome [44]. In cancer cells, CIN modifies the expression of numerous genes, leading to a poorer prognosis of patients with MIN or NIN tumors.

3.3. Microsatellite instability

Microsatellites are small tandem repetitive sequences of DNA located throughout the genome. MIN arises due to the malfunctioning of DNA mismatch repair system. This may result in the development, shrinkage, deletion, and random insertion of microsatellites [45]. The MMR system recognizes and attaches to the mismatch, and deletes the erroneous nucleotide and

http://dx.doi.org/10.5772/65429

maintains the genome integrity. MIN has been recognized in several cancers, including colorectal, ovarian, lung, endometrial, and gastric [46]. Till now, five MIN markers have been suggested for disease screening in patients prone to Lynch syndrome. MIN is generally observed in approximately 15% of all colorectal cancer patients, which contain both hereditary and sporadic forms. Tumors with MSI are reported to show better prognosis than nonMSI tumors [46].

4. Molecular basis of the MMR system

Microsatellites are small repetitive sequences dispersed in whole genome, which contain mono, di, trinucleotide, or tetra nucleotide repeats like $(A)_n$ or $(CA)_n$. Most of these repeats are precisely predisposed to accumulation of mutations, mainly due to the DNA polymerases, which cannot bind DNA competently at DNA synthesis period. Generally, observed errors in microsatellites are base–base mismatches, which escape the DNA polymerases proofreading activity, and insertion–deletion loops, which form DNA hairpins [47]. These unpaired nucleotides arise when the initial nucleotide and template strand separates and incorrectly reanneals in a microsatellite. Insertions or deletions in microsatellites situated in exonic regions causes frameshift mutations, which may lead to truncations of protein [47].

The MMR system is accountable for the recognition and correction of errors that occur in microsatellites. The major proteins involved in MMR system are MLH1, MSH2, MSH3, MSH6, and PMS2, and interact as heterodimers. When a mismatch is identified, MsH2 associates with either MSH6 or MSH3 (forming Mutsα and Mutsβ complexs), and MLH1 couples WITH PMS2, PMS1, or MLH3 (forms MutLα, MutLβ, or MutLγ complexes) [48]. Muts and a MutL complexes recognizes mismatches and mutations, and interacts with the replication factor C. Exonuclease 1 and proliferating cell nuclear antigen participate in the excision of mismatches [48]. As a final step, resynthesis and relegation of the nucleotide strand is done by DNA polymerase δ and DNA ligase. Variations in the genes responsible for the identification step lead to gathering of mutations in DNA, which may results in MSI. This has been recognized in various cancers, including CRC, gastric, endometrial, and few other carcinomas, such as glioblastoma and lymphomas [2].

5. Detection of MSI

Several techniques that are available to detect tumors with MSI are well established and are being used as a clinical diagnostic tool. Microsatellite repeats specific to MSI are being detected by PCR amplification. This can also be determined by comparing the length of nucleotide repeats in tumor cells and adjacent normal cells. This analysis was initially performed using polyacrylamide gels and radiolabeled primers; later on, this analysis has been made easier with fluorescent primers and capillary electrophoresis. In the 1990s, a microsatellite markers panel, known as the Bethesda panel, with appropriate sensitivity and specificity to diagnose

MSI CRC has been developed. This panel includes five microsatellite loci: two mononucleotides (BAT25 and BAT26) and three dinucleotides (D5s346, D2s123, and D17s250) [2].

Few researchers and clinicians have expanded this MSI panel to 10 markers. Three different MSI groups have been established based on the instability criteria: MSI-high (MSI-H), indicating instability at two or more loci; MSI-low (MSI-L), indicating instability at one locus; and microsatellite stable (MSS), indicating no loci with instability [49]. In most of the patients MSI-low cases only show instability for dinucleotide markers, so the analysis of dinucleotides alone may lead to the misclassification of MSS or MSI-L colorectal cancer as MSI-H. In contrast to this, mononucleotides BAT25 and BAT26 are nearly monomorphic, MSI determination could be easy using these markers in the absence of normal tissue [50]. Hence, MSI panel has an appropriate set of markers for MSI detection. These days commercial kits include a majority of mononucleotide markers with improved sensitivity [51].

MSI can also be detected by gene expression analysis methods. Immunohistochemical analysis of MMR proteins has become a standard procedure to detect MSI in the diagnosis centers and as an alternative to the genetic testing of Lynch syndrome [52]. Antibodies against MMR pathway proteins such as MLH1, MSH2, MSH6, and PMS2 will give a clear awareness about the mechanism and functioning of the MMR system [15]. Variation in functionality of one or more MMR genes is diagnostic, and concludes about the gene which is most probable to have a mutation or which gene got inactivated. Elucidation of the Immunohistochemistry (IHC) pattern may give more benefit for the dependent expression of heterodimers in the diagnosis of CRC as described by Vilar and Gruber [2]. They reported that CRCs that are deficient of expression of MLH1 and PMS2, but gain expression of MSH2 and MSH6, show scarcity in the expression of MLH1. In this state, deficiency of expression of PMS2 is simply a result of the inactive MLH1. Whether the absence of MLH1 is initiated by promoter hypermethylation that leads to inactivation of the gene or a germline mutation that causes Lynch syndrome need more exploration, but Immunohistochemistry (IHC) results direct the evaluation to concentrate on *MLH1* than the other MMR genes.

6. Conclusions

Genetic instability and microsatellite instability are the most common characteristics of colorectal cancer. Microsatellite instability is a subclass of CRC, which is reported to show a clear histopathological and therapeutic profile compared to other molecular subtypes. Various advanced methods have been developed in the past two decades for the detection of MSI. The molecular basis of MSI in cancer is still being explored. Recent findings revealed that MSI is caused due to mutations in genes coding for kinases. Further studies are required to identify the molecular basis of MSI and also to develop more cost-effective diagnosis and prognosis methods.

Acknowledgements

The project was financially supported by King Saud University, Vice Deanship of Research Chairs.

Author details

Narasimha Reddy Parine[1*], Reddy Sri Varsha[2] and Mohammad Saud Alanazi[1]

*Address all correspondence to: reddyparine@gmail.com

1 Genome Research Chair, Department of Biochemistry, College of Science, King Saud University, Riyadh, Saudi Arabia

2 Dept of Biotechnology, Sreenidhi institute of Science and Technology, Hyderabad, India

References

[1] Ferguson LR, Chen H, Collins AR, Connell M, Damia G, Dasgupta S, Malhotra M, Meeker AK, Amedei A, Amin A, Ashraf SS. Genomic instability in human cancer: Molecular insights and opportunities for therapeutic attack and prevention through diet and nutrition. Semin Cancer Biol. 2015:S5–S24. doi: 10.1016/j.semcancer.2015.03.005

[2] Vilar E, Gruber SB. Microsatellite instability in colorectal cancer—The stable evidence. Nat Rev Clin Oncol. 2010; 7:153–162. doi: 10.1038/nrclinonc.2009.237

[3] Ogino S, Goel A. Molecular classification and correlates in colorectal cancer. J Mol Diagn. 2008; 10:13–27 doi: 10.1002/cjp2.31

[4] Peltomäki P. DNA mismatch repair and cancer. Mutat Res Rev Mutat. 2001; 488:77–85. http://dx.doi.org/10.1016/S1383-5742(00)00058-2

[5] Boland CR, Goel A. Microsatellite instability in colorectal cancer. Gastroenterology. 2010; 138:2073–2087. e2073. doi: 10.1053/j.gastro.2009.12.064

[6] Strimpakos A, Syrigos K, Saif M. Pharmacogenetics and biomarkers in colorectal cancer. Pharmacogenomics J. 2009; 9:147–160. doi: 10.1038/tpj.2009.8

[7] Fearon ER, Vogelstein B. A genetic model for colorectal tumorigenesis. Cell. 1990; 61:759–767. doi: http://dx.doi.org/10.1016/0092-8674(90)90186-I

[8] Lengauer C, Kinzler KW, Vogelstein B. Genetic instabilities in human cancers. Nature. 1998; 396:643–649. doi: 10.1038/25292

[9] Hoeijmakers JH. Genome maintenance mechanisms for preventing cancer. Nature. 2001; 411:366–374. doi: 10.1038/35077232

[10] Lothe RA, Peltomäki P, Meling GI, Aaltonen LA, Nyström-Lahti M, Pylkkänen L, Heimdal K, Andersen TI, Møller P, Rognum TO, Fosså SD. Genomic instability in colorectal cancer: Relationship to clinicopathological variables and family history. Cancer Res. 1993; 53:5849–5852.

[11] Charames GS, Bapat B. Genomic instability and cancer. Curr Mol Med. 2003; 3:589–596.

[12] Jass J. Classification of colorectal cancer based on correlation of clinical, morphological and molecular features. Histopathology. 2007; 50:113–130. doi: 10.1111/j.1365-2559.2006.02549.x

[13] Goel A, Boland CR. Epigenetics of colorectal cancer. Gastroenterology. 2012; 143:1442–1460. e1441. doi: 10.1053/j.gastro.2012.09.032

[14] Schofield MJ, Hsieh P. DNA mismatch repair: Molecular mechanisms and biological function. Annu Rev Microbiol. 2003; 57:579–608. doi: 10.1146/annurev.micro.57.030502.090847

[15] Harfe BD, Jinks-Robertson S. DNA mismatch repair and genetic instability. Annu Rev Genet. 2000; 34:359–399. doi: 10.1146/annurev.genet.34.1.359

[16] Armaghany T, Wilson JD, Chu Q, Mills G. Genetic alterations in colorectal cancer. Gastrointest Cancer Res. 2012; 5:19.

[17] Al-Kuraya KS. KRAS and TP53 mutations in colorectal carcinoma. S Saudi J Gastroenterol. 2009; 15:217. doi: 10.4103/1319-3767.56087

[18] Walther A, Johnstone E, Swanton C, Midgley R, Tomlinson I, Kerr D. Genetic prognostic and predictive markers in colorectal cancer. Nat Rev Cancer. 2009; 9:489–499. doi: 10.1038/nrc2645

[19] Lao VV, Grady WM. Epigenetics and colorectal cancer. Nat Rev Gastroenterol Hepatol. 2011; 8:686–700. doi: 10.1038/nrgastro.2011.173

[20] Noushmehr H, Weisenberger DJ, Diefes K, Phillips HS, Pujara K, Berman BP, Pan F, Pelloski CE, Sulman EP, Bhat KP, Verhaak RG. Identification of a CpG island methylator phenotype that defines a distinct subgroup of glioma. Cancer Cell. 2010; 17:510–522. doi: 10.1016/j.ccr.2010.03.017

[21] Payne CM, Crowley-Skillicorn C, Bernstein C, Holubec H, Bernstein H. Molecular and cellular pathways associated with chromosome 1p deletions during colon carcinogenesis. Clin Exp Gastroenterol. 2011; 4:75–119. doi: 10.2147/CEG.S17114

[22] Albertson DG, Collins C, McCormick F, Gray JW. Chromosome aberrations in solid tumors. Nat Genet. 2003; 34:369–376. doi: 10.1038/ng1215

[23] Ashktorab H, Schäffer AA, Daremipouran M, Smoot DT, Lee E, Brim H. Distinct genetic alterations in colorectal cancer. PloS ONE. 2010; 5:e8879. doi: 10.1371/journal.pone.0008879

[24] Migliore L, Migheli F, Spisni R, Coppedè F. Genetics, cytogenetics, and epigenetics of colorectal cancer. J Biomed Biotech. 2011: 1–19; http://dx.DOI.org/10.1155/2011/792362

[25] Ilyas M, Straub J, Tomlinson I, Bodmer WF. Genetic pathways in colorectal and other cancers. Eur J Cancer. 1999; 35:1986–2002. http://dx.DOI.org/10.1016/S0959-8049(99)00298-1

[26] Cunningham JM, Boardmann L, Burgart LJ. Microsatellite instability. Mol Pathol Early Cancer. 1999: p 405–426. IOS press, Amsterdam, Netherlands. S. Srivastava, DE. Henson and A. Gazdar et al. eds.

[27] Burrell RA, McGranahan N, Bartek J, Swanton C. The causes and consequences of genetic heterogeneity in cancer evolution. Nature. 2013; 501:338–345. doi: 10.1038/nature12625

[28] Lee J-K, Choi Y-L, Kwon M, Park PJ. Mechanisms and consequences of cancer genome instability: Lessons from genome sequencing studies. Annu Rev Pathol Mech. 2016; 11:283–312. doi: 10.1146/annurev-pathol-012615-044446

[29] Trautmann K, Terdiman JP, French AJ, Roydasgupta R, Sein N, Kakar S, Fridlyand J, Snijders AM, Albertson DG, Thibodeau SN, Waldman FM. Chromosomal instability in microsatellite-unstable and stable colon cancer. Clin Cancer Res. 2006; 12:6379–6385. doi: 10.1158/1078-0432.CCR-06-1248

[30] Wilding J, Bodmer W. Genetic instability. Oxford Textbook of oncology; 3 edition 2016. 72 p. ISBN-13: 978-0199656103 Oxford University Press; United Kingdom

[31] Wang H, Liang L, Fang J, Xu J. Somatic gene copy number alterations in colorectal cancer: New quest for cancer drivers and biomarkers. Oncogene. 2016; 35(16):2011–2019. doi: 10.1038/onc.2015.304

[32] Lassmann S, Weis R, Makowiec F, Roth J, Danciu M, Hopt U, Werner M. Array CGH identifies distinct DNA copy number profiles of oncogenes and tumor suppressor genes in chromosomal- and microsatellite-unstable sporadic colorectal carcinomas. J Mol Med. 2007; 85:293–304. doi: 10.1007/s00109-006-0126-5

[33] Timmermann B, Kerick M, Roehr C, Fischer A, Isau M, Boerno ST, Wunderlich A, Barmeyer C, Seemann P, Koenig J, Lappe M. Somatic mutation profiles of MSI and MSS colorectal cancer identified by whole exome next generation sequencing and bioinformatics analysis. PloS ONE. 2010; 5:e15661. doi: 10.1371/journal.pone.0015661

[34] Pino MS, Chung DC. The chromosomal instability pathway in colon cancer. Gastroenterology. 2010; 138:2059–2072. doi: 10.1053/j.gastro.2009.12.065

[35] Kinzler KW, Vogelstein B. Lessons from hereditary colorectal cancer. Cell. 1996; 87:159–170. http://dx.DOI.org/10.1016/S0092-8674(00)81333-1

[36] Grady WM, Carethers JM. Genomic and epigenetic instability in colorectal cancer pathogenesis. Gastroenterology. 2008; 135:1079–1099. doi: 10.1053/j.gastro.2008.07.076

[37] Weng W, Feng J, Qin H, Ma Y. Molecular therapy of colorectal cancer: progress and future directions. Int J Cancer. 2015; 136:493–502. doi: 10.1002/ijc.28722; doi: 10.1002/ijc.28722

[38] Fearnhead NS, Wilding JL, Bodmer WF. Genetics of colorectal cancer: hereditary aspects and overview of colorectal tumorigenesis. Br Med Bull. 2002; 64:27–43. doi: 10.1093/bmb/64.1.27

[39] Roper J, Hung KE. Molecular mechanisms of colorectal carcinogenesis. Molecular Pathogenesis of Colorectal Cancer, edited by K.M. Haigis. Springer, New York; 2013. pp. 25–65. doi: 10.1007/978-1-4614-8412-7_2

[40] Okugawa Y, Grady WM, Goel A. Epigenetic alterations in colorectal cancer: Emerging biomarkers. Gastroenterology. 2015; 149:1204–1225. e1212. doi: 10.1053/j.gastro.2015.07.011

[41] Vogelstein B, Papadopoulos N, Velculescu VE, Zhou S, Diaz LA, Kinzler KW. Cancer genome landscapes. Science. 2013; 339:1546–1558. doi: 10.1126/science.1235122

[42] Iyama T, Wilson DM. DNA repair mechanisms in dividing and non-dividing cells. DNA Repair (Amst). 2013; 12:620–636. doi: 10.1016/j.dnarep.2013.04.015

[43] Pikor L, Thu K, Vucic E, Lam W. The detection and implication of genome instability in cancer. Cancer Metastasis Rev. 2013; 32:341–352. doi: 10.1007/s10555-013-9429-5

[44] Rowley, Janet D. "The critical role of chromosome translocations in human leukemias." Annual review of genetics 32, no. 1 (1998): 495–519.

[45] Woerner SM, Kloor M, von Knebel Doeberitz M, Gebert JF. Microsatellite instability in the development of DNA mismatch repair deficient tumors. Cancer Biomark. 2006; 2:69–86.

[46] Lynch HT, de la Chapelle A. Genetic susceptibility to non-polyposis colorectal cancer. J Med Genet. 1999; 36:801–818.

[47] Kunkel TA, Erie DA. DNA mismatch repair*. Annu Rev Biochem. 2005; 74:681–710. doi: 10.1146/annurev.biochem.74.082803.133243

[48] Kariola R, Raevaara TE, Lönnqvist KE, Nyström-Lahti M (2002) Functional analysis of MSH6 mutations linked to kindreds with putative hereditary non-polyposis colorectal cancer syndrome. Hum Mol Genet 11:1303–1310

[49] Weisenberger DJ, Siegmund KD, Campan M, Young J, Long TI, Faasse MA, Kang GH, Widschwendter M, Weener D, Buchanan D, Koh H. CpG island methylator phenotype

underlies sporadic microsatellite instability and is tightly associated with BRAF mutation in colorectal cancer. Nat Genet. 2006; 38:787–793. doi: 10.1038/ng1834

[50] Murphy KM, Zhang S, Geiger T, Hafez MJ, Bacher J, Berg KD, Eshleman JR. Comparison of the microsatellite instability analysis system and the Bethesda panel for the determination of microsatellite instability in colorectal cancers. J Mol Diagn. 2006; 8:305–311. doi: 10.2353/jmoldx.2006.050092

[51] Salto-Tellez M, Yan B, Wu RI, Pitman MB. Tumors of the gastrointestinal system. Mol Pathol. 2015; pp. 200–221. doi: 10.1586/14737159.2015.1033603

[52] Lynch PM. Current approaches in familial colorectal cancer: A clinical perspective. J Natl Compr Canc Netw. 2006; 4:421–430.